BIOLOGICAL STRUCTURE AND FUNCTION 4

THE PITUITARY GLAND

BIOLOGICAL STRUCTURE AND FUNCTION

THE PITUITARY GLAND

A comparative account

R. L. HOLMES

Professor of Anatomy
University of Leeds

J. N. BALL

Reader in Comparative Vertebrate Endocrinology
University of Sheffield

CAMBRIDGE

AT THE UNIVERSITY PRESS

1974

Published by the Syndics of the Cambridge University Press
Bentley House, 200 Euston Road, London NW1 2DB
American Branch: 32 East 57th Street, New York, N.Y. 10022

© Cambridge University Press 1974

Library of Congress Catalogue Card Number: 73–75856

ISBN: 0 521 20247 7

Printed in Great Britain
at the University Printing House, Cambridge
(Brooke Crutchley, University Printer)

CONTENTS

To
Dr GRACE E. PICKFORD
Pioneer in
Comparative Endocrinology

PREFACE

In this text we have tried to survey in a general way the structure and function of the pituitary gland throughout the vertebrates, believing a broadly based comparative approach on these lines to be a timely one. Overall, a limited selection from a very great body of published work has had to be made; but certain historical aspects, on which present knowledge is necessarily based, have been discussed. Detailed considerations of the glands of individual species have been introduced to illustrate general principles rather than to present a definitive description: anyone wishing to study particular aspects of the pituitary must anyway consult the original published papers. The list of references is also selective, but could, we hope, provide a starting point for wider reading on any particular aspect of this complex organ. The extensive bibliographies in the handbooks of Romeis and Diepen, in *La Cytologie de l'Adénohypophyse* (Benoit, J. and Da Lage, C., eds., 1963) and the three-volume Butterworths set edited by the late G. W. Harris and B. T. Donovan offer much larger lists of works published up to the mid-1960s.

We are happy to express our thanks to Mrs Barbara Whitehead and Miss J. Healey for a great deal of typing, and to Mr R. K. Adkin and Mr D. Hollingworth for photographic work; also to Dr Bridget I. Baker for stimulating discussions about many aspects of the pituitary.

R.L.H.

J.N.B.

ABBREVIATIONS

AB	Alcian blue
ACTH	Adrenocorticotropic hormone (corticotropin)
ADH	Antidiuretic hormone (vasopressin in mammals)
AF	Aldehyde fuchsin
Aliz B	Alizarin blue
Aliz BT	Herlant's Alizarin blue tetrachrome
AVT	Arginine vasotocin
CAH	Chrome-alum haematoxylin
CRF	Corticotropin releasing factor
CSF	Cerebrospinal fluid
EM	Electron microscope
ENG	Elementary neurosecretory granules
FSH	Follicle stimulating hormone
GIH	Growth hormone inhibiting hormone or factor
GRF	Growth hormone releasing factor
GtH	Gonadotropic hormone
ICSH	Interstitial cell stimulating hormone
IT	Isotocin or ichthyotocin
LGV	Large granular vesicles
LH	Luteinising hormone
LRF	Luteinising hormone releasing factor
LTH	Lactotropic hormone, lactotropin (sometimes called prolactin)
MIF	MSH-inhibiting factor
MSH	Melanocyte (or melanophore) stimulating hormone
NLT	Nucleus lateralis tuberis
NSM	Neurosecretory material
OG	Orange G
PAS	Periodic acid–Schiff
PbH	Lead haematoxylin
PIF	Prolactin inhibiting factor
PON	Preoptic nucleus
PTO	Propylthiouracil
PVN	Paraventricular nucleus
RER	Rough endoplasmic reticulum
RF	Releasing factor
RNA	Ribonucleic acid
STH	Somatotropic hormone, somatotropin (= growth hormone)

TRF	Thyrotropic hormone releasing factor
TSH	Thyroid stimulating hormone, thyrotropic hormone, thyrotropin
SO-H	Supraoptico-hypophysial system
SON	Supraoptic nucleus
VP	Vasopressin
VP:O	Vasopressin: oxytocin

Greek Letters denoting Cell-types

α	alpha
β	beta
γ	gamma
δ	delta
ϵ	epsilon
η	eta
κ	kappa

EXPLANATION OF COLOUR PLATE

(A)   Pars distalis of a mole stained by PAS–AB–OG. Acidophils, AB+ cells and chromophobes; in the centre of the field a streak of PAS+ colloid can be seen.

(B)   Pars distalis of the jird, *Meriones libycus*, stained by PAS–AB–OG, to show the variety of cells in a single field.

(C)   The pituitary of a potto stained by PAS–AB–OG. The pars intermedia lies across the centre of the field and shows light and dark cells and red-stained colloid. Part of the infundibular process containing blue-stained NSM appears at the bottom of the figure and part of the pars distalis at the upper border.

(D)   Section through the supraoptic nucleus of a dog stained by PAS–AB–OG. Many of the neurons, particularly those to the left are heavily stained with AB, demonstrating their content of NSM, but other neurons are only lightly stained with this dye. On the right lies a group of the characteristic vesiculated neurons.

(E)   Sagittal section through the pituitary gland of the teleost fish *Poecilia latipinna*, stained by azan, anterior to the right, hypothalamus top left, base of cranium below. Note the mass of LTH cells (red), with strands of faintly pink ACTH cells along posterior border, forming the rostral pars distalis. The blue gonadotropes form the ventral part of the proximal pars distalis, and above them are the STH cells (orange) mixed with a few TSH cells. The pars intermedia forms a very thin rim to the posterior neurohypophysis.

(F)   Section of isolated pituitary gland of the trout, *Salmo gairdneri*, stained by alizarin blue tetrachrome, lateral to midline, anterior to the left. The LTH cells (pink-orange) are arranged in follicles, forming the rostral pars distalis; the proximal pars distalis lies behind, and contains yellow STH cells and blue gonadotropes. The rather few TSH cells lie in the rostral zone, but cannot be seen in this photograph. The large neuro-intermediate lobe forms the ventral (lower) half of the gland.

(G)   Rostral pars distalis of *Poecilia latipinna* to the right, proximal pars distalis to the left, stained by alizarin blue tetrachrome. The red-brown LTH cells on the right; a group of intrusive pars intermedia PAS+ cells in the middle (blue), then a band of grey ACTH cells, with characteristically elongated nuclei. To the left, yellow STH cells. Note the neurohypophysial processes with capillaries containing erythrocytes (orange).

(H)   Part of the neuro-intermediate lobe of the eel, *Anguilla anguilla*, stained by lead haematoxylin, showing pars intermedia cells arranged around a neurohypophysial process. Note the magenta PAS+ cell, and the black PbH+ cell, with its characteristic club-shape and in contact with the neuro-intermediate junction.

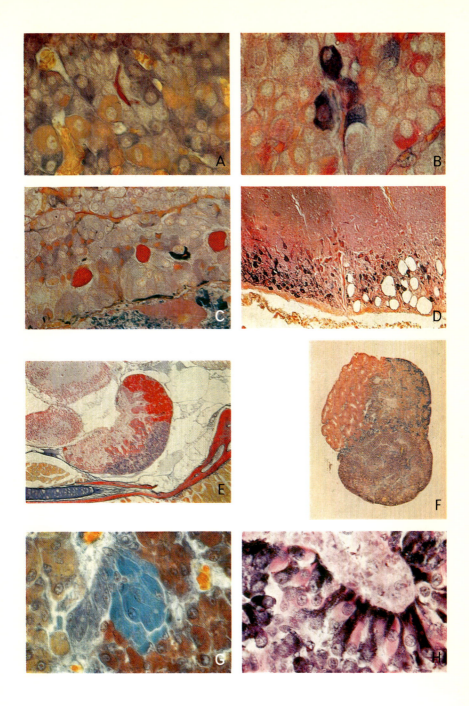

INTRODUCTION

Early ideas relating to the function of the pituitary stemmed from Aristotle's view that the brain served to cool the body, secreting one of the four humours, the phlegm or pituita. This was thought to pass via the pituitary gland through the cribriform plate of the ethmoid bone into the nasal cavity. Although Vesalius, perhaps the leading anatomist of all time, held a different view of the route taken by this mucus (see Singer, 1952) the general idea was apparently accepted until the seventeenth century, when it was asserted by Schneider, and again by Richard Lower, that catarrhal secretions originated in the nasal passages, not the brain. After this time the pituitary was described in various anatomical texts, but little was known of its true function until towards the end of the nineteenth century.

From about 1840 onwards, however, evidence was accumulating which, from a viewpoint of later years, can be seen as providing clues to the gland's activity. Reports were published of such observations as the occurrence of obesity, sexual infantilism, and acromegaly (a secondary excessive growth of parts of the skeleton) in patients with tumours of the gland; and gigantism was observed to be associated with tumours developed in still-growing individuals. But appreciation of the full extent of the role of the pituitary in the body's economy could only be achieved when an experimental approach, involving surgical interference with the gland, became possible early in the present century.

The position of the gland, lying in a hollow in the base of the skull completely overlaid by the brain, inevitably makes it difficult to approach in the living animal. The earliest attempts were on dogs, and it was found that removal of the gland was soon followed by death, although damage to other structures might well have contributed to this. Harvey Cushing in 1909 drew attention to the interrelationship between the pituitary and other ductless glands, and together with his colleagues, increased understanding of the gland by a combination of clinical observations and experimental studies (see Cushing, 1912). Aschner (1912) also published results of removal of the pituitary of dogs, and noted that cessation of growth and genital infantilism followed the operation. Although similar work continued, the way was not really clear for large-scale experimental studies on mammals until 1926, when P. E. Smith described a technique for hypophysectomy of rats, a small, cheap and readily available animal, which also offered the possibility of uniform inbred colonies allowing controlled comparative studies.

Before the turn of the century physiological experiments involving the injection of extracts of the gland were being carried out, and Oliver and Schäfer (1895) noted that this procedure resulted in a rise in blood pressure. They, however, had used an extract of the whole gland, and it was not until extracts of its subdivisions were injected that it became evident that the pressor effect was caused by some constituent of the posterior lobe (Howell, 1898).

Our present understanding of the functions of the pituitary gland has been achieved through an enormous amount of observational and experimental work. Initially, as already indicated, pathological changes in the gland were associated with various clinical disorders. Development of appropriate surgical techniques to allow hypophysectomy with survival then enabled the study of the deficiencies resulting from the operation, and Smith (1927) described the full effects of hypopituitarism. Injections of crude extracts of the gland, or implantation of glandular tissue as in the experiments of Smith (1927, 1930) which indicated something of the relationship between the pituitary, the other endocrine glands and the reproductive system, were followed by the purification of active principles and their analysis, with the ultimate aim of synthesis. The assessment of activity of such principles was first made possible by studying the effects of their injection into pituitary-deficient animals, but now more sophisticated and sensitive in-vitro methods are available.

Morphological studies progressed with functional ones, and by the application of a wide variety of cytological and other techniques it has become possible to understand to a large extent the morphological basis of function in the various parts of the gland. In recent years the way in which the anterior pituitary is controlled by the central nervous system has become clear in outline, although the details are still only partially understood. Furthermore, it is now apparent that the role of the endocrine system in general, and of the pituitary in particular, is not limited to post-natal life, and that the gland plays a major part in fetal growth and development of mammals as well as of other species. Major contributions to knowledge in this regard have been published by Jost over a number of years (see Jost, 1966). Among the techniques used by him was that of fetal hypophysectomy; although he employed the apparently somewhat crude technique of decapitation *in utero*, he was nevertheless able to show for example that the fetal pituitary gland is essential for the normal development of the reproductive system, and that this action is exerted at a specific and critical time in fetal development. More recently a more refined technique for fetal hypophysectomy has been described, in which the gland is destroyed by a coagulating electrode inserted from the lateral aspect of the skull, leaving the bulk of the intracranial tissues undamaged.

The experimental work accompanying the earlier clinical investigations had inevitably stimulated interest in the pituitary gland of laboratory mammals, especially that of the rat, rabbit and guinea-pig. While a good deal of the subsequent work on these animals has been aimed at the solution of clinical problems, to a growing extent the 'laboratory mammals' have been investigated simply in order to elucidate fundamental endocrine physiology, with no thought of direct clinical applications. The knowledge gained in such work forms the foundation of endocrinology as a branch of biology, distinct from practical medicine. From the early years of this century, the boundaries of 'pure' endocrinology have been extending to include more and more of the tens of thousands of non-mammalian vertebrates; even before the surgical skills of P. E. Smith had established the laboratory rat as a central character in the pituitary story, study of the gland in lower vertebrates was well under way with work on amphibians. In 1916, P. E. Smith and B. M. Allen had independently devised a technique for removing the adenohypophysial anlage in young frog tadpoles, and their work provided the first conclusive evidence for any vertebrate of a regulatory relationship between the pituitary gland and the development of the thyroid, gonads and adrenal cortex. Since those pioneer years, the science of comparative endocrinology – embracing endocrine mechanisms in all animals, not just man and the living vertebrates – has expanded enormously, and a considerable part of this body of information relates to the pituitary gland.

In retrospect, it is possible to discern certain landmarks in the progress of comparative endocrinology, and to see how valuable has been the interaction of information gained from widely different animals. For example, during the 1930s, B. A. Houssay and his students in Argentina worked not only on mammals, but also on amphibians, and they obtained information on the metabolic role of the endocrine glands, including the pituitary, in the toad *Bufo arenarum*. This information served to guide much of the later work in this field on mammals and man. Because of the role it plays in adaptive colour changes in amphibians, we know far more about the pars intermedia from work on frogs and toads than from work on mammals; were it not for this information from the lower vertebrates, the mammalian pars intermedia would be even more enigmatic than it actually is.

Attention was drawn to the avian pituitary when Riddle showed in 1933 that the pituitary principle which earlier had been found to initiate and maintain milk secretion in mammals was the same as that which caused growth of the pigeon crop-sac (Riddle, Bates and Dykshorn, 1933). Riddle called the active factor *prolactin*, and the response of the pigeon crop-sac provided a rapid, specific and sensitive means of detecting and measuring prolactin (lactotropic hormone) in pituitary extracts, and so led in 1937 to its crystallisation, the first pituitary hormone to be isolated as a pure, or nearly pure, protein.

During the 1930s, information was accumulating about the fish pituitary, some of it coming from the growing practice on Brazilian fish farms of injecting fish pituitary material in order to induce spawning in fishes reared for food, which otherwise would not breed. Similar methods were developed in Russia during this period, to induce spawning in sturgeons in attempts to improve the yield of the important sturgeon fisheries. In France and Canada, interest in the economically important migrations of salmon gave impetus to fundamental studies on the pituitary and other endocrine glands of teleost fishes, studies which have continued in these countries from the 1940s to the present day. The fish pituitary may be said to have come into its own, scientifically speaking, with the publication in 1957 of one of the germinal works in comparative endocrinology, *The Physiology of the Pituitary Gland of Fishes* by G. E. Pickford and J. W. Atz. This book critically reviewed the whole field of pituitary studies on fishes and amphibians, and it undoubtedly was the stimulus for the great burgeoning of research on the pituitary of lower vertebrates which started in the 1950s, much of it in Pickford's own laboratory, and which has occasioned a large part of this book.

The following account of this complex gland is necessarily selective; merely to list the titles of published works on the pituitary would require a book larger than this one. A brief introductory outline of the general structure and function of the gland is followed by chapters on specific aspects of the mammalian pituitary, introduced where appropriate by historical considerations. The subsequent chapters deal in turn with the gland in each of the non-mammalian vertebrate groups. It might seem more logical to begin at the beginning with the cyclostomes, and then to climb up the evolutionary ladder to the mammals. But the mammalian pituitary is known more completely than any other, and it seems to us easier for the reader if he comes to the relatively poorly-understood gland of lower vertebrates with the mammalian pituitary in mind. Not that we intend to imply that within every fish or frog there lurks a rat pituitary waiting to be discovered; on the contrary, one point that emerges in this comparative survey is the variety of specialisations that the gland has undergone during evolution. The pituitary gland, diagnostic feature of living vertebrates as it is, occurs in the most primitive living 'fishes', as well as in man, but it is less conservative than it looks at first sight.

1

A GENERAL CONSIDERATION
OF THE PITUITARY GLAND

The pituitary gland is both structurally and functionally the most complex of the organs of internal secretion. It occurs throughout the vertebrates, in cyclostomes, fish, amphibians, reptiles, birds and mammals. The subneural gland of sea squirts (*Urochordata*) has morphological features suggestive of its homology with the pituitary gland of higher forms, and Willmer (1970) has even suggested that a forerunner of the pituitary can be recognised in the invertebrate nemertine worms.

In all of the vertebrate classes the gland shows remarkable similarities in its overall morphology; but it is structurally highly specialised, and there are considerable differences in detail between the different classes and even between closely related species. Structural complexity is equalled by that of the gland's secretions and of the mechanisms by which these are controlled.

In all forms the pituitary gland is derived from ectoderm, and it is always made up of two structurally distinct parts, one derived from buccal epithelium, that is somatic ectoderm, and one from the ectodermal neural tube. Unlike the adrenal gland, in which the intimate association of neural and epithelial components only becomes manifest in the higher vertebrates, the close association of the two divisions of the pituitary is seen even in creatures such as the lamprey (*Petromyzon*), and persists throughout the vertebrates. This association is indeed essential for the function of the epithelial part of the gland, which is to a large extent controlled by the central nervous system.

The mammalian pituitary, here considered as a general model of pituitary structure and function, demonstrates something of the complex, variable and often confusing terminology which the gland has acquired. The two main divisions (fig. 1.1), epithelial and neural, can be conveniently designated as the adenohypophysis and the neurohypophysis respectively. Each consists of several subdivisions, which are not equally evident in all species. The neurohypophysis arises as a downgrowth (sometimes called the saccus infundibuli) towards the oral cavity from that region of the neural tube which later forms the hypothalamus, and retains a connection with this part of the brain by means of a stalk of nerve fibres. The part of the hypothalamus from which this stalk arises is

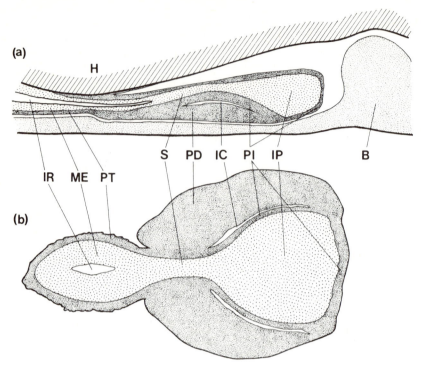

Fig. 1.1. Diagram of (*a*) sagittal and (*b*) horizontal sections through the pituitary gland of a ferret. B, base of skull; H, hypothalamus; IC, intraglandular cleft; IP, infundibular process; IR, infundibular recess; ME, median eminence; PD, pars distalis; PI, pars intermedia; PT, pars tuberalis; S, stalk.

the tuber cinereum; it is bounded anteriorly by the optic chiasma and posteriorly by the mammillary bodies, and lies in the floor of the third ventricle. Between the optic chiasma and the origin of the stalk lies the median eminence of the tuber cinereum. This differs in structure from the rest of the hypothalamus and is properly considered as the proximal part of the neurohypophysis. In some species this specialised zone extends behind the attachment of the stalk, so that the median eminence is not limited to the anterior region. The two other components of the neuro-hypophysis are the stalk of nerve fibres already noted, and a distal enlargement forming the 'posterior' pituitary, made up largely of expansions of the nerve fibres of the stalk in close association with blood vessels. The latter has been called the infundibular process; the stalk of nerve fibres linking it with the hypothalamus is designated as the infundi-bular stem. Hence, the neurohypophysis consists of three main parts: the median eminence in the basal hypothalamus; the infundibular stem made up of nerve fibres; and the infundibular process. The important portal

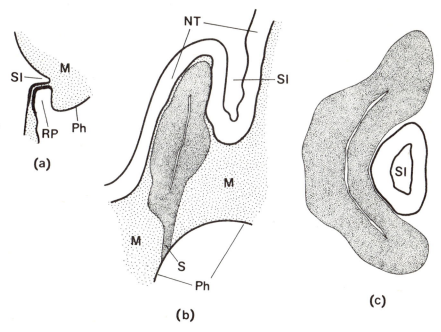

Fig. 1.2. Diagrams of the developing pituitary.

(*a*) Mid-sagittal section through the saccus infundibuli and Rathke's pouch in an early mammalian embryo. Rathke's pouch and the saccus are both wide open.

(*b*) Mid-sagittal section of a later stage of development in a pig embryo. The developing adenohypophysis (dark) contains only a residual lumen and is still connected by an epithelial stalk (S) with the epithelium of the pharynx. It is closely apposed to the hollow neural downgrowth.

(*c*) Horizontal section through the developing pituitary of a slightly later embryo. The adenohypophysis extends laterally and partially embraces the neural process; by this stage the anterior wall of Rathke's pouch has already become thicker than the posterior.

M, mesenchyme; NT, neural tube; Ph, roof of pharynx; RP, Rathke's pouch; SI, saccus infundibuli.

venules (see pp. 99 ff) run down from the median eminence with the nerve fibres of the infundibular stem so that the pituitary *stalk*, referred to as such, consists of both neural and vascular elements. The term 'stem', strictly speaking, should be used to refer only to the *neural* part of this neurovascular structure. Incidentally, an obvious stalk, from which the mass of the gland appears to depend, is not present in all forms (see chapter 2).

During early development the neural downgrowth carries with it a prolongation of the central cavity of the neural tube. In many species this cavity later becomes obliterated; but in some it persists, so that a prolongation of the third ventricle extends for a distance towards, or even into, the infundibulum. Such a cavity is called the infundibular recess, or the recessus hypophyseus.

The nomenclature of the adenohypophysis is derived directly from the association of its three main subdivisions with the neurohypophysis. The whole of this epithelial part of the gland first develops as a pocket of the buccal ectoderm called Rathke's pouch, closely associated with the neural downgrowth (fig. 1.2). Part of the lumen of Rathke's pouch commonly persists, so that a cleft separates the lamina of cells lying apposed to the neural downgrowth from the rest, although the two parts are continuous laterally and above (fig. 1.2). The apposed part develops into the pars infundibularis,* often (and appropriately for many species) called the pars intermedia. Meanwhile two lateral outgrowths of the upper part of the pouch grow forwards and towards the midline, usually joining, and becoming closely applied to the tuber cinereum; these form the pars tuberalis. The anterior wall of the pouch, already at an early stage of development thicker than the posterior, develops into the pars distalis, which constitutes the major epithelial part of the gland.

In pituitaries of some species the ventral parts of the lateral outgrowths of Rathke's pouch which form the pars tuberalis fuse with the pars distalis, and strands of cells derived from the outgrowths can be seen along the anterior-ventral part of the latter. These form the pars tuberalis interna; the superior part, applied to the hypothalamus, is referred to as the pars tuberalis externa. The former should be distinguished from the zona tuberalis (see p. 25), a rostro-medial region of the pars distalis which stains differently from the rest, and which may or may not represent a derivative of those parts of Rathke's pouch giving origin to the pars tuberalis. This, and other subdivisions of both adeno- and neuro-hypophysis, will be considered in the sections devoted to the microscopy of the gland.

The terminology of the various parts of the neurohypophysis and of the adenohypophysis varies considerably in the writings of different authors. The term 'pars anterior', for example, is sometimes used synonymously with pars distalis. 'Pars distalis' in effect refers to the part of the gland which is not so 'juxtaneural' as the other two parts of the adenohypophysis; whereas 'pars anterior' refers to an 'anterior' position-ing of that part of the gland – a true description for man and many other species, but not applicable to the pituitary of all. Purves (1961), however, uses the term 'pars anterior' as the general one of choice, and reserves the term 'pars distalis' for the human gland, in which, he arguably asserts, the pars intermedia has become intermingled with the pars anterior. Purves also proposes a somewhat different terminology for the neurohypophysis. Thus, he divides this into two parts only, a pars

---

* Spatz, Diepen and Gaupp (1948) use the term 'pars infundibularis' for the pars tuberalis.

eminens and a pars nervosa. In the former he includes both the median eminence and the stalk, on the grounds that they have a common vascular pattern (see Green, 1951, and p. 105) and uses 'pars nervosa' for the infundibular process alone.

A common usage, particularly in earlier publications, is to refer to the gland as being made up of anterior and posterior lobes. This has some validity for species in which the lumen of Rathke's pouch persists as an intraglandular cleft, since in such forms the pars intermedia is closely applied to the infundibular process and separates with it when the gland is dissected to form the posterior lobe, leaving the 'anterior lobe', made up of pars distalis (and possibly some pars tuberalis). These terms are not applicable to glands of those species which have no intraglandular cleft.

THE PITUITARY PORTAL SYSTEM

The blood supply is of particular importance in any endocrine gland, since on it depends not only the essential metabolism of the glandular tissue, but also the transport of the gland's secretions to whatever target organs or tissues they influence. In the pituitary gland the vascular system plays a third role in addition to the two basic ones: it serves as a link through which the secretory activity of the pars distalis is controlled by the central nervous system.

A portal vascular system is one in which two capillary beds are linked by veins or venules, so that instead of blood passing from arteries to arterioles to capillaries to venules to veins, and back to the heart, it follows a more extended course, and having passed through a primary set of capillaries to venules or veins is then directed through a secondary vascular bed before passing to the systemic veins.

The pituitary portal system is small; but it is of comparable importance in the animal economy to the enormously larger hepatic portal system. Its precise arrangement varies within wide limits, according to the form of the pituitary gland. Although it is most highly developed in mammals and birds, some form of portal system can be recognised in almost all species having a pituitary gland.

In mammals the arterial blood reaches the pituitary by two sets of vessels, the superior and inferior hypophysial arteries (fig. 1.3). The superior vessels are those predominantly concerned in the blood supply to the adenohypophysis, the inferior with that of the lower part of the neuro-hypophysis, that is the lower stem and the infundibular process itself. As a rule no branches of the superior arteries run directly to the adenohypo-physis, but pass through the pars tuberalis and penetrate the median eminence. Here the blood flows through capillaries arranged in the form of loops, or in the higher mammals complex 'spikes' which penetrate the nervous tissue for up to several millimetres. These capillaries lead into

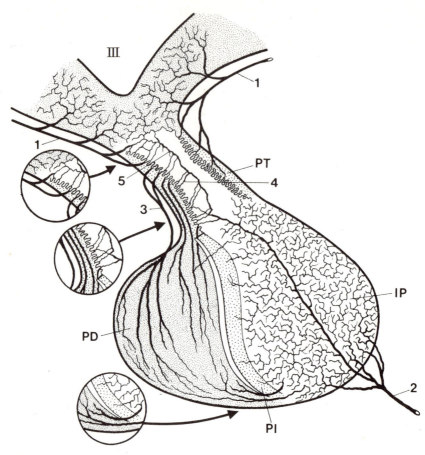

Fig. 1.3. Diagram of the blood supply of the mammalian pituitary gland as seen in a mid-sagittal section through an ink-injected specimen. Insets from above down show anastomoses between hypothalamic capillaries and the portal system; inferior hypophysial vessels and portal system; capillaries of infundibular process and adenohypophysis.

III, third ventricle; 1, superior hypophysial arteries; 2, inferior hypophysial arteries; 3, portal vessels; 4, primary plexus; 5, vessel linking primary plexus and hypothalamic vessels; IP, infundibular process; PD, pars distalis; PI, pars intermedia; PT, pars tuberalis. Reproduced from Holmes, *Symp. zool. Soc. Lond.* **11,** 35–47, by permission of the Zoological Society of London.

portal venules, which leave the median eminence and, lying superficially, pass down the stalk to the pars distalis. Here they open into the second capillary bed in the pars distalis, from which the blood passes into the neighbouring venous sinuses and back into the venous system.

The presence of an anatomical portal system was first described by Popa and Fielding in England and by Pietsch in Germany in 1930, but its full functional significance only became clear later. Perhaps inevitably, before and after the descriptions of this complex vascular system had been published, it was thought that the function of the pars distalis was controlled, as in some other glands, by means of a secreto-motor inner-vation. Many investigators searched for (and apparently found) nerve fibres in the gland, and these are illustrated in many early papers – almost always, however, by drawings. Probably a few nerve fibres do pass into this part of the gland with blood vessels, but most of the so-called nerves seen by the earlier observers were almost certainly reticular fibres, which readily take the deposit of silver which is commonly the agent used to demonstrate nerve fibres histologically. Excellent as many neurohisto-logical methods are, they are never so specific that doubt is entirely lacking as to whether a fibre revealed in a non-neural tissue is a nerve or not. Electron microscopy on the other hand can demonstrate nerves with certainty, and it is significant that, apart from in some fishes, few reports of nerve fibres in the pars distalis have been published, despite the extensive electron microscopic studies of the last fifteen years or so.

SECRETIONS OF THE PITUITARY

The mammalian adenohypophysis secretes at least seven hormonal principles. Six of these are elaborated by cells of the pars distalis; they are:

Thyrotropic hormone (TSH), regulating growth and secretion of the thyroid gland.

Adrenocorticotropic hormone (ACTH), having a similar action on the adrenal cortex.

Somatotropic (or growth) hormone (STH), which controls growth and influences metabolism.

Follicle stimulating hormone (FSH), which is responsible for growth and maturation of ovarian follicles up to the time of ovulation.

Luteinising hormone (LH), which, acting together with FSH, brings about ovulation, and then stimulates the formation and secretion of the corpus luteum.

Lactotropic hormone (LTH), which acts on the mammary gland in mammals. In lower vertebrates this is usually referred to as prolactin.

Apart from STH, all these have a specific target organ, on which their primary action is exerted, and four of these targets are themselves glands of internal secretion, namely the thyroid, adrenal cortex, ovarian follicles and corpus luteum. Although the last three hormones in the list, which are concerned particularly with reproductive activity, are often discussed in terms of their action on the ovaries and mammary glands, they are also secreted by the male pituitary. Thus, FSH acts on the tubules of the testis, stimulating the early stages of spermatogenesis, while LH acts on testicular interstitial cells, located between the tubules, which secrete androgen; hence LH may be referred to as the interstitial cell stimulating hormone (ICSH). The role of LTH in the male is uncertain.

The pars intermedia secretes the hormone intermedin which controls skin colour in lower vertebrates such as amphibians. This is also known as melanocyte (or melanophore) stimulating hormone (MSH). The role of this factor remains something of an enigma as far as the higher mammals, such as man, are concerned (see p. 54). Chemically, it has some affinity with ACTH and exists in two forms. In 1964 C. H. Li reported the isolation from pituitary tissue of yet another factor having both melanocyte stimulating and lipolytic activity, which he called lipotropin (see Li, 1969), but little is yet known of the role of this hormone in relation to the other pituitary principles.

THE NEUROHYPOPHYSIS

The neural part of the pituitary is associated with two hormones, oxytocin, which brings about contraction of smooth muscle in the reproductive tract and of myoepithelial cells in the mammary gland, and antidiuretic hormone (ADH). The latter acts on the distal tubules and collecting ducts of the kidney, increasing the resorption of water from the dilute glomerular filtrate and hence concentrating the urine. Since in high dosage ADH also causes a rise in blood pressure (in mammals), it is sometimes called vasopressin.

The neurohypophysis consists essentially of the distal parts of the processes of neurons whose cell bodies lie in two pairs of hypothalamic nuclei, called supraoptic and paraventricular. These hypothalamic neurons elaborate the two neurohypophysial hormones which then pass via the nerve fibres of the infundibular stem to be stored in the infundibular process. The two factors thus belong to the category of neurosecretory hormones (see p. 71).

CONTROL OF ACTIVITY OF THE PITUITARY

The understanding of the way in which activity of the pituitary is regulated has been arrived at as a result of many experimental studies, some of which are referred to in chapter 6. By way of introduction, however, several dogmatic (and hence not necessarily entirely correct) statements may be made:

1. The secretory activity of the adenohypophysis is to a large extent under the direct control of the nervous system.

2. The pituitary portal vascular system, and not a direct nervous connection, is the major functional link between the adenohypophysis and the central nervous system.

3. The levels of adenohypophysial hormones in the blood play a part in regulating the gland's activity, by means of 'feedback' mechanisms.

4. External environmental factors can modulate pituitary activity via the hypothalamo-portal-adenohypophysial link.

5. Neurohypophysial activity is more immediately dependent on the central nervous system than adenohypophysial, since the infundibular process is largely made up of the expanded terminals of processes of neurons lying in the hypothalamus.

Some endocrine glands, such as the thyroid, can continue to function more or less normally if they are transplanted to some site in the body other than their usual one. The pituitary, however, does not behave in this way; if in the mammal it is transplanted to the capsule of the kidney, for example, a site where it can readily acquire a good blood supply, the animal shows effects which approach those of total hypophysectomy. Thus, there is an almost complete loss of gonadotropic activity, including cessation of reproductive cycles, and a severe reduction in the secretion of STH, ACTH and TSH, with resultant effects on growth and metabolism and atrophy of the adrenal cortex and thyroid. The secretion of lactotropic hormone alone of the six normally secreted by the pars distalis is not reduced, but increased. Cytological changes in the transplanted pituitary gland correspond to the changes in activity (see p. 117), and the only cells which do not undergo marked degranulation and degeneration are those which are thought to secrete LTH. The return of the gland to a position under the median eminence where it can regain a 'portal' supply of blood, however, often results in considerable or even complete restoration of secretory activity.

Division of the pituitary stalk, even if the gland is left in its normal position, may also be followed by a great loss of function of the pars distalis. The results of many such operations have been described in the literature, but the reported effects of the lesion have varied considerably, some observers finding greater or lesser disturbance of function, others virtually no effect. In the light of what is now known, such variance is hardly surprising. Firstly, division of the stalk interferes with the normal blood supply to the pars distalis, and may therefore result in death of a greater or lesser part of the secretory tissue. Secondly, loss of the vascular hypothalamo-hypophysial link removes the pathway through which the central nervous system controls the gland, and in that way also disturbs glandular function. It now seems likely that, in those experiments which revealed no apparent loss of activity or only a transient disturbance, either the stalk had not been completely divided, or the vessels had regenerated. Vascular re-connection can occur within a day or two, but may be prevented by placing an impermeable barrier between the cut ends of the stalk.

It seemed evident from observations such as these that some factor or factors carried in the portal blood might be essential to the gland's activity. In recent years this has been proved to be correct, and a number of potent 'releasing factors' for the adenohypophysial tropic hormones have been isolated from hypothalamic tissue and from blood (McCann and Porter, 1969), and their chemical structure determined. Some of these have now been synthesised.

It has long been appreciated that feedback mechanisms play an important part in controlling adenohypophysial activity. At first the chief mechanism was thought to be one of 'negative feedback'. For example, cells of the pars distalis secrete TSH which acts on the thyroid gland to increase the output of thyroxine; the thyroxine in the blood then acts on the hypothalamo-pituitary axis to inhibit the output of TSH, thus providing a regulatory mechanism to prevent over-stimulation of the thyroid. It is now evident that a complex series of feedback mechanisms operates; Motta, Piva and Martini (1970) discuss these and distinguish four types. The first is a 'long' feedback mechanism, in which the hypothalamus monitors hormones synthesised by peripheral target organs, as in the TSH–thyroid example given above. The second is a 'short' feedback mechanism, in which the tropic hormones themselves are monitored by the hypothalamus. The third is a mechanism by which the hypothalamus monitors the various releasing factors (see p. 126); and the fourth is a mechanism whereby the tropic hormone within the tissue and tissue fluid regulates the release of the tropic hormone.

As for the neurohypophysis, the effects of transplantation or of cutting the stalk were more readily predictable, at any rate in morphological terms, than for the adenohypophysis. When any nerve or tract of nerve fibres is divided, the distal part of each divided fibre (that is that part separated by the lesion from the cell body) degenerates. This happens if the pituitary stalk is divided. Following such a lesion, the nerve fibres passing to the infundibular process atrophy below the point of division. As this occurs, the hormones stored in the process are released. Since the infundibular process normally serves not only as the main site of storage of these principles but also as that of their release into the bloodstream, signs of deficiency appear when the store is exhausted. Most marked is an increase in the output of urine, and a fall in its specific gravity.

The pituitary gland is thus complex in origin and in function, and plays a major role by the direct action of its hormones in reproduction, lactation, growth, metabolism and the conservation of water. Indirectly through the adrenal cortex and thyroid the gland further influences the metabolism of the body. Its gonadotropic hormones, acting on the reproductive glands, control not only maturation and release of the germ cells, but indirectly, by stimulating the secretions of male and female sex hormones, the development of secondary sexual characteristics, reproductive cycles and fertility. The pars intermedia seems to be of particular importance in lower vertebrates, in which adaptation of skin colour to the surroundings may be necessary for survival.

Yet the pituitary gland itself has only a very limited autonomy. Separated from direct association with the central nervous system it loses the greater part of its potency. It is indeed no longer held to be 'the leader of the endocrine orchestra', as it was once popularly described, but a kind of transducer which by means of its endocrine secretions enables the central nervous system to control a wide range of bodily functions. This does not diminish the intrinsic importance of the gland, for without it life is barely possible; but it acts as a member of a neuro-endocrine unit, each part of which is necessary for the function of the whole.

2

COMPARATIVE MORPHOLOGY
OF THE MAMMALIAN PITUITARY

The dual origin of the pituitary gland described in the introduction and the interrelationships of the two components during the whole developmental and growth period clearly play a major part in the determination of the final form of the gland. In this context a few aspects of its embryology are considered.

The two anlagen of the gland, Rathke's pouch and the saccus infundibuli, are commonly described as 'outgrowths', and the concept of two ectodermal pouches which grow together to form the neural-epithelial complex of the fully developed pituitary is one that is commonly found in embryological texts. Martinez (1960) in his thesis, however, noted that this idea is apparently not correct, and drew attention to a detailed study of the formation of the pituitary in the cat by Brahms (1932). This work showed that already at an early stage of development (eleven somites) a 'hypophysial area' could be defined, where the two plates of ectoderm, neural and stomodeal, were already in close contact with each other (fig. 1.2), no mesoderm intervening. The later development of the complex, with the appearance of Rathke's pouch in its typical form, appears to be the result of the drawing out of a diverticulum from the stomodoeum by the ventral bending of the rostral part of the neural tube, the two ectoderms remaining adherent to one another over the hypophysial area. Isolation of the hypophysial area from the future mouth follows, partly at any rate, by extensive proliferation of mesenchyme. This early and close contact between neural ectoderm and that part of the buccal ectoderm which becomes the posterior wall of Rathke's pouch may be essential for the differentiation of a typical pars intermedia (see below).

The relative degrees of development, of extent and of association of the various parts of the pituitary differ considerably in different species of mammals and more so in other vertebrates. The origin of these differences lies in the way in which the complex develops from the two original pouches. Each of the two diverticula is at first a hollow protrusion of the wall of a cavity – Rathke's pouch from that of the stomodoeum immediately in front of the buccopharyngeal membrane, and the saccus infundibuli from that bounding the closed cavity of the neural tube. Early,

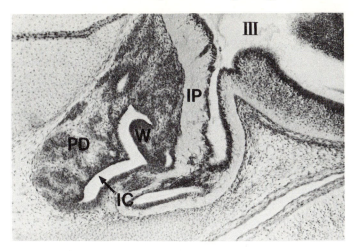

Fig. 2.1. Mid-sagittal section through the developing pituitary gland of a sheep. The infundibular process (IP) has a lumen continuous with the third ventricle (III) and the thickening of the anterior wall of Rathke's pouch giving rise to the pars distalis (PD) is apparent. The cone of Wulzen (W) projects into the intraglandular cleft (IC).

the lumen of Rathke's pouch loses continuity with the future buccal cavity, by obliteration of the lower (oral) part of the pouch. The upper (aboral) part is by this means converted into a closed cavity whose wall remains connected for a time with the oral epithelium by a strand of cells (fig. 1.2). In mammals, but not in all birds, this strand disappears and mesodermal proliferation increases the separation between the developing pituitary and the roof of the pharynx. The cavity of the pouch remains in many species as the intraglandular cleft, and may contain colloid material.

A remnant of the pharyngeal extremity of Rathke's pouch may persist, and develop to give rise to a pharyngeal hypophysis, lying in the roof of the pharynx just behind the nasal septum. Boyd (1956) described this structure as well vascularised and as showing some cellular differentiation similar to that of the pars distalis. It lies of course remote from the hypothalamus, the sphenoid bone intervening, and there was initially no evidence that it was secretory. McGrath (1968), however, published evidence for the occurrence of prolactin (LTH) and growth hormone in pharyngeal hypophyses of human cadavers. More recently (1971) she has published the results of volumetric studies of the pharyngeal hypophysis in a series of human cadavers, and produced evidence indicating that the structure undergoes a significant increase in size after about the age of fifty in women but not in men. She suggests that this might indicate the development of a trans-sphenoidal extension of the hypothalamo-hypophysial portal system, and hence that some controlled function of the pharyngeal hypophysis may begin in women at about this age.

Another feature that has been considered to be derived from Rathke's pouch is the craniopharyngeal canal, a channel passing through the body of the sphenoid. This is constant in some mammals, and is said to be frequent (9 per cent) in human newborn infants, although commonly obliterated later (Arey, 1950). Its occurrence along approximately the line of Rathke's pouch might suggest that it also is a remnant of this structure; but according to Arey this is not so, and the canal is a secondary development which forms during osteogenesis after the obliteration of the oral part of the pouch.

At the time of its formation the walls of Rathke's pouch are uniformly thin, but soon the anterior wall begins to thicken more than the rest. This difference in rate of growth is apparent from an early stage of development (fig. 2.1) and by an extensive proliferation the anterior wall gives rise to most of the pars distalis. As already noted (p. 8) there is in some instances a contribution in the form of a pars tuberalis interna derived from the lateral outgrowths from Rathke's pouch which constantly form the external pars tuberalis.

The posterior wall of the pouch, closely applied to the neural downgrowth, undergoes a certain amount of growth and differentiation, although it remains relatively thin compared with the anterior wall. The differentiation of the pars intermedia, it has been suggested, is dependent on the intimate contact between the posterior wall of Rathke's pouch and the neural downgrowth, the latter probably exerting an inductive influence over the cells of the former. Embryological evidence in favour of such a mechanism is the fact that a pars intermedia only develops when there is close apposition between epithelial and neural elements of the developing pituitary and that the differentiation only occurs in the epithelial component which is in such contact. Furthermore, in birds, in which a typical pars intermedia does not develop, the equivalent wall of Rathke's pouch becomes separated from the neural tissue by connective tissue at an early stage of development. When, occasionally, small areas of contact between the neural tissue and pars distalis occur, these areas develop chromophobic, intermedia-like tissue (see Wingstrand, 1951). Similarly, in those mammals in which connective tissue separates the neurohypophysis from the adenohypophysis, as in the Cetacea, again no pars intermedia is found. There is also considerable experimental evidence supporting the hypothesis of the kind provided by Gaillard (1937) who cultured together anterior and posterior pituitary tissue from young rabbits, and found that the part of the anterior pituitary tissue lying close to neural elements developed to resemble intermedia. This effect was not produced when non-pituitary tissues were substituted for the neural component of the culture (see also the section on Amphibia, p. 237).

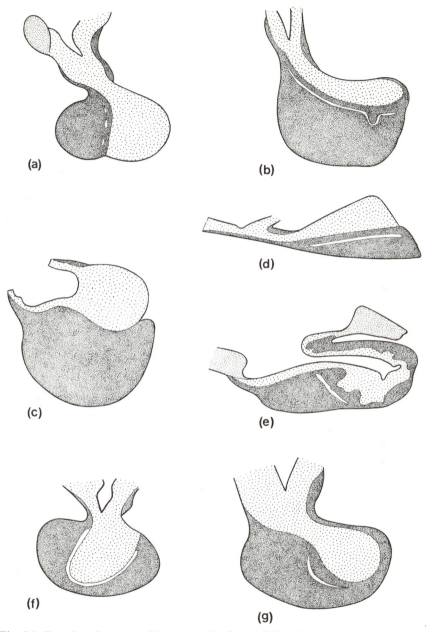

Fig. 2.2. Drawings (not to scale) to show the form of the pituitary gland as seen in the mid-sagittal section, rostral to left, caudal to right. In each drawing the whole adenohypophysis is in dark grey; the bulk of this forms the pars distalis, but the pars intermedia can be distinguished particularly in (*a*) and (*d*) as closely applied to the neural part of the gland. The pars tuberalis forms a collar around the upper part of the stalk and median eminence. (*a*) rhesus monkey; (*b*) ox; (*c*) Indian unicorn; (*d*) rat; (*e*) polar bear; (*f*) opossum; (*g*) sea lion. (Figs. *b, c, e, f* and *g* redrawn from Hanström, 1966.)

GENERAL MORPHOLOGY
MAMMALS

Even within the order of mammals, the pituitary gland often shows great variations in morphology in different species, although many similar forms occur. Detailed descriptions can be found in reviews such as those of Oboussier (1947) and Hanström (1966) as well as in numerous papers by these and other authors (see Hanström, 1966, for references), and here only the main patterns will be described with appropriate examples.

The main features to be noted are summarised as follows:

1. The degree of development of the three parts of the neurohypophysis, the infundibulum, infundibular stem and infundibular process; the extent of persistence of the infundibular recess; and the orientation of the axis in relation to the brain and base of skull.

2. The degree of development of the three parts of the adenohypophysis, pars distalis, pars tuberalis and pars intermedia; the relations of these to the neurohypophysis; and the degree of persistence of an intra-glandular cleft.

3. Any other notable features which distinguish the glands of particular species.

Glands are often described by reference to midline sagittal sections; these give a good idea of many key features, but inevitably fail to give any indication of the overall shape of the gland, the lateral extent of its various components and such features as the extent to which the neural part is enveloped by the adenohypophysis. Such sections do, however, give more information than any other single plane, and will be used here as main reference points.

THE NEUROHYPOPHYSIS

The orientation of the neurohypophysis varies (fig. 2.2) from an axis extending more or less vertically down from the hypothalamus, as in man, to one which is almost horizontal, as in the ferret. Other species such as the rhesus monkey have an axis lying at some intermediate angle; alternatively, the axis may be bent, as in the ox, in which the upper part of the stem and median eminence descends almost vertically from the tuber cinereum, but the lower stem and infundibular process lie horizontally. In man and some monkeys (for example *Macacus rhesus*, fig. 2.2) the stalk is long, and easily divided surgically without direct injury to the pituitary or to the overlying brain. In the ferret, although the stalk is fairly long, because of its horizontal axis, both it and the main part of the pituitary gland are closely overlain by the brain.

In many species the stalk is relatively short. Even when long and free, it is often more or less covered by the pars tuberalis, but a short stalk may lie in a groove in the epithelial tissue of the adenohypophysis or be completely embedded within and surrounded by such tissue. Distinction may then be made into an upper and lower infundibular stem; the latter with its associated vessels may then be referred to as the 'intraglandular stalk'.

An extreme instance of a modified infundibular stem is found in the Rhinoceridae, in which it is apparently completely absent (Oboussier, 1956). In the Indian unicorn (*Rhinocerus unicornis*), for example (fig. 2.2), the median eminence with a large hypophysial recess is continuous directly into the infundibular process so that no true stalk is apparent.

The size of the infundibular or hypophysial recess is also a major variable in relation to the general form of the neurohypophysis. This recess may persist as little more than a slight depression in the floor of the hypothalamus; it may extend down the stem to a variable extent, or less commonly run as far as the infundibular process itself. In some forms the cavity may enlarge within the process so that the latter is in effect a hollow structure (e.g. polar bear, Hanström, 1947). The extent of the recess in the neurohypophysis is of some practical importance in relation to any kind of surgical procedure involving the gland. In the ferret, for example, division of the stalk beyond the extent of the pars distalis must inevitably open the third ventricle, and allow drainage of cerebrospinal fluid through the wound.

THE ADENOHYPOPHYSIS

Pituitary glands in which the neurohypophysis lies more or less horizontally often tend to be more flattened than those with a more vertical axis, and in such glands the pars distalis tends to lie antero-inferiorly, as for example in the ferret (fig. 1.1). In rats (fig. 2.2) the pars distalis lies entirely inferiorly, so that the only part of the neurohypophysis which comes into relationship with the base of the skull is the median eminence and the first part of the stalk arising from it. At the other extreme the pars distalis may lie entirely in front of the neurohypophysis as in *M. rhesus* (fig. 2.2), when it justifies the name pars anterior.

Whatever may be the position of the main mass of the pars distalis, or for that matter of the pars intermedia as well, glandular tissue is not necessarily limited to that position, whether anterior, antero-ventral or ventral, but may extend to surround the neurohypophysis to a greater or lesser extent, as in the opossum (Wheeler, 1943) (fig. 2.2). Horizontal sections are of course necessary to show any such lateral and posterior extensions of the adenohypophysis.

HPG

THE PARS INTERMEDIA

This part of the gland varies considerably in extent; often it consists only of a thin lamina of cells more or less co-extensive with the posterior aspect of the pars distalis, and separated from it by the intraglandular cleft. It may extend further over the infundibular process, either maintaining the same kind of relationship with the pars distalis, as in the dog or, as in the ferret, form a layer of cells on posterior and superior aspects of the process not accompanied by cells of the pars distalis (fig. 1.1). Such an extension may be incomplete, so that in any particular histological section, apparently isolated islands of intermedia cells are seen.

The most notable variant of the mammalian pars intermedia is its complete absence in those Cetacea (whales and dolphins) so far studied. In these forms (see Hanström, 1966, for references) the neural and glandular lobes of the pituitary are separated from each other by a lamina of connective tissue; the pars distalis is a solid mass of epithelial cells and no intraglandular cleft is present. The separation between the two major divisions of the gland is not, however, total, since a process of pars tuberalis extends upwards to form a small expansion about the median eminence and perhaps the upper stem, and thus provides a cellular matrix for the passage of portal vessels to the pars distalis (see p. 113).

In the human pituitary there is no general agreement as to whether the pars intermedia is present or not. It is present during fetal life, and probably largely disappears as a distinct division of the adenohypophysis later. Commonly a layer of colloid-containing cysts remains in its place (fig. 2.3), but in some specimens chromophobic intermedia-like cells can also be seen (the evidence published before 1940 was considered by Romeis (1940)). On balance it seems that true elements of the pars intermedia can be found in the human gland, but that these constitute only a very small part of the whole. In part, however, the posterior wall of Rathke's pouch has probably contributed to basophilic cells which are found within the infundibular process and constitute an additional component of the posterior part of the gland in man, but not apparently to any considerable extent in other animals.

Functional aspects of the pars intermedia are considered later, but some note should be taken here of the considerable variation in the degree of development of this part of the gland. H. Legait (1964) published a table comparing the percentage volume of the anterior, neural and intermediate elements in pituitary glands of over seventy mammalian species. In rodents he found that the proportion of intermedia varied from 0.2 per cent in the garden dormouse to 27 per cent in the jird *Meriones crassus*, and considerable, although lesser, variations occurred in carnivores, primates and others. Legait considered that the size of the

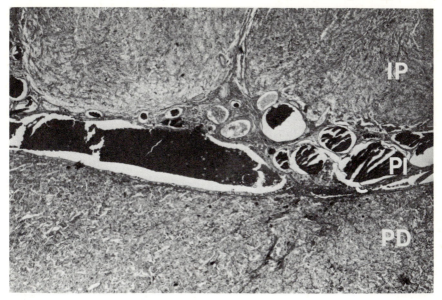

Fig. 2.3. Photomicrograph of the region of the pars intermedia (PI) of the human pituitary gland. Note the colloid-filled cysts. PD, pars distalis; IP, infundibular process.

pars intermedia could be correlated directly with resistance to lack of water, i.e. with life in a desert habitat (see p. 60). Certainly the absence of a pars intermedia in aquatic mammals such as the whales and dolphins would not go against such a view.

THE CONE OF WULZEN

Wulzen's cone, 'a capriciously occurring lobe in the mammalian hypophysis' (Hanström, 1965), was first described by Wulzen (1914) in the pituitary of the ox. It consists of a cone-shaped mass of adenohypophysial tissue which is derived from the posterior wall of Rathke's pouch and extends forward from the pars intermedia, but which has a microscopic structure more akin to that of the pars distalis. It also occurs in the sheep (fig. 2.1) and in a few rare species (see Hanström, 1965). The cone may be continuous with the pars distalis, but can be differentiated from it by being composed of smaller and 'less specialised' cells. The particular interest of this structure is its derivation, since the posterior wall of the pouch does not normally give rise to secretory cells typical of the pars distalis. Perhaps the cone is less influenced by the neural process, which is thought to determine development of the intermedia type of structure, or more strongly influenced by the pars distalis during a critical period of embryogenesis.

THE PARS TUBERALIS

The third component of the adenohypophysis, the pars tuberalis, has already been described as a development from lateral outgrowths of Rathke's pouch, which give rise to a pars tuberalis externa lying on the surface of the tuber cinereum and, in some species, a pars interna which joins the pars distalis. The full extent of the pars tuberalis externa may not be appreciated unless the gland and the overlying hypothalamus are examined together.

In mammals, in contrast to birds (see p. 323), the pars tuberalis externa is usually closely associated throughout its extent with the median eminence and infundibular stem, although it often extends over the tuber, reaching (as in the ferret) the optic chiasma anteriorly, and in some species extending also behind the origin of the stem. Over much of its extent its cells lie around the small arteries and arterioles supplying the primary plexus of the portal vessels, and similarly its extension along the stem forms a cellular sheath for the portal venules themselves. The pars tuberalis is often continuous with the pars distalis, and may appear continuous with the pars intermedia immediately below the tuberal region. Embryologically of course these two latter divisions have distinct origins, and cytologically the two can be readily distinguished (p. 61). In the egg-laying mammals (Prototheria), the spiny ant-eaters and the duck-billed platypus, there is no such continuity. A pars tuberalis externa extends over the surface of the median eminence, but cellular continuity with the pars distalis is achieved only via strands of cells which accompany portal vessels and run to the pars tuberalis interna within the pars distalis. Thus, these lower mammals show a typical porto-tuberal tract, such as is found in birds and many reptiles (see below). The pars tuberalis appears to be lacking in the West African pangolin (Herlant, 1958) and sloths (Wislocki, 1938*a*). The functions of the pars tuberalis are not clear and some possibilities are discussed on p. 62.

CELLULAR PATTERN OF THE PARS DISTALIS

The general disposition of glandular cells within the mammalian pars distalis is one of cords or clumps of cells closely associated with blood vessels, often with large perivascular spaces, best shown in electron micrographs (see fig. 3.4). The glands of some species show a striking arrangement of the cells in follicles, each with a lumen of variable size, often containing PAS-positive colloid. This pattern occurs in the tree shrew, and even more strikingly in the potto (fig. 2.4). Isolated follicles with colloid occasionally occur in glands of species which do not usually have them, such as the monkey *M. rhesus*. A follicular pattern is evident during the proliferative stage of Rathke's pouch.

In the glands of many species, the various types of secretory cell (see

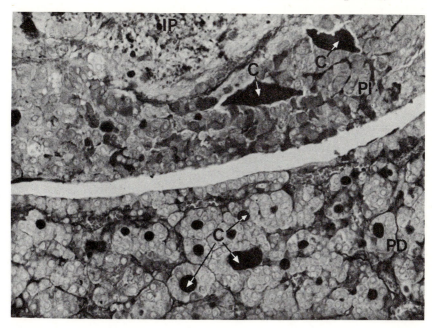

Fig. 2.4. Pars distalis of the potto. Note the colloid (C) in follicles of the pars distalis and pars intermedia. IP, infundibular process; PI, pars intermedia; PD, pars distalis.

pp. 26ff) are not uniformly distributed throughout the pars distalis. In the rat, for example, basophils of different function are differently located (see Purves and Griesbach, 1951). A more striking feature is the presence of a zona tuberalis, such as that described in the rabbit (Dawson, 1937). This consists of a zone situated in the median antero-ventral part of the pars distalis made up almost entirely of basophils and chromophobes. The zone is continuous superiorly with the pars tuberalis. A similar zone, more or less distinct, occurs in other species, such as the rhesus monkey (Dawson, 1948). In the tree shrew, whose pituitary gland is flattened dorso-ventrally, such a non-acidophilic zone lies immediately adjacent to the intraglandular stem, and is continuous with the pars tuberalis.

3

THE CYTOLOGY OF THE PARS DISTALIS

Our present understanding of the relationship between the structure and function of the adenohypophysis, as far as its cytology is concerned, has come from the interpretation of results obtained by applying a number of techniques to the study of both normal glands and those from animals subjected to a variety of experimental procedures designed to alter secretory function; for man, glands from subjects with various pathological conditions have served as 'experimental models'. Up to the later 1940s, most techniques used were essentially based on optical microscopy; at first simple and later more complex dye mixtures were used to stain sections of the gland and distinguish the various types of cell by virtue of their different affinity for the dyes. From the late 1940s onwards, the methods of histochemistry, then becoming popular, began to be applied to pituitary studies. At first this simply involved the use of what were in effect stains having a greater degree of specificity for certain components of the secretory cells – for example, the application of the periodic acid-Schiff (PAS) method for the demonstration of glyco- or mucoprotein, which has now become almost a routine procedure in the study of pituitary cytology. The methods of enzyme histochemistry have also been used, and some techniques of this kind have helped in the elucidation of the function of certain elements of the gland.

Cytological studies were considerably advanced by the general availability of the electron microscope, which provided a means of more certain identification of types of cell on the basis of their fine morphology. Since the shape and range of size of secretory granules is often characteristic for a given (functional) type of cell, this has enabled functional attributions to be made more certainly. The high resolving power of the electron microscope proved particularly useful in the study of cells which stained feebly with dyes, and it became clear that such chromophobes are usually, if not always, simply secretory cells which possess few specific granules, without necessarily being inactive. Electron microscopy has also made possible the correlation, to a greater extent than was possible before, of structure and hormonal activity of the pituitary cells, by applying it to the study of cell homogenates obtained by ultra-centrifugation. Fractions consisting predominantly of one particular size of granule can be obtained; the type of granule can be identified by electron microscopy and its biological activity and its biochemical make-up determined.

The techniques of autoradiography have also been used in the investigation of pituitary function, although, as will be seen in chapter 5, it is our understanding of the neurohypophysis that has in particular been advanced by this technique. Another development, which may provide one of the most specific means of identifying functional cell types, is that of immunofluorescence, whereby protein hormones secreted by the adenohypophysial cells can be localised and identified by a specific antigen–antibody reaction in histological sections.

THE DEVELOPMENT OF STAINING TECHNIQUES

The beginning of understanding of the microscopic structure of the pars distalis dates from the period between 1844 and 1876 when attention began to be paid to the cellular make-up of the gland. Hannover (1844) described the pituitary of several different creatures, including the plaice, frog, hen and man. In the plaice and man, he identified two kinds of cell, although, as was usual during this early period, the features noted were mainly the overall shape and size of cells and their nuclei, and the presence or absence of obvious granulation. The drawings with which Hannover and other authors illustrated their work are not much help in identification of these cell types at the present day. At this time histological techniques were little developed, and although the use of aniline dyes to stain biological material was first described in 1862, these substances did not come into widespread use until about the turn of the century.

Probably the first characterisation of cell types to have some clear affinity with later studies was that made by Flesch (1884), who presented his findings on the anterior pituitary of the horse, dog and man at the 67th meeting of the Société Helvétique des Sciences Naturelles. His sections were stained with osmic acid, eosin, indigo or Weigert's chrome haematoxylin. He described the arrangement of cells in 'cellular tubes' and noted two distinct types, namely large cells with large granules which coloured strongly with his dyes and smaller cells which did not take up the stains. A pupil of Flesch, Lothringer, published further observations in 1886, which were notable for the introduction of the term 'chromophil' for the granular, dark, strongly staining cells similar to those described by Flesch himself.

The next important advance came some six years later with a publication by Schönemann (1892), describing preparations stained with alum haematoxylin and eosin. He noted two types of stainable chromophil cells, coloured red or blue, and designated these as eosinophil and cyanophil respectively. The cells which did not take up dyes to any appreciable extent constitute the chromophobes.

Other early work has been reviewed by Romeis (1940), and papers such as the one by Bailey (1921) refer to many earlier studies. Progress in appreciating the real complexity of the microscopic structure of the adenohypophysis was slow, for two main reasons – firstly, the limitations of the histological techniques then in use, and secondly the lack of precise knowledge of the complexity of the functions of the gland. Increased understanding of the latter has been an important stimulus to cytological studies, so that at the present time, at any rate in the glands of some of the commoner species of mammals, specific hormone secretion can be ascribed to specific cell types, so that the ideal of a functional terminology is possible. In many species, however, functional attributions are uncertain or hypothetical, being based on such characteristics as staining reactions similar to those of cells in other species whose function is known. This problem is considered more fully elsewhere (see pp. 48ff).

Methods of fixation used by early observers tended to be complex, and one of the problems of cytological studies was that too much was preserved in the cells by some of these methods. Mitochondria, for example, which are destroyed by many methods of fixation, persist after some of the 'classical' fixatives and take up acid dyes. Bailey (1921) suggested that the observations of such acidophilic 'granules' among the basophilic* granules of the basophils may have led to the idea that transitional forms between acidophils and the former cell type existed, the amphophil (see Severinghaus, 1938).

Several authors supported the latter theory and considered that the acidophil, basophil and chromophobe were simply different functional states of the same type of cell. Others, however, while noting a variety of transitional forms between chromophobes and eosinophils, and chromophobes and basophils, did not observe any signs of eosinophil–basophil transitions (see Severinghaus, 1938).

Little real advance was made in the differential staining of adenohypophysial cells until the early 1930s, although a considerable variety of dyes had been tried by this time. Bailey gives details of a number of staining schedules, but even using these he was apparently not able to differentiate the cells of the pars distalis (pars buccalis) beyond the granular basophils and eosinophils and the chromophobes.

In the absence of clearly defined ideas of the full function of the pituitary – which were not possible at the time – cytological studies of the pars distalis were sometimes a by-product of investigations directed to other ends. Maurer and Lewis (1922), for example, whose primary interest was in the pars intermedia, stained the pituitary of the domestic pig by

* The terms 'basophil' and 'basophilic' are commonly used by many authors to describe a type of chromophil cell distinct from acidophils, and are so used in this text. The terms are not entirely satisfactory, and the matter is considered more fully on pp. 32ff.

three different methods, acid fuchsin–acid violet, neutral safranin–acid violet, and a neutral gentian method. They employed the technique of staining sections by one method, extracting the dyes after microscopical examination, restaining by the second and repeating the procedure to stain with the third. Thus, the staining characteristics of the same adeno-hypophysial cells stained by different dyes could be studied. Perhaps the most important outcome of their observations was the realisation that the terms oxyphil (acidophil) and basophil are not truly descriptive of cells of the anterior lobe, since a given cell may stain with acid or basic stains. This is an important concept, since it must follow that the use of 'acidophilic' and 'basophilic' can lead to considerable confusion. Maurer and Lewis also claimed to have differentiated five types of cell in the anterior lobe. Three of these were chromophils, two of which were readily recognisable as the eosinophils and basophils described by earlier investigators. Their description of the third type as 'a hitherto undefined cell forming the main mass of the darker band of tissue extending down from the stalk on the anterior surface of the gland' seems to refer to the pars tuberalis. Interestingly, the two authors also described two types of chromophobe; one, with no 'secretion antecedent granules', stained faintly and was found after Helly fixation; the other, observed after formalin fixation, showed diffuse staining of the cytoplasm, and was described as sometimes containing a few large granules which stained with acid violet.

The possibility of considerable advances in pituitary cytology came in 1932 when Cleveland and Wolfe published details of a new technique for staining the anterior lobe of the gland. This was based essentially on a Mallory method, modified in the light of the findings of Biedermann (1927). The latter had used mixtures of acidic and basic dyes, and found that the staining characteristics of pituitary cells varied according to the alkalinity or acidity of the medium in which the dyes were dissolved, and hence that (as already noted) acidophilia and basophilia are not un-changeable characteristics. Cleveland and Wolfe fixed their material in Regaud's mixture, and followed fixation by chromation in 3 per cent potassium dichromate for eight days. Although they refer to this latter procedure as if it were novel, the value of this salt as a mordant seems to have been already well known, as it was used by Benda and others in the early part of the twentieth century (see Romeis, 1940, for references). Later work confirmed the fact that such treatment greatly improves the staining characteristics of the secretory granules of pituitary cells. Cleveland and Wolfe also substituted erythrosin for the acid fuchsin of the original Mallory mixture, and stained the sections with each dye separately, following erythrosin first with orange G in 1 per cent phospho-molybdic acid, and then with aniline blue. Applying their techniques to glands from the sow, dog, white rat and rabbit, they found that it was possible to distinguish four types of secretory cells, namely large pale blue, dark blue with purple-red granules, orange with large granules and those containing yellow-stained granules.

Wolfe and his colleagues (Wolfe, Cleveland and Campbell, 1933) also applied this method of staining more extensively to the dog's pituitary, and in 1933 published a paper in which they described a fourth type of cell. This was one which stained selectively with erythrosin; they referred to it as type II, and thought that it had some characteristics of the basophil. By the end of the 1930s a number of other papers describing types of cell in the pars distalis, in addition to the three classical elements, had been published. The chief studies were still at this time directed towards mammalian glands, although a few studies of the pituitary of birds, reptiles, amphibians and fish had appeared in print.

In 1938 Dawson and Friedgood described a technique by which they were able to differentiate two classes of acidophils in the pars distalis of female rabbits and cats. One class stained red with azocarmine, the other orange with orange G. Their technique resembled that of a number of other authors, in that it was essentially a modification of Mallory's connective tissue stain. Fixation of the specimens was in sublimate-formol, and as a preliminary to staining, sections were post-chromed in 3 per cent potassium dichromate for twelve hours, and stained in a warm acid solution of azocarmine. After washing, the sections were differentiated until only the 'carmine' cells were stained; the sections were then treated with phosphotungstic acid and stained with orange G followed by methyl or aniline blue. The same issue of *Stain Technology* as that containing Dawson and Friedgood's paper carried one by Koneff, also an adaptation of the Mallory–azan method to stain the anterior pituitary gland of the rat.

The species studied by Dawson and Friedgood proved to be not the only ones to show two tinctorially distinct types of acidophil. Thus Dawson (1938) observed them in the opossum's pituitary, and Oldham (1938) found that with the Mallory–azan method some 'alpha cells' (acidophils) in the gland of the armadillo stained with azan, some with orange G. Dawson later reported two types of acidophil in the ferret and monkey, in addition to the rabbit and cat (Dawson, 1942); and two similar types of cell were described in some non-mammalian species, as for example in the garter-snake (Hartmann, 1944.)

During this period some observations were published which suggested that the class of basophilic cells of the pars distalis might also be capable of further differentiation. Hall (1938) described in glands of cattle basophils which stained strongly with aniline blue and whose granules had a strong affinity for haematoxylin, and others which stained weakly. The two types were differently distributed in the gland, the darker cells being widespread throughout the pars distalis, the paler ones largely limited to the central region.

As it became evident that the cytological make-up of the pars distalis was not as simple as at first appeared, a number of problems arose. A fundamental one, which is still only partially solved, was that of homology. As noted, two types of 'acidophil', carmine- or azan-staining, and orange G-staining, are present in a number of species; but similarity of staining reactions does not necessarily indicate similarity of function, and certainly cannot be assumed to indicate the secretion of identical (or even similar) hormones. But before this problem can even be considered, an even more fundamental one has to be faced, namely that of relating the descriptions published by various authors of the cytology of the adeno-hypophysis of different, or indeed sometimes of the same, species. The main source of variance, apart from the inevitable subjectivity of the authors themselves, lies in the fixation and staining procedures; minor variations in the techniques of dehydration and embedding, although possibly significant, are likely to be of much less importance.

Baker (1958) has considered in detail the effects of different fixatives, whether simple substances such as formalin, or mixtures, on tissues. Leaving aside the illogical composition of some fluids, it is clear that the final appearance of a stained section is greatly influenced by the fixative used – its constituents, the time it is allowed to act, and the after-treatment of the tissue. Other factors, such as the speed of penetration of fixative into the tissue, or whether exposure to the fixative is by immersion alone or by perfusion, affect the quality of preservation.

Many simple and complex solutions have been used to fix pituitary tissue, but the best all-round results, as far as the differential staining of the adenohypophysis is concerned, seem to have been obtained by two, sublimate-formol and Helly's solution (Zenker-formol). Post-chromation, already referred to, has been employed by some authors, particularly after the sublimate-formol mixture, as means of improving the stainability of cytoplasmic granules.

Staining, the final crucial step in the preparation of microscopical preparations, must also be precisely controlled and standardised if comparative studies are to be undertaken. The concentration of the dye in the staining solutions and the time of staining are factors which can be easily regulated. Some variables may, however, be beyond the control of the investigator. Thus, dyes purporting to be the same, but produced by different manufacturers, may vary considerably in constitution, and hence in the colour they produce; even different batches from the same source may suffer this defect. Further, the cells of the pituitary of one species may not stain so readily, or the same shade, as those in another, making even simple tinctorial comparisons difficult, and modifications of techniques may have to be made to obtain satisfactory results. For example, Hartmann, Fain and Wolfe (1946), in a study designed to re-examine the question of a fourth cell type in the dog's pituitary, which had been first described by Wolfe, Cleveland and Campbell in 1933, modified Dawson and Friedgood's (1938) azocarmine technique by increasing the time of staining in the solution of azocarmine to $2\frac{1}{2}$ hours at 56 °C – and incidentally noted that the technique was successful with tissue fixed in sublimate-formol, but not with that fixed in Regaud's mixture, containing only potassium dichromate and formalin.

Examples already given, as well as many others, had made it abundantly clear by 1940 that simple division of the cells of the pars distalis into three types, two chromophil and one chromophobe, was not an adequate classification; nevertheless, no description of the full range of cells had so far been published. Knowledge of the secretory functions of the gland had progressed considerably by this time, but cytological studies, not being able to provide a full correlation between cell types and the hormones secreted, had not kept pace. Since that time many studies based on differential staining techniques have appeared. Increasingly, the methods used have been refined, and although the affinity of some types of cell for particular stains still plays an important role in studies of the adenohypophysis, methods based on a few histochemical techniques which distinguish cells according to the chemical characteristics of certain of their constituents have become increasingly used.

BASOPHILIA

Reference has already been made (p. 29) to the finding that the cells designated as acidophils and basophils do not under all conditions show a selective affinity for acid and basic dyes respectively. Maurer and Lewis (1922), in their paper already referred to, noted that chromophil cells (they used the terms eosinophil or oxyphil for acidophils) would stain with either acid or basic dyes. Bailey and Davidoff (1925) referred to this observation; and in an attempt to avoid the erroneous implication of naming cells acidophils and basophils, suggested that it would be preferable to speak of their secretory granules as α (acidophilic) and β (basophilic) types – the cells containing the appropriate granule can then be designated α or β respectively. Many other authors have commented on this problem. Feyel (1939), for example, who used Pappenheim's stain on the pituitaries of guinea-pigs fixed in Helly's mixture, stated that she never observed cells which were entirely basophil, but acidophil cells with abundant 'chrondriome' associated with basophil inclusions. Hartmann, Fain and Wolfe (1946) also referred to this matter, and commented that many stains used for the differentiation of cells of the anterior pituitary contain only acid dyes, so that the terms acidophilic and basophilic are virtually meaningless.

From 1940 onwards papers were published which explained the reason why the staining reactions of the secretory granules and those of other constituents of the cytoplasm did not necessarily correspond. Desclin (1940) noted cells in pituitary glands of lactating rats which stained deeply with toluidine blue, and found that such cells, in contrast to normal basophils, were poorly stained by the Mallory technique or Mann's methyl blue. Treatment of sections with ribonuclease removed the stainable material, which was thus shown to contain RNA, which is not a constituent of normal basophil granules.

Dempsey and Wislocki also contributed to this topic in an important paper published in 1945. They pointed out that the original descriptions of acidophils, cyanophils (i.e. basophils) and chromophobes were based on sections stained with eosin–methylene blue and haematoxylin and eosin (Schönemann, 1892), that is, on the use of stains with an affinity for nucleic acids which revealed substances possessing true chemical basophilia. They further noted that aniline blue, a component of some trichrome stains, is a sulphated acid and acts as an acid dye, so that it is irrational to use this dye to show basophilia; indeed, it fails to stain the strongly basophilic nucleoli. Dempsey and Wislocki further showed that the basophilia revealed by eosin–methylene blue or eosin–toluidine blue in the pituitary disappeared after treatment of the sections with ribonuclease. They concluded that the variations in the amount of aniline blue-stainable material in the pars distalis in different stages of activity might be due to variations in an acidophilic protein matrix, or alternatively to acidophilic formed products of secretion.

Abolins (1952) used pyronin to reveal areas of high concentrations of RNA in the cytoplasm of cells in the guinea-pig's pituitary, and also by the use of ribonuclease noted that most RNA occurred in acidophilic areas. Peterson and Weiss (1955) used an acid dye, fast green, and basic methylene blue to study this problem using glands of cats, rats, rabbits, guinea-pigs and mice. They found that the acidophil granules stained intensely with fast green at a low pH, and only moderately with the basic dye at high pH; basophil granules were strongly stained with the basic dye at a high pH, although only in glands of the guinea-pig, rabbit and cat. Basophilia due to the ergastoplasm, present in almost all cells, could be demonstrated by staining with the basic dye at a much lower pH than that required for staining of the basophil granules; ribonuclease digestion removed this ergastoplasmic basophilia, but basophil granules were unaffected by such digestion – and hence contained no RNA. The authors, however, favoured the retention of the terms acidophil and basophil on the grounds that granules of these two types can be differentiated by staining at a controlled pH, even though both types of granule are amphoteric.

The use of certain histochemical techniques, notably periodic acid-Schiff (PAS) staining, have now diminished the importance of many of the stains formerly used in the identification of basophil granules (see p. 367). Acidophils, however, are still usually identified by their affinity for certain dyes, particularly orange G, which are not selective in a histochemical sense. True basophilia is not dependent on the staining properties of either class of granule, but on that of cytoplasmic ribonucleoprotein located in free ribosomes or rough endoplasmic reticulum; but neither the precise role of RNA in the synthesis of protein, nor the ultrastructural morphology of cells was known at the time when many studies of basophilia, such as those referred to above, were being made. From present knowledge it is easy to appreciate that cytoplasmic basophilia conferred by abundant rough endoplasmic reticulum (the old 'ergastoplasm') or free ribosomes is quite distinct from any tinctorial property of the secretory granules. More than this, cells lacking all secretory granules, and hence designated as chromophobes, may nevertheless have strongly basophilic cytoplasm, a feature noted, among other authors, by Foster and Wilson (1952). Furthermore, Deminatti (1959) observed that a numerical increase in secretory granules is associated with a decrease in cytoplasmic RNA, and suggested that chromophobes may be sites of intense protein synthesis, while the presence of granules does not necessarily indicate the same order of activity, but perhaps a storage phase.

The disparity between the amount of cytoplasmic RNA and secretory granules is of relevance in a consideration of certain tumours of the anterior pituitary. Some of these, classed as chromophobic, are rich in cytoplasmic RNA. They may not, as was once thought, be inactive, but rather so active that the secretory granules are ejected from the cells as soon as they are formed, so that the cytoplasm is filled with the organelles associated with secretory activity (endoplasmic reticulum and Golgi apparatus) but almost devoid of the end-products of this activity.

NAMING OF CELL TYPES

Most staining methods which have been used to differentiate the various types of cell in the adenohypophysis stain the secretory granules, and it is largely on their staining properties that differentiation and classification of the various types has been made. These granules contain the hormones of the gland, probably associated with some kind of carrier substance. At the time when many of the studies of pituitary cytology were published there was uncertainty about the precise function of the various types of cell, and this, coupled with the inter-specific variations, as well as intra-specific ones arising from differences in preparative techniques and in the state of activity of different glands, inevitably led to some confusion in terminology.

The introduction of a Greek alphabetic nomenclature method of designating cells by Bailey and Davidoff in 1925 was an attempt to avoid such difficulties. Much of the more recent use of this terminology, however, stems from the description of the cytology of the human pituitary by Romeis (1940) in his monograph, based on the microscopic appearance of the granules after staining with kresofuchsin or resorcin–fuchsin and counterstaining with azan. Later investigators, attempting to repeat the work of Romeis, found that the former stains had apparently lost their particular properties, and it has not been possible either to repeat the studies precisely or to apply his technique to a wide range of other species.

The cell types described by Romeis were thus based essentially on the human gland using particular and later unrepeatable techniques. Furthermore, his classification of cell types was essentially a morphological and tinctorial one based on his particular material. Application of the original nomenclature to glands of different species, stained by different dyes, or the application of the same nomenclature to cells identified by completely different methods of staining, as by Herlant (1960), could only lead to the confusion which is likely to beset anyone attempting a comparative study of the literature on adenohypophysial cytology. Happily, the complexities of staining and nomenclature have been carefully discussed by Purves (1966), whose chapter should be read by anyone concerned with cytological studies of the pituitary gland.

There is a general feeling that ideally a nomenclature for cells of the adenohypophysis should be a functional one, in which each cell could be named according to the type of its secretory activity. An International Committee was established in 1963 to consider the problem, and its findings were published two years later (van Oordt, 1965).

The proposed names were as follows:

Somatotropic or STH cells;
Lactotropic or LTH cells (i.e. those producing prolactin);
Corticotropic or ACTH cells;
FSH cells and ICSH cells (for the two gonadotropic or GTH cells), secreting follicle stimulating and luteinising/interstitial cell stimulating hormone respectively;
Thyrotropic or TSH cells;

and for the pars intermedia cells secreting melanophore stimulating hormone:

Melanotropic or MSH cells.

It was realised that it is not yet always (indeed, for all but common species, not often) possible to be certain of the function of a given cell type; and hence, that there is a need for a morphological name by which to refer to cells whose function is not known beyond any doubt. The Committee came to the conclusion, however, that it was 'not practical to insist on a morphological terminology based on a restricted number of

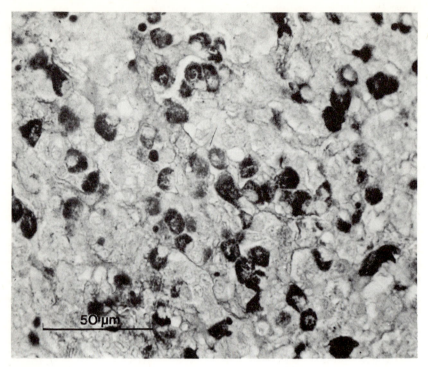

Fig. 3.1. PAS+ gonadotropic cells in the pars distalis of the ferret in the pro-oestrous period. From Holmes (1964a). Reproduced by permission.

standardized techniques'. Until the function of different types of cells is known for a given species, morphological criteria must suffice, but homologies with the findings in other species can only be tentative ones.

Descriptive studies must still, however, be based on the appearance of different types of cell after particular staining methods. Probably one of the most important developments in pituitary cytology during the past twenty-five years has been the application of the periodic-acid–Schiff (PAS) technique. This reaction stains carbohydrate-containing material in tissues, and depends on the fact that after a preliminary weak oxidation by periodic acid, carboxyl groups present in the carbohydrate molecules are converted to aldehydic ones. The sections are then exposed to a solution of fuchsin which has been decolorised by sulphur dioxide to leucofuchsin; this colourless compound attaches to the carbohydrate, forming a red colour – it is thought by combining with adjacent exposed aldehyde groups.

The application of the method to the pituitary depends on the fact that certain of the adenohypophysial cells contain glyco- or mucoprotein material – that is, protein–carbohydrate complexes, which, reacting after partial oxidation with the Schiff's reagent, stain pink or red. This stainable material appears to be closely associated, if not identical with, some of the hormones secreted by the pars distalis, namely TSH, FSH and LH (fig. 3.1).

As with most histochemical techniques, the specificity of a positive result cannot be taken for granted. The PAS reaction will stain polysaccharides, mucopolysaccharides, mucoproteins and glycoproteins, as well as some other substances (see Pearse, 1968). Therefore, for strict histochemical application of this technique controls and the careful standardisation of all its stages, as described by Pearse, are essential. The simplest control procedure, to eliminate the staining of glycogen, is to treat the sections with diastase (or saliva) before carrying out the PAS reaction.

McManus (1946) first noted that in sections treated by the PAS reaction to demonstrate mucin, certain pituitary cells contained stained granules. Catchpole (1947) applied the technique specifically to the pituitary, and found positive granules in some cells of the pars distalis. Pearse (1948, 1949) used the method extensively, and Purves and Griesbach (1951) applied it to the localisation of thyrotropic and gonadotropic cells in the rat. In 1952 Pearse suggested that cells of the pars distalis shown to contain muco- or glycoprotein, i.e. PAS-positive materials, should be designated 'mucoid cells' – a class which includes definitive 'basophils', but also extends more widely to include cells not clearly basophil which contain some PAS-positive material.

The PAS technique has proved to be of great value in studies of the pituitary. It is simple to carry out, gives readily reproducible results, and can be used in combination with most other staining methods (see colour plate). Variations in PAS staining (its intensity, the precise shade of red coloration) and the size, shape and position of the cells enable some degree of differentiation of different cell types to be made within the PAS+ group.

For some years the dye aldehyde fuchsin (AF) was popular as a stain for the adenohypophysis. The technique was introduced by Gomori (1950) for staining elastic tissue and he noted that among other structures it also stained certain pituitary basophils, apparently those which took up resorcin–fuchsin. Aldehyde fuchsin proved to be a somewhat unreliable stain to use, and did not always give good results. Halmi applied the method to staining the pituitary gland of the rat, and showed that it could be used to distinguish, in an apparently specific manner, between two kinds of basophil (Halmi, 1950). This differentiation into AF+ and AF− cells was considered by Halmi also to be directly comparable with that obtained by Romeis (1940), combining resorcin–fuchsin with azan, to distinguish β and δ cells; as already noted, it had proved difficult to obtain satisfactory results by repeating the technique of Romeis, and the AF technique as described by Halmi (1952a) seemed to be more reliable.

Halmi (1950) had clearly distinguished two types of basophil, and by means of removal of various target endocrine organs, attempted to ascribe a function to each of the two types. The β cells, generally irregular in outline and more numerous in the core of the gland, were AF+ while the more rounded δ cells, most numerous in the anterior-median and dorsal part, were AF−. Following thyroidectomy Halmi observed numerous hyperplastic vacuolated cells which, as they were AF−, he thought were δ cells; β cells also regressed after thyroidectomy but after castration were not generally affected, while increase in numbers, hypertrophy and vacuolation of δ cells again occurred.

Halmi concluded that the δ cells probably secreted both FSH and TSH, and thought it possible that the β cells were concerned with the secretion of ACTH. Later (Halmi, 1952*b*) he realised that AF− cells could arise by degranulation of β cells, and expressed agreement with the findings of Purves and Griesbach (1951) who, applying the PAS staining technique to glands of normal rats and of rats treated to produce variations in the output of gonadotropins and TSH, concluded that the centrally placed cells (equivalent to Halmi's β cells) were thyrotropes, the peripherally placed (δ) cells the gonadotropes. Thus, as pointed out by Purves and Griesbach (1951), thyrotropes are AF+ and PAS+, gonadotropes AF−, PAS+.

The AF technique has been used to stain pituitary glands of species other than the rat; for example, Yamada *et al.* (1960) found AF+ cells, apparently equivalent to the β cells of the rat, in the mouse. Usually, however, aldehyde fuchsin has been used together with other techniques such as PAS. It must be repeated, however, that a staining characteristic *per se* cannot be assumed to indicate the function of the cell type. Serber (1958), for example, concluded from her studies of the hamster pituitary that in this species the gonadotropic cells are AF+, while the thyrotropic ones are AF−. Furthermore, the staining reaction is not necessarily a specific one; for example, the use of permanganate oxidation as a preliminary step results in the staining of both β and δ granules with aldehyde fuchsin in cells of the rat pituitary (see Purves, 1966), and Herlant and Racadot (1957) found that when a preliminary oxidation is used, the intensity of staining also varies with the length of time for which this is allowed to act.

A dye which has proved both useful and reliable in pituitary studies is the copper phthalocyanine derivative Alcian blue. This dye, used at a low pH, stains neurosecretory material in sections previously treated with a strong oxidising agent (Adams and Sloper, 1956, and see p. 73). According to the authors the specificity of staining depends on the oxidation of the cystine or cysteine groups in neurohypophysial hormones to acidic groups with which the dye combines. The technique was successfully applied to the staining of adenohypophysial cells by Adams and Swettenham (1958). These authors used performic acid for the preliminary oxidation; staining with acid Alcian blue was followed next by the PAS procedure and sections were finally counterstained with orange G. Two types of basophil granule could be distinguished, coloured by Alcian blue and Schiff's reagent respectively. If the preliminary oxidation with performic acid was omitted, both types of granules were PAS+. As the similarity of these results to those obtained using aldehyde fuchsin on the rat's pituitary was not clear, Adams and Swettenham designated the two types of granules as S and R. The authors used a number of other histo-chemical staining techniques on their material, and concluded that the staining of S granules with Alcian blue indicated that they were rich in sulphur-containing amino acid (i.e. cystine), while the R granules con-tained polysaccharide resistant to extraction by performic acid. Herlant (1964) considers that the staining with Alcian blue after oxidation may be attributable to the presence of acid groups in the mucoproteins.

Histochemically-based staining methods have proved particularly useful for differentiating several categories of mucoid cells, but have not so far contributed similarly to the staining of acidophil elements. Barrnett and his colleagues showed that the latter type of cells reacted more strongly for sulphydryl and disulphide groups than other adenohypo-physial cells (Barrnett and Seligman, 1954; Ladman and Barrnett, 1956), but differential staining methods still provide the simplest way of demon-strating these cells. In 1960 Herlant published a report of two techniques which have proved valuable in the differential staining of all adeno-hypophysial cell types. One of these schedules essentially differentiates mucoid cells by acidified permanganate–Alcian blue followed by PAS staining, which allows a final staining with orange G for acidophils; the other uses an erythrosin–Mallory–alizarin blue sequence (Herlant's tetrachrome). Results from these and other studies have appreciably advanced our understanding of the cytology of the pituitary, although clearly they must be associated with experimental studies (see pp. 49 ff) if functional attributions are to be made with certainty.

At the present time, the chromophil cells of the pars distalis can be broadly divided into two groups, made up of 'acidophils' on the one hand, and mucoid cells on the other. These two groups correspond broadly, but not precisely, to the acidophils and basophils of earlier classifications. Acidophils contain granules made up of simple protein, while the mucoid elements contain muco- or glycoprotein; hence Herlant (1964) proposed the term 'serous' cells for acidophils. Many studies have shown that several types of acidophil can be differentiated, by the use of appropriate stains, within the group which stain with orange G, eosin and similar acid dyes; as already discussed (p. 33) the granules have amphoteric properties.

ACIDOPHILS

Initially all classed as α cells, acidophils were later subdivided. One class is now known to be concerned with the secretion of growth hormone, STH. As already noted, Dawson and Friedgood (1938) distinguished a second category of acidophils, which had an affinity for azocarmine, and which they called carminophils. In the rabbit and cat Friedgood and Dawson (1940) observed that these cells increased greatly in number after mating, and considered that this indicated that the cells secreted LH. The cells were also found to be numerous during lactation, and several authors, including Pearse (1951), came to the conclusion that they were in fact concerned with the secretion of prolactin (LTH). Herlant, however, on the basis of the results of PAS–OG staining, considered that Dawson and Friedgood's carminophils in fact secreted LH, not LTH. In 1964 he reported that in the rat two types of acidophils apart from STH cells could be identified and that one of these was concerned with the secretion of ACTH. He equated this with the ϵ cell of Romeis.

It seems reasonably certain that in many species the cells secreting LTH are acidophilic. Again, a major problem has been the clear distinction of these cells from STH cells, as granules of both types of cell have an affinity for the same dyes. They have been distinguished (Saunders and Rennels, 1959) by making use of a selective affinity of rat STH cells for azocarmine, and of LTH cells for orange G, or in many species (Herlant, 1960) for orange G and erythrosin respectively. But fixation is critical, as is final differentiation, and the methods leave much to be desired.

The cellular site of origin of ACTH was disputed for many years and at various times acidophil, basophil and chromophobic cells were associated with this hormone. The evidence now seems to point to cells containing acidophilic granules, but of such a small size and sparsity that the cells may appear as chromophobes. Among evidence in favour of such a designation is the structure of ACTH-secreting tumours (Furth and Clifton, 1958). Recently Pelletier and Racadot (1971), in a combined light and electron microscopic study, described them as virtually chromophobic and of irregular shape, but containing sparse small granules visible with the electron microscope (see p. 60).

BASOPHILS

In general the distinction between the various categories of mucoid cells has offered fewer problems than that of the acidophils. Three tropic hormones are known to be glycoprotein in nature (see Barrnett, Siperstein and Josimovich, 1956): TSH, FSH and LH. The cells producing FSH have been equated with the δ cells, already described as being AF – and

PAS+. These are classic basophils, often concentrated in the antero-median parts of the pars distalis. There is evidence that the PAS+ material in these cells is at any rate closely associated with the hormone. Barrnett *et al.* (1956), for example, extracted FSH from pituitaries and found that the positive PAS reaction was then absent. Castration leads to hypertrophy and vacuolation of these cells in the rat (Purves and Gries-bach, 1951), explicable on the basis of their over-activity when freed of the restraint of the feedback effect of gonadal hormones.

There is now abundant evidence that FSH and LH are distinct entities (see for example Li, 1949) and although a dual cellular origin has been questioned from time to time, it seems clear that in the commoner species each hormone is secreted by a distinct type of cell. Purves and Griesbach (1954, 1955) suggested that in the rat distinct FSH- and LH-producing cells could be demonstrated. It is now evident that difficulties and contra-dictions in the definition of any LH-secreting cell lie partly in the fact that species differences in this respect are considerable. In some species the granules of LH-producing cells are acidophilic, but they are also, to a variable degree in different species, PAS+. Furthermore, LH-secreting cells are not necessarily present at all times, appearing in some species only at the breeding season or during gestation. The combined PAS reactivity and acidophilia is responsible for the characteristic 'brick red' colour of these cells after PAS–OG staining, as was described by Herlant (1956) in the pituitary of the pregnant bat.

ULTRASTRUCTURE OF THE PARS DISTALIS

The increasing availability of electron microscopes from the early 1930s onwards enabled a new approach to be made to pituitary cytology. The technique has, as its main advantage, that of greatly increased resolution over that of the optical microscope. Hence, finer details of the structural relationships of intracellular organelles to each other can be studied, and cells characterised by their ultrastructural morphology. Furthermore, the relationships of cells to each other, and to other tissue components such as blood vessels and nerves, can be precisely determined.

Ultrastructural studies are subject to the same limitations as those of optical microscopy. Notably, the structure of tissues is revealed only as they were at the moment of fixation; hence, the attribution of function must depend on the building up of a serial picture from many different samples; here the same techniques to modify the activity of the gland as those used for many years by optical microscopists (see pp. 49ff) must be employed. Electron microscopy is, however, subject to even more serious limitations than optical, chiefly in that only a relatively minute amount of tissue can be examined. Using optical microscopy, for example, it is not difficult to examine whole pituitary glands in serial sections, and to make differential cell counts sampling all parts of the specimens. With electron microscopy, such extensive sampling is hardly possible. Electron microscopy has, however, contributed to our understanding of both structure and function of the adenohypophysis. Considering first the purely structural aspects, the various categories of secretory cells can be recognised. Perhaps the most valid criteria applied are the size and shape of the secretory granules, but other factors such as the shape of the cell, its size and position relative to blood vessels and the general features of its cytoplasm are all useful.

The earliest attempt to study the anterior pituitary with the electron microscope appears to be that made in 1949, by Fernandez-Moran and Luft. Ultramicrotomes for cutting sections of adequate thinness to permit transmission of the electron beam were at that time not readily available, and the work was based on the study of smears and surface replica adhesion preparations. The authors were able to observe spherical granules 100–250 nm in diameter and thought they could also detect some signs of ultrastructure within these, but more detailed studies were not possible.

In 1953 Rinehart and Farquhar, in the first of a series of studies of the rat pituitary, described the ultrastructural appearances of the three classical types of cell. Chromophobes had relatively clear cytoplasm with no, or very few, granules; acidophils contained cytoplasmic granules with a maximum diameter of 350 nm; basophils contained finer granules, with maximum diameters of 140–200 nm. At this time the authors were not able to subdivide this latter category of cells. Changes in various cytoplasmic elements, notably in the Golgi apparatus, with different phases of activity, were also described.

The next year the same two observers published further observations (Farquhar and Rinehart, 1954a, b). The first of these papers described the gland of female rats at various times after ovariectomy; the second, the glands of thyroidectomised animals. Correlation of optical and electron microscopic appearances was achieved by examining with the light microscope thick (i.e. 1 μm) sections cut from the blocks adjacent to thin sections used for electron microscopy, parts of the same structures being included in both the thick and thin sections.

This work led to the identification of two types of basophil which respond differently (in structural terms) to castration. One type showed an initial increase in its content of mitochondria and granules, then progressed to vacuolation accompanied by loss of granules. By seventy-five days after castration, 'signet ring' cells were formed, with a peripheral rim of cytoplasm surrounding one or more large central vesicles. The other type of basophil underwent a different type of change, developing a 'filigree' appearance of the cytoplasm with vacuolation. The authors considered that the first of these types of cell was probably that responsible

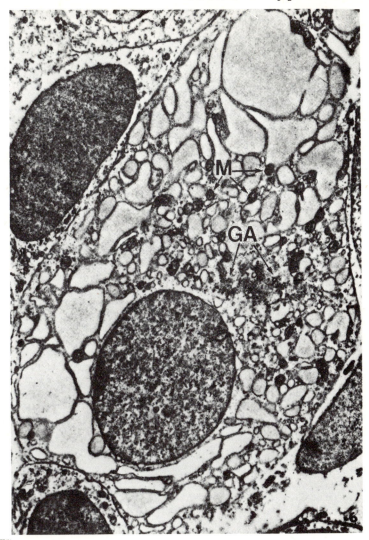

Fig. 3.2. Ten-day thyroidectomy basophil in rat pars distalis. Note the extensive vesiculation of the cytoplasm. M, mitochondria; GA, Golgi apparatus. From Farquhar and Rinehart (1954*b*).

for the secretion of FSH, the second for LH. They also observed two distinct types of acidophil, one with rounded granules, the other with larger elliptical ones – both types of granule, however, being larger than the granules of basophils. The authors suggested the possibility that the first of the two types of acidophil might be responsible for the elaboration of STH, while the second might secrete one of the other hormones, ACTH or LTH.

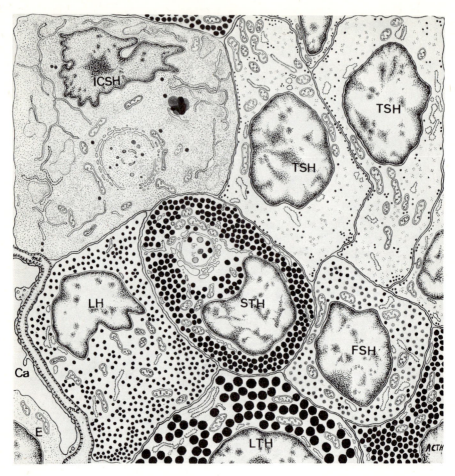

Fig. 3.3. Diagram of the ultrastructure of the various types of cells secreting tropic hormones in the mink (*Mustela lutreola*) (see list of abbreviations for key). Reproduced by permission from Azzali and Romita, L'Ateneo Parmense – *Acta Bio-Medica* XIII, 1971, p. 286.

The second study enabled the authors to distinguish not only the thyroidectomy cells (fig. 3.2), but also the normal thyrotropes, which they described as angular cells, containing ill-defined granules smaller than those found in gonadotropic cells. Hence, three distinct types of 'basophil' could be distinguished, two concerned with gonadotropic secretion and one with that of TSH.

Since these fundamental papers, electron microscopy has naturally been used to study the pituitary glands of many different species. Notable among the numerous publications are those of Barnes on the mouse (1962), and Girod on the monkey (*Macacus sylvanus*) and other species, summarised to that date in Girod (1966) and elsewhere. As with optical microscopy, it is now possible to identify in some species the types of cells concerned with the elaboration of each of the six hormones of the pars distalis (fig. 3.3).

Electron microscopy has also shown that the pars distalis contains cells apparently distinct from both connective tissue and secretory elements. These are agranular, bear microvilli and occasional cilia and occur in follicles; they may be identical with other elements which do not form follicles and which have been designated as stellate cells (see Farquhar, 1971). Farquhar originally (1957) associated such agranular cells with the secretion of ACTH, but now considers that there is good evidence for the origin of this hormone from small-granule-containing cells. She also notes (1971) that the stellate cells can act as phagocytes. Harrison and Young (1969) observed in the pituitary of the dolphin a close association between stellate cells and perivascular channels, suggesting a role in transport of hormones to capillaries (see chapter 15).

The pattern of vascularisation of the hypothalamo-hypophysial system is considered in detail later (see pp. 101ff). Electron microscopy, however, has clarified some points bearing on the precise relationship of cells to vessels. In the pituitary, as in other endocrine glands, this relationship is clearly of great importance, since the vascular route is the only one by which the secretory products can pass to influence their target organs. Furthermore, the various releasing factors coming from the hypothalamus travel in the portal blood to influence the secretory cells. Particular attention was paid to the vessels by Rinehart and Farquhar (1955) and Farquhar (1961). Essentially the pars distalis is permeated by capillaries lined by endothelium which is generally very thin (*c.* 20–30 nm) except in the region of the endothelial cell nuclei; it frequently shows pores, such as those described in other endocrine glands, bridged by a thin membrane. The endothelium is closely apposed to a basement membrane (fig. 3.4), which consists of two parts, an endothelial and a parenchymal one closely applied to the cell membrane of the secretory cells. In some areas these two components are fused to form a single thick basement membrane, but often they are separated by a perivascular space of variable width containing acid mucopolysaccharides (Rinehart and Farquhar, 1955), together with various connective tissue elements, both cells and collagenous fibrils. The surface of the parenchymal cells is often irregular, so that their surface area is increased, and processes of the cells may project into the pericapillary space between the two basement membranes, either devoid of basement membrane or only partially covered by it. Farquhar also showed that release of granules from the secretory cells takes place by a process of exocytosis into the perivascular space (fig. 3.4), a feature which has been confirmed by later observers.

Much of the literature on the pituitary designates the vascular bed of

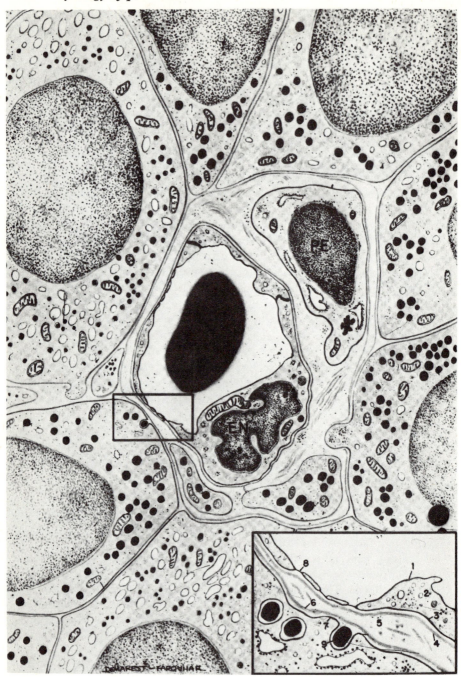

Fig. 3.4. Diagram of the relationships of pituitary cells to capillaries. Note the lower inset showing the process of exocytosis of granules into the pericapillary space. From Farquhar (1961).

the pars distalis as sinusoidal. Sinusoids are vessels such as those of the liver, generally of larger diameter than capillaries, with a discontinuous lining of phagocytic and non-phagocytic cells, compared with the continuous endothelial lining of capillaries. Farquhar (1961) noted that the small vessels of the anterior pituitary met none of these criteria and as shown earlier (Rinehart and Farquhar, 1955) their lining is not phagocytic. Hence, they should be considered as capillaries, not sinusoids.

HORMONE CONTENT OF GRANULES

Although considerable progress in the attribution of secretion of specific hormones to specific types of cell had been made by the combined use of experimental techniques and differential staining for optical microscopy, the electron microscope, used in conjunction with ultra-centrifugation techniques, enabled such relationships to be determined with greater precision. Catchpole (1948) and McShan and Meyer (1949) examined by bioassay for gonadotropic activity the various fractions obtained by centrifugation of homogenised pituitaries of rats and sheep. They found that the bulk of such activity was associated with large granule fractions, shown by electron microscopy to contain, among other elements, mitochondria.

More precise studies were made possible by improved techniques of differential gradient centrifugation and by using electron microscopy to identify the constituents associated with the various active substances. For example Hartley, McShan and Ris (1960) used pituitary glands of rats castrated for 6–10 weeks to ensure a high content of gonadotropin. They homogenised the anterior parts of the glands and by means of repeated differential and gradient centrifugation and microfiltration obtained a fraction which was shown by bioassay to contain most of the gonadotropic activity. Electron microscopy of a pellet finally obtained showed it to be made up mainly of granules measuring 200 nm in diameter. Similar studies were reported by Perdue and McShan (1962), who also included analysis for succinic dehydrogenase and phosphatases as a control for the degree of contamination of the fractions with microsomal, mitochondrial and other cytoplasmic elements. The authors again used electron microscopy to classify their fractions, and found that gonadotropin and a lesser amount of thyrotropin was associated with a small-granule (*c*. 200 nm) fraction. Similar techniques have been used to investigate the other tropic hormones. Isolation of secretory granules has also been achieved by the use of column chromatography, again the morphology of the fractions being determined by electron microscopy (Hymer and McShan, 1962; McShan, 1971).

EXPERIMENTAL TECHNIQUES IN THE STUDY OF THE FUNCTIONAL CYTOLOGY OF THE ADENOHYPOPHYSIS

However specific the methods of staining, such as those discussed above, may be for individual types of adenohypophysial cells, those techniques *alone* cannot be used to ascribe specific functions to the cells. A variety of experimental techniques have been used together with cytological studies to this end, and the commoner ones are briefly considered here.

FLUORESCENT ANTIBODY STUDIES

The use of immunofluorescence techniques is in effect the application of a particularly specific form of staining to enable the various protein hormones to be localised to specific cells. The technique, which was first used to demonstrate pneumococcal antigen in tissues (Coons, Creech, Jones and Berliner, 1942), depends essentially on the fact that dye molecules can be linked to molecules of antibody and still leave the antibody able to react in an antigen–antibody reaction. The basic steps in the application of this principle to studies of the pituitary gland are:

1. Preparation of antibody to an appropriate antigen (i.e. one of the pituitary hormones) by repeated injection of the antigen into a suitable animal.
2. Labelling of the antibody with some substance detectable microscopically. Fluorescein isocyanate, which fluoresces brilliantly in ultraviolet light, has commonly been used for this.
3. Exposure of histological sections to the solution of labelled antibody.

Provided that the labelled antibody is specific for a given antigen (hormone), and that the latter has not been inactivated or washed out of the sections, an antigen–antibody reaction will occur, and a fluorescent complex will be formed at the sites of this reaction. Using fluorescence microscopy, such sites can be accurately determined and by comparing a treated section with an adjacent one stained by a conventional method, such as PAS, the particular hormone can be localised to a given cell type.

This technique offers the possibility of identification of cells containing (secreting) specific hormones with considerable precision, always provided of course that the reaction is specific, and that there has been no change in localisation of hormone during preparation. The problems inherent in the application of the technique were discussed by Coons (1956).

Not all work based on this method has been accepted as clearly demonstrating cell–hormone relationships. An early application of the technique to the pituitary was made by Marshall (1951), who attempted to determine the cellular origin of ACTH using a labelled antibody prepared against a fairly crude preparation of corticotropin. He concluded that on the evidence obtained ACTH is elaborated in basophil cells. His findings have not been generally accepted, however, on the grounds that the results were due to some non-hormonal protein in his preparation of antibody (see Purves, 1961). Nevertheless, a number of useful contributions to pituitary cytology have resulted from the use of this technique. Della Corte and Biondi (1964) refer to earlier work and describe their own studies, in which anti-FSH antibody (pig) was localised in most but not all the cells identified as type β, suggesting that these elaborated FSH. The identification was made by staining the sections by a PAS method after photographs of the distribution of fluorescence had been taken. Midgley (1964) localised LH antibody to lightly PAS-positive cells in the human pituitary; and a number of authors have similarly localised the production of STH to acidophils (e.g. Leznoff *et al.* 1960), although generally only a proportion of the acidophils have shown fluorescence. The technique has also been extended to the target organs for the tropic hormones; for example Greenspan and Hargadine (1965) localised TSH in cells of the thyroid gland.

AUTORADIOGRAPHY

Studies of the adenohypophysis using autoradiographic techniques have yielded information of less significance than has the application of the technique to the neurohypophysis (see pp. 74 ff). Deminatti (1961*a*) administered ^{35}S di-sodium sulphate to guinea-pigs and reported an intense incorporation of radioactive material in cells with the histochemical properties of thyrotropes. In another study (1961*b*) this author correlated the intensity of the radioactivity with the degree of pyroninophilia (i.e. true basophilia) of the cells. He considered that chromophobes were sites of intense protein synthesis, which was negligible in chromophils. Ford *et al.* (1961) observed that the pars intermedia showed less activity than the 'anterior lobe' after the injection of ^{35}S-cystine, although Deminatti (1961*b*) had found considerable activity in both nucleus and cytoplasm of cells of the pars intermedia.

ENDOCRINE ABLATIONS

The output of pituitary tropic hormones is controlled largely by means of the negative feedback effect of the hormones secreted by their target glands (p. 14). If this feedback effect is removed then there is no such curb on secretion, and in the absence of other suppressive factors the cells secreting the tropic hormone concerned become over-active. This hyperactivity is reflected in the morphology of the secretory cells and in their staining reactions.

Procedures of this kind have been used extensively in attempts to identify the adenohypophysial cells concerned with each of those tropic hormones which act on specific target glands. Thus gonadectomy has been used to study the origins of the gonadotropic hormones FSH and LH/ICSH; thyroidectomy for TSH; and adrenalectomy for ACTH. Lactotropic hormone (prolactin) and STH, which do not act specifically to bring about the secretion of other hormones, cannot be so readily studied by this sort of investigation.

There are, however, differences in the reaction of the gland to ablation of target endocrines according to the species of animal concerned. The gonadotropic and thyrotropic cells of the rat respond in a very characteristic way. Addison in 1917 described the effects of castration on the pituitary gland of this animal as essentially an increase in size of basophils leading, two months or more after the operation, to the development of vacuolated basophils. These are the 'castration' or 'signet ring' cells, and their changed morphology represents their response to the loss of the restraining influence of the sex steroids on their activity. Purves and Griesbach (1955) combined cytological studies with hormonal assays of 'castrate' pituitaries and suggested that a distinction could be made between cells secreting FSH and those secreting LH. Typical 'castration' cells do not occur in all species. For example, although gonadectomy is followed by changes in granulation of basophils in the pituitary gland of the palm squirrel, the 'signet ring' forms seen in rats do not occur (Dhaliwal and Prasad, 1965); neither were such cells found in the ferret (Holmes, 1963*a*).

Thyroidectomy brings about a similar kind of response to that following gonadectomy, which was described by Trautmann (1915) in the goat, and Kojima (1917) in the rat, and has been frequently confirmed by other observers since the publication of these early papers. These include Severinghaus, Smelser and Clark (1934), who made no clear distinction between thyroidectomy and castration cells, Reese, Koneff and Wainman (1943), and Purves and Griesbach (1954). The latter authors described degranulation as occurring rapidly after thyroidectomy and the early development of vacuolated cells. Surgical removal of the thyroid is not essential to study the effects of loss of thyroid hormones since destruction may be brought about by the use of radio-iodine.

Even destruction or blocking of single elements of the endocrine system does not, however, necessarily produce clear-cut changes in pituitary cytology. In thyroid deficiency, for example, acidophils also show changes, notably degranulation (Eayrs and Holmes, 1964); this is hardly surprising, since any change in the secretion of a metabolically active hormone such as thyroxine must affect general metabolism and hence to some extent the other components of the endocrine system. Removal of target organs (gonads) which are influenced by more than one tropic hormone may also bring about results which are difficult to interpret, as reference to work already noted shows. The widespread metabolic effects of the adrenal cortical hormones no doubt contributed to the difficulty in attributing the secretion of ACTH to a specific adeno-hypophysial cell type. Reese, Koneff and Akimoto (1939), for example, found that adrenalectomy in rats was followed by degranulation and other changes in both acidophils and basophils, although some basophils showed early enlargement of the Golgi zone, an organelle known to play a major part in secretory activity). The uncertainty of the attribution, as it existed to about 1960, has been summarised by Purves (1961). Purves ends his summary by referring to a then recent paper by Farquhar (1957) in which she had described a sixth cell type in the pituitary gland of the rat, a cell with no granules, occurring throughout the pars distalis in a follicular pattern, and associated with colloid. Since that time further studies have identified corticotropes more certainly (see Pelletier and Racadot, 1971).

Similar principles to those used in the ablation of target organs are involved in experiments in which hormonal secretion is altered by either administering hormones, or blocking their effect. For example, injection of thyroxine will result in decreased activity of the thyrotropes, while treating an animal with a blocking agent such as propylthiouracil, which prevents the synthesis of thyroxine, will have a similar effect to thyroid-ectomy.

CYCLICAL CHANGES

Another approach to the interpretation of the functional cytology of the pituitary is to correlate the microscopic appearance of the gland with different phases of some pituitary-controlled cyclical activity. For example, reproductive cycles, determined by the cyclical release of gonadotropic hormones from the pituitary, are accompanied by cytological changes in the cells secreting these hormones. Cyclical changes in the gland can be observed even in animals such as the rat, with its polyoestrous pattern of recurrent short cycles. In seasonally breeding species, the changes are extended over much greater periods of time. In the vole, for example, Clarke and Forsyth (1964) found that during the breeding season cells filled with PAS+ granules were numerous, but in the non-breeding (winter) season PAS+ material was present only in the walls of large intracellular vesicles. Assays showed a high content of gonadotropin in the glands of males during the breeding season, but not in winter. Such observations provide suggestive if not conclusive evidence that the granular PAS+ cells are gonadotropes. Similar cytological changes occur in the pituitary of the ferret (Holmes, 1963*a*). Increase in PAS+ cells in a hibernator, the ground squirrel, was correlated with increased gonadal and thyroid activity by Hoffman and Zarrow (1958).

'ABNORMAL' GLANDS

The pituitary glands of dwarf mutant mice possess no acidophils (Smith and MacDowell, 1930; Bartke, 1964), a finding which suggested (or rather seemed to reinforce) the association between this type of cell and the secretion of STH. In common with other (pathological) pituitary states, however, the glands of these animals are deficient not only in STH, but also in other tropic hormones – hence, the assumed relationship is not a clear-cut one.

TUMOURS OF THE ADENOHYPOPHYSIS

In man the functional cytology of the pituitary has necessarily had to be derived largely from the study of glands in relation to various patho-logical states. Pituitary tumours associated with an excess secretion of a tropic hormone have indicated the probable type of cell normally secreting it. Studies of tumours have also added to our knowledge of functional cytology in animals.

Tumours of the adenohypophysis are still usually classed, according to their cytology, as acidophil, basophil or chromophobe. There is abundant evidence to associate excessive growth in man either before epiphysial closure (gigantism) or after (acromegaly) with over-activity of acidophils and the presence of an acidophil tumour. Rarer are basophil adenomas which may be associated with Cushing's disease (Cushing, 1932), although this disease also occurs with no evidence of such a tumour. Chromophobe adenomas frequently give rise to signs of hypopituitarism; not only may they be non-secretory, but they also destroy surrounding pituitary tissue by pressure.

Tumours of the pituitary are particularly common in old animals of certain species and strains. Saxton and Graham (1944), for example, found that chromophobe adenomas developed in 60 per cent of male and 30 per cent of female Wistar rats aged more than 600 days. Such spon-taneous tumours are commonly but not invariably chromophobic (Holmes and Mandl, 1961) and are often associated with tumours and hyperplasia of the mammary glands (Howell and Mandl, 1961).

Pituitary tumours can also be induced experimentally (see Furth, 1955). Reference has already been made to the changes which occur in the pars distalis after castration or thyroidectomy, and if such hormone-deficient animals are kept for long enough, tumours of the appropriate tropic cells may develop. Long-term administration of oestrogen may also induce tumours, as may exposure of animals to whole-body radiation. Trans-plantable strains of tumour cells can be isolated, some producing a single factor, such as an adrenocorticotropic one, others a mixture, for example one of thyrotropic and growth factors.

As Furth (1955) described, the cytological characteristics of tumours producing particular hormones often do not resemble those of the cells known to secrete these factors in normal glands. Tumours, whether spontaneous or induced, often appear largely chromophobic. Study of their cells by electron microscopy shows, however, that they are not necessarily either completely devoid of granules, or lacking in morphological criteria of activity. Schelin (1962) found that cells from chromophobe adenomas of human pituitary glands could be recognised as either degranulated acidophils or basophils with features associated with little secretory activity, such as a small Golgi zone and little rough endoplasmic reticulum. Cells of chromophobic adenomas of senile rats associated with mammary hyperplasia could be identified as large-granule-containing acidophils (the type associated with the secretion of LTH) and also showed morphological signs of intense activity (Holmes, 1964*a*) including extensive rough endoplasmic reticulum. Such cells are chromophobic simply because they fail to store their secretory granules. Schelin also found that in adenomas removed from patients with clinically active acromegaly sparsely granulated, but morphologically active, acidophils predominated. Cells of thyrotropic pituitary tumours in mice (Lundin and Schelin, 1964) which were chromophobic or amphophil by optical microscopy, were seen by electron microscopy to resemble thyroidectomy cells, with sparse granulation, extensive Golgi zones and greatly developed rough endoplasmic reticulum.

4

THE PARS INTERMEDIA
AND PARS TUBERALIS

It has already been noted that the pars intermedia is not present in all species. It is present, in a variable degree of development, in most but not all mammals, in reptiles and amphibia, while it is absent in birds. In some vertebrates such as teleost fishes and elasmobranchs the intermedia closely interdigitates with nervous tissue of the neurohypophysis, forming a complex referred to as the neuro-intermediate lobe (see pp. 149, 196).

More is known about the function of the pars intermedia in non-mammals than of most other vertebrates (see p. 270). In these the principle secreted, intermedin (also known as melanocyte or melanophore stimulating hormone (MSH)) (Zondek and Krohn, 1932) has a clear-cut dual action on certain pigment-containing cells, the chromatophores, bringing about dispersion of their contained pigment, usually melanin, throughout the cell – hence causing darkening of the skin, and in the longer term increasing the amount of pigment in the cells. Such changes play an important part in the colour adaptation of many lower vertebrates to their background.

Such creatures have both a pars intermedia and chromatophores. Birds and mammals, however, do not have chromatophores, and birds and some species of mammals also lack a pars intermedia. Nevertheless intermedin, or at any rate some substance with a similar effect, has been isolated from the pituitary gland of birds (the pars distalis) as well as from that of mammals.

The role of the pars intermedia in higher vertebrates, notably mammals and man, in which changes in pigmentation of the skin are not effected in the same way as for lower vertebrates, is far from clear. As Parker (1950) pointed out, however, it need not necessarily be assumed that the pars intermedia, or rather its hormone, MSH, has the same function in all animals, even though it occurs in the pituitary glands of higher vertebrates. The fact that Lerner and McGuire (1961) found that repeated injections of MSH did bring about darkening of the skin, particularly facial, of medium coloured negroes, in itself demonstrates an effect, not a function. Mammalian pars intermedia contains two peptide substances, α-MSH and β-MSH; each shares some basic chemical structure with the ACTH molecule (see Harris, 1960), and this is emphasised by the obser-

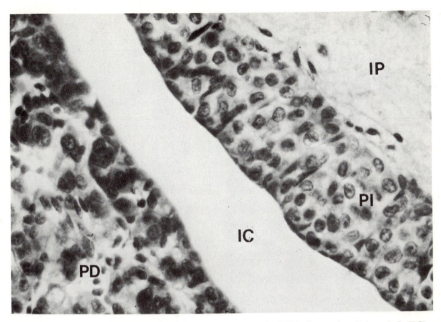

Fig. 4.1. Photomicrograph to show the pars distalis (PD), intraglandular cleft (IC), pars intermedia (PI) and infundibular process (IP) of the ferret. Note rounded and elongated cells in the pars intermedia.

vation that ACTH produces pigmentation. Lerner (1966) briefly considered some of the possible roles for MSH in higher vertebrates, and in the absence of an unequivocal demonstration that MSH is primarily concerned with pigmentation in mammals, many recent attempts have been made to associate it with other roles. It has been shown to have effects on nervous activity and behaviour (e.g. Sandman, Kastin and Schally, 1971); associated with various aspects of reproductive activity (e.g. Taleisnik and Tomatis, 1968) and has also been found to have a wide range of effects outside these two systems (see review by Howe, *J. Endocr.* in press).

STRUCTURE OF THE MAMMALIAN PARS INTERMEDIA

The varying degrees of development of the pars intermedia in different species have already been noted (p. 22). It is closely associated with the neurohypophysis and, in forms where a hypophysial cleft persists, is largely separated from the pars distalis by the cleft. When such a cleft is not present, cells of the pars intermedia may mingle with those of the pars distalis (Beato, 1935). There is usually a more or less continuous basement

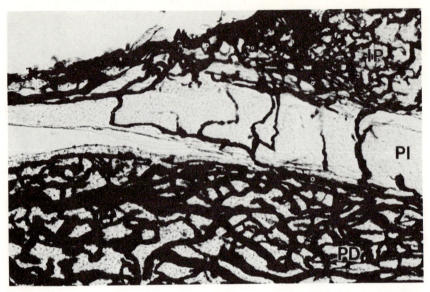

Fig. 4.2. Transverse section of an Indian-ink-injected pituitary gland of a rat. Note the vessels crossing the pars intermedia (PI) linking the much denser capillary beds of the pars distalis (PD) and infundibular process (IP). Reproduced by permission from Duvernoy (1958).

membrane between the intermedia and the neurohypophysis but this is often defective in parts, and penetration of intermedia cells into the neural tissue occurs, notably in man (Romeis, 1940), but also in other species.

The cells of the pars intermedia are commonly arranged in several layers, giving the appearance of a stratified epithelium (fig. 4.1 and colour plate). In some species a kind of lobulation has developed, groups of cells being separated by membranous septa (see, for example, Hanström, 1952). 'Follicles' may occur, and often, as in the ferret (Holmes, 1960) contain amorphous PAS+ material. The intermedia is relatively avascular compared with other divisions of the pituitary gland. There is commonly a vascular layer at the junction between the intermedia and neuro-hypophysis, within the membrane forming the boundary between the two zones. Vessels do extend into the intermedia or pass across it, but they are generally sparse (see Duvernoy, 1958, and fig. 4.2). In lobulated forms small vessels lie in the septa at the periphery of the lobules. The presence of a persistent intraglandular cleft prevents the direct passage of vessels between the pars distalis and pars intermedia, but vessels may traverse the zones of continuity where the derivatives of the rostral and caudal walls of Rathke's pouch join. The low degree of vascularity of the pars intermedia seems hardly to accord with an endocrine function.

INNERVATION

The pars intermedia differs from the pars distalis in yet another way, in that it is penetrated by nerve fibres. Such fibres, arising from the neural lobe, were described by Cajal in 1894 and later observed in many studies of the innervation of the adenohypophysis (see pp. 95ff). Pines (1926), for example, described fibres passing to the pars intermedia, as well as to the posterior lobe, from what are generally recognised as the supraoptic nuclei of the hypothalamus. The literature contains a number of descriptions of nerve fibres in the mammalian pars intermedia (Croll (1928) in the rabbit; Hair (1938) in the cat; Brooks and Gersh (1941) in the rabbit and rat, and Ribas-Mujal (1958) in the ox). Hillarp and Jacobsohn (1943), using a methylene blue technique, demonstrated a rich innervation in the rat. Green, who so strongly denied the presence of nerve fibres in the pars distalis, noted their presence in the pars intermedia of the cat and rat (1951) and of the Cebus monkey (1952). Methods for staining neurosecretory fibres have been found to reveal typical beaded fibres passing between the cells of the intermedia (e.g. Bargmann, 1949), although Ortman (1954) suggested that such beads might indicate only neurosecretory material which had diffused from the neurohypophysis, and not necessarily nerve fibres.

Nevertheless, it seemed clear, on the basis of light microscopic studies, that the pars intermedia of a number of widely different species does contain a significant number of nerve fibres, most of which end within it rather than passing to some other destination. It seemed possible also that there might be at least two kinds of nerve fibre present – 'normal', which can be demonstrated by metallic impregnation techniques, and neurosecretory, which can be shown by methods used for staining neurosecretion (see pp. 73–4). Thus, Stutinsky (1958) found both 'normal' and neurosecretory nerve fibres in the pars intermedia of the ox, horse and pig, although he noted that neurosecretory fibres need not necessarily be filled with NSM and might then appear as 'typical' nerve fibres.

The likelihood of at any rate a dual innervation was increased by the results of studies using fluorescent techniques for the demonstration of catecholamines and related substances, such as 5-hydroxytryptamine. These compounds are thought not to occur in neurosecretory neurons, so that the demonstration of both neurosecretory and aminergic nerve fibres, even if not shown together in the same section, is a strong indication that more than one type of nerve fibre is present. Enemar and Falck (1965) showed that aminergic fibres constitute a rich terminal innervation in the pars intermedia of the frog, and shortly afterwards reports of similar kinds of findings in mammalian glands suggested that the possibility of a dual or even more complex innervation was not confined to amphibians (see Baumgarten, Björklund, Holstein and Nobin, 1972, for references).

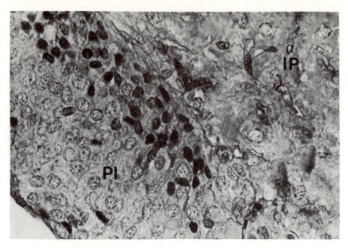

Fig. 4.3. Photomicrograph of the pars intermedia (PI) of a rat. Note cells with large pale-staining nuclei and smaller cells with dense nuclei. IP, infundibular process.

Studies with the electron microscope had already indicated that neurosecretory nerve fibres from the neurohypophysis penetrate the mammalian pars intermedia and come into close association with the cells (Kurosumi, Matsuzawa and Shibasaki, 1961; Ziegler, 1963). It was later shown that fibres containing small dense-cored vesicles, measuring up to *c.* 100 nm in diameter and usually considered to be associated with catecholamines, also entered this part of the gland; the aminergic character of these fibres was later confirmed by Baumgarten *et al.* (1972).

CYTOLOGY

Although the pars intermedia is relatively simple in its cytology as compared with the pars distalis, it is not structurally homogeneous (fig. 4.1). Commonly at least two types of cell can be distinguished by optical microscopy. One, the more numerous, appears rounded or cuboidal, with a round or oval nucleus, which may be large and pale staining or smaller and darker (fig. 4.3). The other, which has been called 'ependymal', has less cytoplasm, is elongated in form and has an elongated nucleus. The term 'ependymal' should not be taken as indicative of the derivation of the second type of cell, only of its shape.

Trautmann (1911) described light and dark cells in the pars intermedia of the rat, and this has been confirmed by later authors. Kurosumi, Matsuzawa and Fujie (1962) also noted two such types in the rat, but found that in preparations stained by PAS they could make no clear distinction between them, as there was a continuous gradation of one to the other. It is of interest also that they found that dark cells could not be distinguished after certain fixatives, Zenker-formalin, formalin and Carnoy's solution – an observation which may accord with that of Porte *et al.* (1971) (see below).

Raftery (1969) observed two types of cell in the pars intermedia of the ox, and noted that the cells probably equivalent to the 'ependymal' elements described by others (his 'type II') were more strongly PAS+ than the chief type, the latter giving a variable reaction, which was not abolished by pre-treatment with diastase, and hence not due to the presence of glycogen. The ependymal type of cell stains strongly with pyronin (Holmes, 1960) at any rate in the ferret, and pyronin staining of the intermedia became more intense after division of the pituitary stalk (see below).

The surface of the pars intermedia adjoining the intraglandular cleft may be covered with a single layer of low cuboidal cells; this is clearly evident in some rodents such as the jird, *Meriones libycus*, the rat and the ferret (fig. 4.1). Kurosumi *et al.* (1962) were able to distinguish clearly such a marginal zone of flattened cells in the rat, some of which were ciliated.

The presence of at least two types of parenchymal cell in the mammalian pars intermedia has been confirmed by electron microscopy. Kurosumi, Matsuzawa and Shibasaki (1961) and Ziegler (1963) described light and dark cells, the latter having a well-developed Golgi zone and many free ribosomes, while the Golgi zone was less developed in the light cells. Kobayashi (1965) observed that the light cells in the rat were filled with numerous clear vesicles 150–350 nm in diameter and small dense granules within a well-developed Golgi zone. Clear vesicles were few or absent in dark cells.

The relationship of the light and dark cells to each other has frequently been discussed by other authors. Romeis (1940) considered that the two forms represented different functional states of the same cell type. Duchen (1962) observed an increase in the number of dark cells after giving hypertonic saline to rats and considered the two types to be essentially the same.

A number of other observers have noted striking changes in the intermedia following experimental procedures. Kobayashi (1964) considered that variations in electron density of secretory granules brought about by dehydration indicated that the function of the intermedia, whatever this might be in mammals, was controlled by neurosecretory material of the posterior pituitary. The same author later (1965) thought changes following stress and adrenalectomy to be indicative of 'a close functional correlation' between the pars intermedia and the adrenal cortex – an interesting hypothesis in view of the already-mentioned overlap in molecular structure between MSH and ACTH.

This idea was recently taken further by Porte *et al.* (1971), who also studied the pars intermedia of the rat. They found that two types of fixation gave strikingly different results; after using glutaraldehyde, the chief cells of the intermedia appeared rich in electron-dense secretory granules, whereas after fixation using osmium tetroxide these granules were largely transformed into more or less empty vesicles. A second type of cell, smaller in size, contained smaller granules (*c.* 100–130 nm) which were resistant to osmium fixation. Porte and his colleagues noted that the latter cells resembled certain cells of the pars distalis, namely those believed to secrete ACTH and TSH, and suggested that they may in fact secrete ACTH, which unlike the ACTH of the pars distalis can be released under neurosecretory control. Stoekel *et al.* (1971) later described a zone of cells in the mouse in the rostral part of the pars intermedia surrounding the stalk which on the basis of reactive changes after adrenalectomy they considered to secrete ACTH. These cells (which also occur elsewhere in the intermedia) are in direct contact with nerve fibres of the stalk and also closely related to the portal vessels, so that they could be the first to contact CRF in the portal blood. Further evidence may confirm the hypothesis put forward by Porte *et al.* (1971) that there may be a dual system for the secretion of ACTH, one governed by the posterior pituitary and one by the hypothalamus by means of CRF.

Despite ideas such as this, which might provide a key to the role of the pars intermedia in mammals, problems remain. The histochemical studies of Raftery (1969) suggest that the tissue is metabolically active, as indeed it must be if it is elaborating one or more hormonal principles. After extensive studies the Legaits (Legait and Legait, 1964; Legait, 1964) suggested that the size of the pars intermedia in mammals is related to the ability to survive in arid surroundings, and that the tissue is larger in desert-living species. In amphibians, however, the pars intermedia is largest in those species in which the colour change mechanism is most highly developed. Further, the authors suggest that the volume of the intermedia decreases in states of increased hypothalamic activity, as in dehydration and lactation, and increases in states of reduced hypothalamic activity. Certainly interference with the hypothalamo-neurohypophysial system may markedly affect the pars intermedia. Transection of the pituitary stalk in ferrets resulted in a marked increase in the cellular content of RNA of the intermedia cells (Holmes, 1961*a*), possibly indicative of increased activity. Although no hypertrophy of the pars intermedia was found in this study, a later one in which the stalk was transected in monkeys (Holmes, 1962) gave unequivocal evidence that a true as well as a relative hypertrophy of the intermedia occurred, together with the anticipated shrinkage of the infundibular process and a variable but usually marked diminution in size of the pars distalis, following the interruption of the portal vascular supply.

The low epithelium covering the luminal surface of the pars intermedia

was studied histochemically and electron microscopically by Vanha-
Perttula and Arstila (1970). They concluded that this layer of cells, which
lines the whole of the cleft, is more likely to transport rather than to
secrete material, and suggested that the colloid which is often present in
the cleft may originate in the anterior lobe.

THE PARS TUBERALIS

Despites its widespread, although not universal, occurrence in mammals,
birds, reptiles and amphibians, and the presence of a probable homologue
in elasmobranchs, but not in other fishes and amphibians, the significance
of this part of the pituitary complex remains less understood than that of
any other. Although absent in sloths (Wislocki, 1938*a*), in most mammals
it is in contiguity with the main mass of adenohypophysial tissue. Its
extension around the stalk and on the inferior surface of the hypothalamus means that most of it is damaged, or left behind, when the gland
is dissected free from the base of skull and hypothalamus, and this no
doubt accounts in part for the relatively scant attention hitherto paid to
its structure, compared with that devoted to the rest of the gland. Furthermore, the pars tuberalis is so intimately involved with the origin of the
portal vessels that its selective destruction without severely damaging the
blood supply to the pars distalis is not possible.

The extent of understanding of the pars tuberalis was briefly reviewed
by Atwell (1938), who concluded that 'the pars tuberalis remains an
enigma'. It must be admitted that the same comment largely applies
today, although more information on the cytology of this part of the
gland is now available. It is made up of cellular cords and follicles which
often contain colloid interspersed with a variable amount of connective
tissue. It is generally extremely vascular and arterioles and venules run
through it or lie at the junction of the tuberalis with the surface of the
hypothalamus. The venules are those forming the portal system of vessels.

The cells are generally described as chromophobic, and although
granular cells resembling those of the pars distalis may occur, the majority
appear to be of the former type. With appropriate stains, they have been
shown in several species to contain cytoplasmic RNA (Allanson, Foster
and Menzies, 1959; Holmes, 1960). Harris (1955) suggested that the cells
of the pars tuberalis merely served as a bed for the vessels; but since the
presence of RNA suggests synthetic activity, this idea should not be
accepted without further study. Recently electron microscopy (Cameron
and Foster, 1972) has shown that in the rabbit two main types of cells are
present; the most numerous contains small (*c*. 100 nm) cytoplasmic
granules and abundant polyribosomes. The second type (interstitial cell)
has long processes which encircle cells of the first type. Nerve fibres have
been reported penetrating the pars tuberalis (see p. 99).

Some evidence has been published indicating that at any rate some of the cells of the pars tuberalis may contain, and hence possibly secrete, LH. Midgley (1966), using an immunohistochemical technique, localised this hormone in cells of both the pars anterior and pars tuberalis, which were found to be both AF+ and PAS+. Legait (1969) injected extracts of pars tuberalis into male and female prepubertal rats, and reported a decrease in volume of the pars tuberalis, stimulation of testicular interstitial tissue in males and of ovarian luteal tissue in females, and also concluded that the pars tuberalis secretes LH. The tuberalis is also closely associated with the tanycytes of the basal hypothalamus (see pp. 92 ff) and may play a part in their activity. Much further work is, however, needed before this part of the adenohypophysis can be understood.

5

THE NEUROHYPOPHYSIS

I. THE SUPRAOPTICO-HYPOPHYSIAL SYSTEM

In contrast to the epithelial adenohypophysis, the posterior part of the pituitary, derived from the neural downgrowth, consists essentially of neural elements and blood vessels, cells making up only a small proportion of its bulk. The earliest observations on its structure, however, described cells, with or without processes, which were thought to resemble ganglion cells (Luschka, 1860; Peremeschko, 1867). Later the Golgi impregnation technique was applied to the organ, and revealed elements which Berkley (1894) considered to be nervous and glial, and which Retzius (1894) recognised as glial. The cells of the neurohypophysis are considered in more detail below.

Early reference to the passage of nerve fibres into the infundibular process seems to have been made by Krause (1876). Ramon y Cajal (1894) described and illustrated a large tract of fibres entering the process in a young mouse, and considered the lobe to be a sensory organ. Cajal's findings were supplemented by those of later authors, among them Tello (1912) who refers to a number of other publications, and Pines (1926). Some authors did not accept Cajal's view; Herring (1908), for example, thought that most of the fibres were processes of glial cells, and that the few true nerve fibres present in the infundibular process were largely derived from bundles accompanying blood vessels – a view which persisted into the 1920s (see Cowdry, 1922). It must be admitted that problems of differentiating between nervous and non-nervous fibres were considerable (and, as discussed later with reference to the pars distalis, persisted until recently) and that Tello and Pines described an appreciable innervation of the anterior as well as the posterior pituitary. Later studies left no doubt that the posterior pituitary was indeed a richly innervated organ, the fibres largely reaching it via the stalk (see, for example, the papers on the ox by Bucy (1930) and on the rabbit and rat by Brooks and Gersh (1941)). Rasmussen (1938) found that in the monkey (*Macacus rhesus*) the stalk contained at least 40,000 nerve fibres, and considered these to be too many simply to innervate the number of cells present in the infundibular process.

The origin of at any rate the bulk of fibres entering the infundibular process was ascribed to the hypothalamic neurons lying above the optic chiasma, designated as the supraoptic nuclei (Cajal, 1894; Pines, 1926; Greving, 1926*a*, *b*). Contributions from other groups of hypothalamic neurons were described, and Greving's (1928) proposal that the paraventricular nuclei contributed was confirmed in a series of studies by Roussy and Mosinger (see Diepen, 1962, for references). The latter authors suggested that fibres were also derived from tuberal nuclei. The acceptance of a hypothalamic origin does not of course exclude the passage of other nerve fibres into the neurohypophysis along blood vessels, although these were described by Dandy (1913) as few in number and difficult to demonstrate.

One of the great advances in our understanding of the structural and functional importance of the neurohypophysis was achieved in the second half of the 1930s by Fisher, Ingram, Ranson and other co-workers. In a series of papers and a monograph they published the results of studies which not only confirmed to a great extent the neural connections of the infundibular process, but also demonstrated the crucial role played by the neurohypophysis in the control of water metabolism. Their work, summarised in the monograph (Fisher, Ingram and Ranson, 1938), involved the placing of lesions in the supraoptico-hypophysial (SO-H) system of cats and monkeys, so that a variable proportion of the nerve fibres passing down the infundibular stem was destroyed. They found that lesions of these tracts were followed by degeneration of the median eminence, supraoptic neurons and the infundibular process, and it seemed clear that the supraoptic neurons constituted a major source of the infundibular fibres. The disturbance of water metabolism resembled diabetes insipidus, a pathological condition which occurs in man, characterised by the excretion of large amounts of dilute urine. The syndrome showed a typical pattern of onset. Damage to the SO-H system was shortly followed by an increased output of urine and a fall in its specific gravity. This the authors called the 'transient phase' of polyuria. It was succeeded by a period of normal output, the 'normal interphase' which in turn was succeeded by a secondary long-lasting polyuria, the 'permanent phase'. The severity of the diabetes insipidus could be directly correlated with the amount of damage to the SO-H system, and, as shown later, with changes in the circulating levels of antidiuretic hormone (ADH), one of the two active substances released from the posterior pituitary (see below).

A second function of the neurohypophysis is the secretion of the hormone oxytocin. This resembles ADH in chemical structure, being also an octapeptide, but its chief action is on the reproductive tract rather than the kidney. In mammals, oxytocin causes contraction of the smooth muscle of the uterus, particularly during parturition. It also acts on the contractile epithelial elements of the mammary gland, bringing about the ejection of milk, and forming the hormonal component of this neuro-

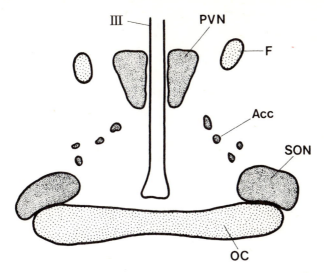

Fig. 5.1. Diagram of a coronal section through the hypothalamus of a rat to show the disposition of the magnocellular neurosecretory nuclei. Note scattered groups of similar (accessory) neurons (Acc) lying between the two major nuclei.

SON, supraoptic nucleus; PVN paraventricular nucleus; F, fornix; OC, optic chiasma; III, third ventricle.

hormonal reflex (see review by Sawyer, 1961). A comparable but chemically distinct analogue of the mammalian neurohypophysial hormones, vasotocin, occurs in birds and other non-mammalian vertebrates (see Sawyer, 1961).

ANATOMY OF THE (NEUROSECRETORY) HYPOTHALAMO-NEUROHYPOPHYSIAL SYSTEM

The hypothalamic components concerned with the activity of the pituitary gland may be considered as two systems, although they are not completely separate either structurally or functionally. The first, concerned with the control of the activity of the adenohypophysis, is considered on pp. 88ff. The second is the neurohypophysial system, whose function has been briefly described above.

The hypothalamic components of this system consist, in mammals, of two paired nuclei, supraoptic and paraventricular. The term 'supraoptic' describes the anatomical position of these nuclei in the basal hypothalamus, where they straddle the optic chiasma and the beginning of the optic tract on each side (Le Gros Clark, 1938) (fig. 5.1). Rostrally they extend on to the lateral aspect of the tract; according to Le Gros Clark they may, in many mammals, extend down into the anterior wall of the infundibulum, and Diepen (1962) describes an extension of this kind in

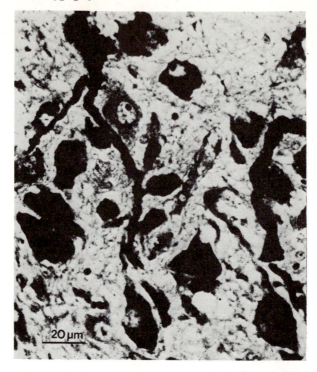

Fig. 5.2. Photomicrograph of supraoptic neurons in the hypothalamus of the dog stained with CAH. Note that some cells stain densely and others less so, indicating variations in the content of NSM. Reproduced from Das Zwischenhirn-Hypophysensystem, by W. Bargmann. Springer-Verlag, 1954, by permission of the author and publishers.

the fox. The rostral and caudal parts of each nucleus may be completely distinct from each other, but they are often linked by a strand of cells lying above the optic fibres. In the hedgehog (Holmes, 1961*b*, and unpublished observations) the supraoptic nucleus is formed of deep and superficial parts, the former lying in the customary position above the optic nerve fibres, the latter lying below these superficially on the basal surface of the hypothalamus.

The cells of the nucleus are large, and contain not only coarse granules of Nissl material, but NSM which can be demonstrated by specific staining techniques (fig. 5.2). The amount of NSM varies not only with the state of activity of the hypothalamo-neurohypophysial system, but also with the species (see Diepen, 1962, for references to studies of different species). Furthermore, there is commonly considerable variation in content of NSM between the cells of a single nucleus, so that neurosecretory stains may colour some cells intensely, while leaving others virtually unstained.

The paraventricular nuclei are situated more dorsally than the supra-optic, and lie medially on either side of the midline cleft of the third ventricle (fig. 5.1). In coronal sections each nucleus is usually seen to be wider dorsally and to taper as it passes inferiorly deep to the ependymal lining of the ventricle. In sagittal sections the cells of the nucleus form a flattened plate lying parallel to the surface. Some authors have described the paraventricular nucleus as being made up of two components, a small-celled (parvicellular) and a large-celled (magnocellular) division. In the rat Gurdjian (1927) distinguished a medial small-celled region from a lateral region of closely-packed neurons, which he described as being medium-sized rather than large; Westwood (1962) described a large-celled component in the ferret, lying dorsolaterally and a small-celled one lying ventromedially, blending with the paraventricular cell mass. Others, however, such as Clark (1938) described only one type of cell, whose nucleus was larger than most others in the hypothalamus. The para-ventricular nucleus was referred to by earlier authors as the 'nucleus filiformis' and other names have also been used; Solnitzky (1939) lists named nuclei which he considered to be homologous with the cell masses in the pig which he called nucleus filiformis.

Probably only the large-celled components of the paraventricular nuclei are homologous with the supraoptic neurons, and they can be grouped with the latter as the 'magnocellular' hypothalamic nuclei. Apart from the morphological similarity of the constituent neurons, it is only among the magnocellular component of the paraventricular nuclei that a marked cell loss occurs following section of the pituitary stalk or hypophysectomy. But although extensive degeneration of the supraoptic neurons follows such lesions, the changes in the magnocellular paraventricular component do not affect all the cells. Frykman (1942), for example, found that about 35 per cent were involved, while smaller more lightly staining neurons, assumed to form part of the parvocellular component of the nucleus, seemed to persist. A smaller proportion of neurons degenerates if a part of the neurohypophysis is left behind.

Frykman also noted that only the magnocellular part of the para-ventricular nuclei is reasonably well defined; the smaller paler staining neurons show no clear-cut limit to their extent and blend with diffusely arranged periventricular cells. Even the large-celled elements, in both supraoptic and paraventricular nuclei, are not, however, sharply delimited. Authors have described characteristic cells scattered between the two nuclei (see Diepen, 1962) and reference has already been made to the two major divisions of the supraoptic nucleus which are joined by a tract of cells extending over the upper aspect of the optic tract. A recent study (Bandaranayake, 1971) has emphasised the fairly extensive distribution of 'accessory' elements of the supraoptic and paraventricular groups of neurons, and concluded that such accessory cells account for some

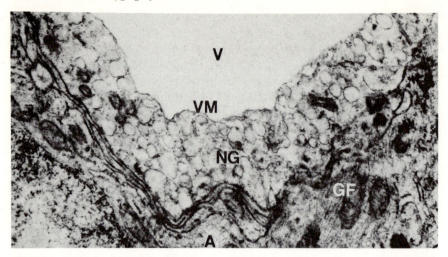

Fig. 5.3. Electron micrograph showing part of a vesiculated neuron in the supra-optic nucleus of a dog. Part of the large vacuole (V) is bounded by a thin band of cytoplasm containing neurosecretory granules (NG). Outside the neurons lie axons (A) and glial fibres (GF). VM–vesicular membranes. From Zambrano and De Robertis (1967), by permission of Springer-Verlag.

8.2 per cent of the total content of the hypothalamic magnocellular nuclei.

The neurohypophysial system of the dog differs from others in that a small proportion (not more than 0.2 per cent, according to Jewell, 1953) of neurons of the supraoptic and paraventricular nuclei are vacuolated (colour plate). The vacuoles vary in size, some reaching 200 μm in diameter, and are often surrounded by such a thin rim of cytoplasm that some authors have considered them to be extracellular spaces. A later study with the electron microscope, however, has confirmed that the vacuoles are indeed neuronal (Zambrano and De Robertis, 1967; fig. 5.3). Jewell noted that the vacuolated neurons contain NSM, and that although they were presumed to belong to the hypothalamo-hypophysial system, hypophysectomy resulted in only a small reduction in their number, despite a great overall loss of neurons. High lesions of the supraoptico-hypophysial tracts, however, were followed by a marked loss of vesiculated cells. The distribution of vesiculated neurons does not appear to be uniform throughout the magnocellular nuclei, and most were found in the posterior division of the supraoptic nucleus, fewest in the paraventricular. Electron microscopic studies showed that the vesicles contained no formed elements, but that the surrounding cytoplasm was packed with vesicles of diameter *c.* 230 nm. Although these contained little if any electron-dense material, they were called by Zambrano and De Robertis 'neurosecretory granules', and were considered to represent

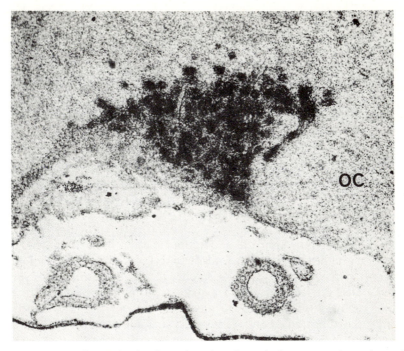

Fig. 5.4. Autoradiograph of a frontal section through the supraoptic nucleus of a rat 5 hours after subarachnoid injection of ³⁵S-DL-cysteine into the cerebrospinal fluid. Numerous silver grains overlie the supraoptic neurons, indicating selective concentration of radioactive material in the cells. The optic chiasma (OC) lies to the right of the supraoptic nucleus. From Sloper, Arnott and King (1960).

an early stage in the formation of the typical electron-dense membrane-bound inclusions found in the nerve fibres of the infundibular process (see pp. 77ff). These authors suggested that vacuolated cells are formed as a result of intracytoplasmic cytolysis, and did not agree with the view (Jewell and Verney, 1957) that they function as osmoreceptors for the regulation of the release of antidiuretic hormone.

Connections of the magnocellular nuclei

It has already been noted that processes of supraoptic neurons pass, via the infundibular stem, into the infundibular process. Even after transection of the stalk at a high level near its origin from the tuber cinereum, however, some supraoptic neurons fail to show degenerative or chromatolytic changes. This indicates that a small proportion of the neurons have processes which do not enter the infundibular stem, and probably end either in the region of the tuber cinereum or in other parts of the hypothalamus.

Although changes in the paraventricular neurons after lesions of the stalk or after hypophysectomy have been noted by numerous observers (see Olivecrona, 1957, for references) not all of these attempted to estimate the proportion of cells involved. Frykman (1942), whose work has already been referred to, was the first to make a quantitative study. Other observers such as Pickford and Richie (1945) and O'Connor (1947), all of whom used dogs as experimental animals, found considerably higher percentages of degenerated cells after lesions of the hypothalamo-neurohypophysial system than the 35 per cent reported by Frykman after hypophysectomy; Pickford and Richie, for example, reported a figure of 84 per cent. It seems likely that this much higher figure might be due to the fact that the lesions were placed at a higher level in the system, and did not damage only those cell processes which passed down to the stalk and into the infundibular process.

In 1928 Greving described fibres from the paraventricular nuclei as passing ventrally towards the supraoptic nuclear masses, but he was uncertain whether or not they ended there or passed further into the supraoptico-hypophysial tract. Laruelle (1934) confirmed Greving's observations, but also described a second component of the paraventricular pathway which extended along the wall of the third ventricle towards the tuber cinereum. Fisher, Ingram and Ranson (1938) considered that most of the paraventricular neuronal processes ran towards the supraoptic nuclei and that most of them terminated there; if this is so, lesions of the supraoptic nuclei should result in degeneration of an appreciable proportion of paraventricular cells. Some of the experiments reported by Olivecrona (1957) bear strongly upon this problem. He found that in the rat only 25 per cent of magnocellular neurons in the paraventricular nuclei survived section of the pituitary stalk; furthermore, the effects of intrahypothalamic lesions suggested that no major component of paraventricular processes passed to the region of the supraoptic neurons, since localised lesions of these latter nuclei were not followed by any reduction in the number of paraventricular cells. Also, lesions placed close to the paraventricular nuclei on the lateral side produced little degeneration, indicating that the fibres do not run laterally for any appreciable distance. Olivecrona came to the conclusion that the fibres pass slightly outwards and downwards towards the tuber cinereum. Lesions of the paraventricular nuclei considered to be complete were followed by the loss of about 20 per cent of the supraoptic neurons.

Neurosecretion

The hypothalamo-hypophysial system of mammals is a major neurosecretory system. The precise definition of neurosecretion has given rise to difficulties, particularly since secretion, in the sense of the elaboration and release of transmitter substances, is a general property of neurons. One definition (not now universally applicable; see Knowles and Bern, 1966; Bern, 1967) distinguishes non-neurosecretory neurons from neurosecretory ones by the fact that the latter produce hormones which are liberated into the bloodstream of a neurohaemal organ. This, with the added feature that material associated with the secretions is stainable within the neurons and their processes, is appropriate for the system under consideration, in which stains for neurosecretory material, as well as the usual metallic impregnation techniques, can be used to study the disposition within the hypothalamus of the fibres passing to the neurohypophysis.

The mammalian hypothalamo-neurohypophysial system may be said to be both a neural system, in that processes of hypothalamic neurons pass via the infundibular stem to terminate in the infundibular process, and an endocrine system. Hormones (as distinct from neurotransmitter substances) are synthesised in the perikarya of these neurons, and travel distally along their processes to be stored in the infundibular process until released into the blood passing through its vessels. The neurosecretory material (NSM) can be demonstrated both histologically and electron-microscopically (fig. 5.5) since it has a more or less defined morphology at the ultrastructural level.

Confusion has arisen about the distinction between neurosecretory hormones and neurohumours. Neurons produce 'transmitter' substances, acetylcholine and noradrenaline, for example, which are released (secreted) by the neurons at synapses, where they bring about a change in the physical state of post-synaptic membranes necessary for the transmission of the nerve impulse. Transmitter substances also may be associated with submicroscopic structures which can be demonstrated by electron microscopy, and, using selected techniques (such as fluorescence microscopy, for catecholamines), sometimes by optical microscopy. Is the formation and release of such substances then neurosecretion? Some authors think that this is so, and would even extend the concept of neurosecretion to include such elements as cells of the pineal body, derived from cells with a potentially neural line of development, which secrete melatonin. It is perhaps logical, however, to differentiate neurohumours from neurosecretory hormones, at any rate as far as the vertebrates are concerned, on criteria based on the time of action of the active principles – phasic (short acting) for neurotransmitter substances, and tonic (long acting) for neurosecretory hormones.

As has already been discussed, by the mid-1940s there was considerable evidence associating the hypothalamo-neurohypophysial system of neurons with the secretion of ADH. In addition, various observers had noted amorphous 'colloid' stainable material associated with this system (e.g. Popjak, 1940). The theory then in fashion was that this colloid was

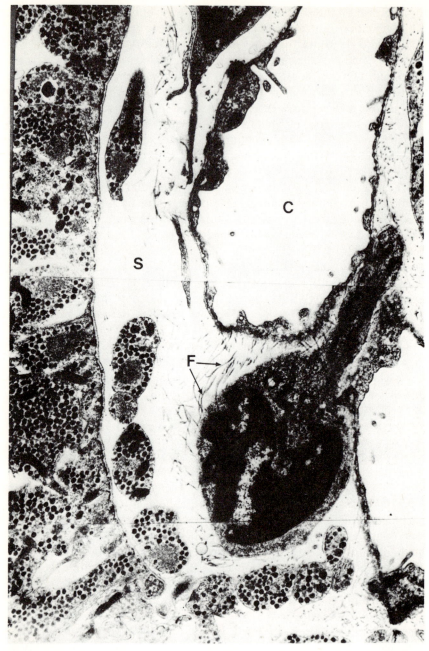

Fig. 5.5. Electron micrograph to show the relationship of neurosecretory fibres to blood vessels in the neurohypophysis of the jird. At the top of the figure is the lumen of a capillary (C) surrounded by pericapillary space (S). Nerve fibres containing dense and lucent vesicles abut on the pericapillary space or project into it; the space also contains collagen fibrils (F) and a fibroblast.

passing from the pituitary to the hypothalamus, a view reminiscent of the original ideas on the direction of flow of blood in the pituitary portal system (see p. 100). The centripetal theory of flow of colloid was not universally held, however, and Palay (1945), from studies of the catfish, proposed a preoptico-hypophysial direction of flow of droplets of material which could be stained with acid fuchsin.

Further development of ideas depended to some extent on the availability of a reliable method of staining NSM in the hypothalamo-hypophysial system. This came with the publication by Bargmann in 1949 of a crucial paper in which he described the application of Gomori's chrome-alum haematoxylin technique, originally used to stain islet cells in the pancreas, to the hypothalamus and pituitary. By this technique 'colloid' material was shown to be present throughout the whole of the hypothalamo-hypophysial system. Furthermore, the demonstration (Ortmann, 1951; Hild and Zetler, 1953a, b) that hormonally active material could be extracted from tissue over the extent of the distribution of CAH staining, including the two hypothalamic nuclei, supported the hypothesis that both the hormones and the stainable NSM were formed in the hypothalamus and transported, via the pituitary stalk, to the infundibular process for storage (Bargmann and Scharrer, 1951; Bargmann, 1951). This view is now generally accepted.

Stainable NSM and hormonal activity

Following the publication of Bargmann's (1949) paper already referred to, CAH was used to study many different neurosecretory systems. Since the chemical basis underlying its use was not clear, however, and since it was known to stain non-neurosecretory material, the equation of CAH (Gomori)+ material with NSM was not universally accepted. Other methods of staining were tried, among these aldehyde fuchsin (see p. 37). In successful preparations this stains NSM intensely; the technique is not always reliable, however, and furthermore, aldehyde fuchsin has affinities for non-neurosecretory material such as lipofuscins, which commonly occur in neurosecretory neurons.

Biochemical studies (see Van Dyke, Adamsons and Engel, 1955, for references) had shown that the neurohypophysis contained material rich in sulphur; accordingly, Barrnett and Seligman (1954) applied to the hypothalamus a histochemical technique for the demonstration of sulphydryl and disulphide groups. Although they obtained intense staining of supraoptic neurons, other, non-neurosecretory hypothalamic neurons also stained. Sloper (1955) obtained greater specificity by using a modified thioglycollate–ferric ferricyanide technique (Adams, 1956). Later, the technique based on the oxidation of cysteine to cysteic acid by performic acid, followed by staining with Alcian blue at a low pH, was applied

(Adams and Sloper, 1956). Provided control (unoxidised) sections are also stained this is a satisfactory way of demonstrating hypothalamic NSM, and although again the method is not completely specific, it has proved most useful for the study of the distribution and concentration of NSM in sections.

Since both oxytocin and ADH contain sulphydryl and disulphide groups, it seemed likely that NSM stained by methods specific for these groups also demonstrated the distribution of the hormones. This is not necessarily so, since carrier substances, neurophysins, are also present in the system, and these also contain sulphur (see Lederis and Jayasena, 1970); furthermore, there is not always a significant correlation between the amount of stainable NSM and the amount of hormone which can be extracted from a tissue, although many studies (for example, those of Hild and Zetler, 1953*a*, *b*) have shown that dehydration, whether by with-holding water or by the injection of hypertonic saline, is accompanied by depletion of both NSM and ADH from the infundibular process. Such changes suggest that depletion occurs because of the need for all available (stored) antidiuretic hormone to conserve the diminished water reserve of the animal.

Dehydration brings about depletion of NSM in both the infundibular processes and the hypothalamic neurons. Bachrach (1957) found that in rats NSM reappeared on the first day after dehydration, and increased in amount up to the sixth day. Dehydration was also found by Bachrach and Koszegi (1957) to be accompanied by an almost total loss of cytoplasmic RNA in the neurons, and by hypertrophy of their nucleoli; the latter finding at any rate is indicative of increased cellular activity. Dehydration is also associated with an increase in neuronal acid phosphatase (Rinne and Kivalo, 1958), again suggesting increased synthetic activity.

Autoradiographic studies

The presence of sulphur-rich material in the neurohypophysis made possible the application of autoradiographic techniques to studies of this system. Goslar and Schultze (1958) gave a yeast preparation containing ^{35}S-cystine and ^{35}S-methionine to rabbits and rats by stomach tube. The rabbits were killed eight, the rats three hours later and autoradiographs of the hypothalamus and pituitary prepared. A high concentration of radioactive material was found in neurons of the supraoptic and para-ventricular nuclei, although other hypothalamic neurons also showed considerable accumulation of material. The infundibular process showed very little activity compared with the adenohypophysis, doubtless (see below) because of the relatively short time the animals were allowed to survive after administration of the ^{35}S-containing material.

Studies using ^{35}S-DL-cysteine gave more precise labelling, and Arnott and Sloper (1958) found that injection of this substance directly into the cerebrospinal fluid gave better results than intraperitoneal injection. Within 30 minutes neurons of the supraoptic and paraventricular nuclei showed a concentration of active material greater than that in the surrounding hypothalamic tissue. Fuller reports of such studies (see for example Sloper, Arnott and King, 1960) gave a clear indication of the dynamic aspects of the production of NSM. Following subarachnoid injection, labelled material was rapidly taken up by neurons of the supraoptic nuclei (fig. 5.4) and to a lesser extent by those of the magnocellular parts of the paraventricular nuclei; other neurons in the brain stem and elsewhere showed appreciable uptake, and radioactivity appeared early in the pars distalis. Nine and a half hours after injection, however, the concentration of radioisotope in the infundibular process exceeded that in the pars distalis, but only after injection of labelled cysteine, not of methionine. Sloper and his colleagues considered that these results were in favour of the hypothesis put forward by Bargmann and Scharrer (1951), namely that the formation of posterior pituitary hormones occurs in the regions of the supraoptic and paraventricular nuclei, whence they subsequently pass, via the infundibular stem, to be stored in the infundibular process.

Further studies were reported by Ficq and Flament-Durand (1963). Again using rats, ^{35}S-methionine and ^{35}S-cystine were injected. The authors noted better localisation of activity to the supraoptic and paraventricular neurons with cystine than with methionine, and also observed the late (10 hours or more) appearance of activity in the distal parts of the neurohypophysis. Animals dehydrated for one month by giving 2 per cent sodium chloride in drinking water showed a higher uptake of radioactive material by the supraoptic nuclei; at 10 hours, activity in the infundibular process of dehydrated rats was greater than in that of normal animals, while at 24 hours this situation was reversed, indicating a more rapid production and turnover of synthesised material in the dehydrated animals.

Ficq and Flament-Durand also applied the same techniques to hypophysectomised rats. They found that although radioactivity could be demonstrated 30 minutes after injection in the remnants of the atrophied paraventricular and supraoptic nuclei, there was none in the stump of the stalk at this time. At 24 hours, however, the stump showed radioactivity in sites where droplets of NSM could be shown by CAH staining, providing further evidence for a proximo-distal flow of NSM.

The suggestion that dehydration greatly increases the rate of turnover in the hypothalamo-neurohypophysial system of material which is closely associated or identical with ADH has been supported by more recent studies (Talanti, 1971). Estimating radioactivity in different parts of the system 0.5, 6 and 24 hours after injection of labelled cysteine, he found that dehydration increased the rate of uptake of material into the hypo-thalamic nuclei, as well as into the neurohypophysis, but also increased the rate of turnover. In control animals counts increased progressively from 0.5 to 6 to 24 hours, while in dehydrated animals, even in the neurohypophysis, there was a fall between 6 and 24 hours.

Further evidence in favour of a proximo-distal flow of NSM has been obtained from other studies, notably experiments in which the pituitary stalk has been transected, and the animal allowed to survive for a time after the operation. This lesion affects both the adeno- and neuro-hypophysis, the former largely by interference with its blood supply (see pp. 13–14), the latter by division of the nerve fibres, whose segments lying distal to the lesion degenerate. This latter change does not occur for some days, however (about four days in the ferret, Holmes, 1961*a*), after which stainable NSM disappears distal to the lesion. In small animals the possibility of trauma to the infundibular process during the operation cannot always be ruled out, due to the shortness of the stalk and the sometimes difficult access. Larger animals enable transection to be carried out with little likelihood of such direct trauma. Holmes (1963) described the results of a series of stalk transections carried out in monkeys (*M. rhesus*), in which after transection a barrier of aluminium foil or poly-thene was placed between the cut ends in some of the animals. In each instance the transection was associated with atrophy of the infundibular process, an increase in its cellularity and a complete loss of NSM in animals allowed to survive the operation for between 6 and 52 weeks. Although no precise data on the time of disappearance of NSM following transection of the stalk were obtained, one animal killed at the presumed onset of the 'permanent' phase of polyuria, 10 days after operation, showed only slight traces of NSM in the infundibular process, suggesting that the onset of this phase of polyuria coincided with the exhaustion of 'usable' ADH stored in the process and normally available from there.

Examination of the median eminence in most of these animals showed an accumulation of NSM above the lesion in some instances, in amounts considerably in excess of normal. Such an accumulation again suggests that a proximo-distal flow of NSM normally occurs. In some specimens in which the cut ends of the stalk were not separated by a barrier, beads of NSM were present below the line of transection, and in one instance extended into the atrophic infundibular process. The characteristic 'string of beads' arrangement of the droplets was reminiscent of that found in neurosecretory nerve fibres, and hence raised the possibility that regenera-tion of such fibres across the lesion could occur. It should also be noted that in all specimens the supraoptic and paraventricular nuclei contained numerous apparently healthy neurons, some of which contained small amounts of NSM.

Ultrastructural studies

Many studies of NSM, based on observations using optical microscopy, describe it as arranged in 'droplets', often aligned to give a 'string of beads' appearance. A further characteristic feature of the neurohypophysis is the occurrence of NSM in quite large, usually rounded accumulations (up to several micrometres in diameter), commonly known as Herring bodies. Initially, it was thought that the secretory material formed a sheath on the outside of the nerve fibres, a view which persisted into the 1950s, as in Bodian's schema of the neurohypophysis of the opossum published in 1951. Electron microscopy, however, enabled the precise relationship between the bounding membranes of neuronal processes and contained material to be clearly determined.

In a paper published in 1955 Green and van Breemen described in the infundibular process of the rat and some other mammals the presence of electron-dense granules with diameters between 0.1 and 0.0625 μm. These did not lie free in tissue spaces but were enclosed by membranes, and the authors believed that they were located within processes of pituicytes, in nerve fibres or in structures shed from the surface of cells. Similar granules were also seen in Herring bodies. Examination of the tractus hypophyseus (stem) showed smaller granules within its nerve fibres. The authors considered that the larger granules in the neural lobe were related to 'Gomori substance', that is CAH-staining NSM, and examination of their micrographs in the light of later studies leaves no doubt that they had demonstrated neurosecretory granules.

In the same year Palay (1955) published an abstract describing the electron microscopic appearance of the infundibular process of normal, hydrated and dehydrated rats. He described closely packed nerve terminals, abutting on the capillaries of the process, which contained numerous small round membrane-bound electron-dense granules, measuring about 100 nm (0.1 μm) in diameter, and clusters of smaller vesicles, 30 nm in diameter. The dense granular material disappeared in dehydrated animals. These observations were later extended and enabled Palay (1957) to formulate a general plan of the structure of the neurohypophysis. According to him, nerve fibres passed down the infundibular stem enclosed in a protoplasmic sheath provided by the pituicytes. They entered the infundibular process in a 'hilar' zone where their sheath was lost, and terminated by dividing in a 'palisade' zone into several short branches which enlarged to form terminals closely applied to capillaries. In the stem and hilar regions the fibres measured c. 0.5 μm in diameter, and contained long delicate tubules of 20–30 nm with occasional dilatations. The terminals of the fibres in the palisade zone measured 1–1.5 μm in diameter, and contained mitochondria, 'synaptic vesicles' (the small membranous inclusions, c. 30 nm in diameter) and vesicles of about

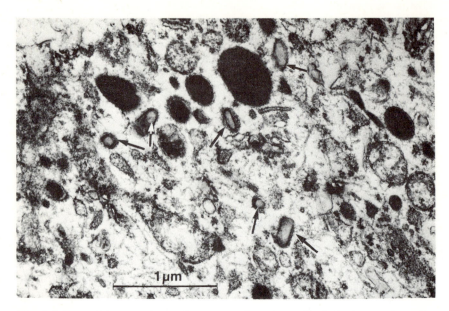

Fig. 5.6. Part of the cytoplasm of a supraoptic neuron of a hedgehog to show the crystal-like bodies (arrows). Reproduced from Holmes (1965), by permission of Springer-Verlag.

100 nm in diameter containing electron-dense material; these inclusions correspond in distribution to stainable NSM. This has remained an acceptable description of the basic structure of the mammalian neuro-hypophysis; furthermore, many of the features can be recognised in non-mammalian species.

At the time of publication of this paper the magnocellular hypo-thalamic nuclei of mammals had not been studied with the electron microscope. In 1962, however, Murakami published a description of supraoptic neurons of the mouse, observing that they contained a well-developed Golgi apparatus and osmiophilic granules. Some of these, which he called type II, were of the order of 400–600 nm in diameter, and closely bounded by a membrane. Smaller granules (type I) measured about 100–200 nm and usually there was a clear zone between the osmiophilic dense core and the bounding membrane. The two types of granules seemed to be distinct, no transitional forms being found, and the author considered that the smaller ones were the same as the elemen-tary neurosecretory granules in the distal parts of the neurohypophysis. Other studies have supported this suggestion; for example it has been possible to demonstrate in the perikarya of supraoptic neurons of the hedgehog (Holmes, 1965; fig. 5.6) the characteristic elongated crystal-like inclusions found in the infundibular nerve fibres of this animal (Holmes and Kiernan, 1964).

Such ultrastructural observations are in accordance with the ideas of proximal (perikaryal) synthesis of NSM, its subsequent transport distally, its storage and the ultimate release of the neurosecretory hormones into the blood passing through the infundibular process; but acceptable though this general hypothesis remains, on both functional and morphological grounds the system is more complex than was at first apparent. Functionally it is now established that the proximal parts of the neurohypophysis, including the median eminence and that part of the stalk containing those vascular complexes which drain by one or other set of portal vessels to the pars distalis (see pp. 101ff), are concerned with hypothalamic regulation of the activity of the adenohypophysis, while the distal part (infundibular process) has been seen to be concerned with the storage and release of the two neurohypophysial hormones, ADH and oxytocin.

The first published studies of the ultrastructure of the mammalian infundibular process referred to above described essentially only two types of vesicular inclusion in the nerve fibres. One, a large (*c.* 200 nm) round electron-dense granule, usually seen to be membrane-bound and losing its density in dehydrated animals, the second a small (*c.* 30–50 nm) electron-lucent vesicle, commonly designated 'synaptic' since a morphologically similar structure commonly occurs at synaptic endings. Later work has indicated that at least four types of inclusion are commonly found. In addition to the two noted above there is a large (*c.* 200 nm) electron-lucent vesicle, which is not necessarily a depleted form of the dense granule, and a small (less than 100 nm) electron-dense, membrane-bound granule (Holmes, 1964*b*; Rodríguez, 1971). In some species additional types of inclusion occur; nerve fibres of the infundibular process of the hedgehog contain dense membrane-bound bodies which in cross section measure some 125 nm and appear hexagonal, and in longitudinal section have the shape of an elongated hexagon up to 300 nm long (fig. 5.7); these were called 'crystal-like' bodies by Holmes and Kiernan (1964). Associated with these were found electron-dense inclusions about 200 nm in diameter, made up of small dense granules bounded by a membrane. The other types of inclusion described above also occur (Campbell and Holmes, 1966). Since these publications, confirmatory evidence for the occurrence of crystal-like inclusions in neurohypophysial nerve fibres of the hedgehog and other species has been published and high-resolution electron micrographs have also shown something of the internal structure of such inclusions (fig. 5.8; Bargmann and von Gaudecker, 1969).

The variety of granular and vesicular inclusions which occur within the nerve fibres of the infundibular process poses the problem of functional

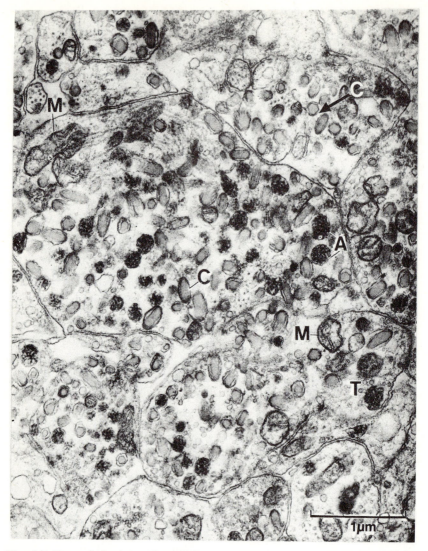

Fig. 5.7. Part of the infundibular process of the hedgehog as seen by electron microscopy. The fibres contain a variety of inclusions including crystalline bodies (C) and mitochondria (M). Reproduced from Holmes and Kiernan (1964*b*), by permission of Springer-Verlag.

associations, notably the relationships of the various inclusions to the processes of synthesis, storage and release of the posterior lobe hormones. This cannot be solved by morphological studies alone, but only by considering also biochemical and physiological data.

Initially the activity of the posterior lobe principles was ascribed to a

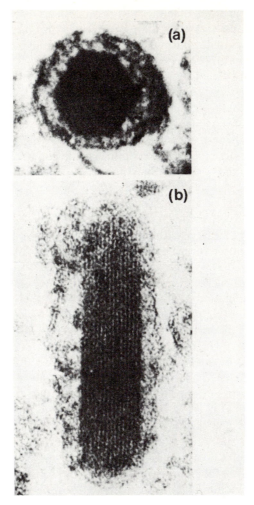

Fig. 5.8. Electron micrograph of crystalline bodies in neurohypophysial nerve fibres of a hedgehog in (*a*) transverse and (*b*) longitudinal section. Note the longitudinal striated pattern in (*b*). Reproduced from Bargmann and von Gaudecker (1969), by permission of the authors and Springer-Verlag.

single compound. In 1942 van Dyke and his colleagues isolated a protein from the neural lobe of ox pituitaries, which had oxytocic, antidiuretic and pressor activities. They considered this to be a pure substance, and calculated its molecular weight to be approximately 26 000. A single pure hormonally active substance might be expected, within a given species, to maintain a fixed ratio of its different activities, in this case vasopressor–antidiuretic and oxytocic actions. It became clear, however, that this ratio (VP:O) did not remain constant at all phases of an animal's life. Dicker and Tyler (1953*a*) found that the VP:O ratio of the posterior pituitary (taken as 1 in adults) was less than 1 in fetuses and puppies, increasing with age; and was greater during lactation. In a second paper (Dicker and Tyler, 1953*b*) the authors reported similar findings in rats, guinea-pigs, cats and humans.

Acher and his colleagues went on to split the van Dyke protein from ox pituitaries into two hormonally active factors, with oxytocic and vasopressor activity, and an inert protein, neurophysin (Acher, Chauvet and Olivry, 1956). Furthermore, they confirmed the work of Dicker and Tyler using rats, and concluded that under some conditions (immaturity, lactation) the synthesis and secretion of the oxytocin occurs independently of that of vasopressin. Furthermore, it now appears that at least two carrier neurophysins occur, one for each hormone (Ginsburg, Jayasena and Thomas, 1966).

Independent synthesis and/or release of the two hormones suggests both a separate source for each, and distinct 'carrying' mechanisms. The fact that neurons of two neurosecretory nuclei, the supraoptic and the magnocellular part of the paraventricular, send processes to the infundibular process, suggested that each nucleus (or rather each pair) was responsible for the elaboration of one of the hormones. Evidence in favour of such a hypothesis could be derived by several means: the hormone content of hypothalamic tissue samples containing only cells of one or other of the nuclei could be determined, and, if selective destruction of either pair of nuclei were possible, the loss of one of the two hormones would suggest that it was elaborated in that nucleus.

Some estimations of the distribution of hormone in the nuclei have been made, using, for obvious reasons, large animals. Adamsons *et al.* (1956) carried out assays of the two hormones and derived VP:O ratios for the supraoptic and paraventricular nuclei of the camel. They found VP:O ratios of just over 2 for tissue including the supraoptic nucleus and of *c.* 0.25 for that including paraventricular cells, although both hormones were present in each nuclear region. Lederis (1962) reported results of similar studies on sheep, finding VP:O ratios of 3.3 in supraoptic and 0.7 in paraventricular nuclei.

Olivecrona (1957), as part of his extensive study of the structure and function of the magnocellular nuclei of the hypothalamus of the rat, already referred to, destroyed the paraventricular nuclei bilaterally. He found that such lesions had no effect on the volume of urine excreted, but were associated with decreased oxytocin in the neural process without a similar fall in vasopressin. He concluded that the paraventricular nuclei are not necessary for the formation of vasopressin, but that they are important for the formation of oxytocin. The next year Duggan and Reed (1958) reported that lesions of the paraventricular nuclei (again in rats) were followed by a fall in the level of oxytocin in the blood. On the basis of his own work and that of other authors, Lederis believes that distinct ADH- and oxytocin-producing neurons exist (Lederis and Jayasena, 1970).

There is evidence from several studies that neurosecretory stains such as CAH demonstrate the carrier neurophysin rather than the hormones ADH and oxytocin themselves (Sloper, 1954; Acher, 1958) and the success of techniques to show sulphydryl groups as neurosecretory stains may depend on the fact that neurophysins as well as the hormones contain such groups. A major problem, however, has been that of determining hormone-granule specificity at the ultrastructural level: in other words, is each hormone associated with a specific type of granule?

As already noted, Palay (1957) associated loss of electron-dense inclusions directly with dehydration and consequent demand for hormone. Certainly, dehydration does bring about release of ADH, as do other stimuli such as stress and ether (but not chloroform) anaesthesia, and additional demand for hormone is also associated with loss of stainable NSM (judged by optical microscopy). Assessment of the degree of granulation using the electron microscope, however, is less easy, since it is not practicable to survey a whole organ by this means, and furthermore any changes brought about in the neurohypophysis by various stimuli may not be uniform throughout the organ, so that general assumptions based on the study of electron micrographs of small samples may be in error. Nevertheless dehydration does seem to be associated with a loss of electron-dense material from infundibular nerve fibres, and Palay's (1957) report has been confirmed by many later studies. Bodian (1963) found that in the opossum loss of electron density occurred rapidly, within 30 minutes of the injection of a hypertonic solution of urea, but noted that it was not uniform, Herring bodies retaining their stainable NSM. By contrast, Barer and Lederis (1966) found that ether anaesthesia for 30 minutes caused extensive loss of electron-dense material both from nerve fibres and Herring bodies. Similar changes are brought about by suckling in the glands of lactating animals (Monroe and Scott, 1966).

Initial attempts to determine the morphological criteria for the presence of hormone were not entirely successful. Schiebler (1952) applied the technique of ultra-centrifugation to the homogenised posterior pituitary of cattle and obtained a granular fraction which was CAH +. Electron microscopic examination of this material showed a wide range of size of the granules, and Schiebler concluded that hormone was associated with mitochondria. Barer, Heller and Lederis in 1963 published a report of an extensive study of a similar kind. They obtained by differential centrifugation of homogenised rabbit neurohypophysial tissue a fraction rich in granules, and showed by electron microscopy that these resembled the 'neurosecretory' inclusions in sections of 'intact' neurohypophysis. Furthermore, they showed that half of the total hormone content of their material was contained in the granular fraction. This confirmed earlier studies associating hormone with granules (Lederis and Heller, 1960).

A further stage of this work was an attempt to identify two types of granule, one associated with each of the two posterior lobe hormones. Unlike, for example, the hedgehog, there was no clear indication from electron microscopy of more than a single type of large electron-dense granule. Using density gradient centrifugation followed by assay of particle-containing fractions, the authors obtained some evidence that oxytocin particles were slightly denser than those containing vasopressin (ADH).

While there is thus fairly strong evidence that the granules do contain the posterior lobe hormones, the loss of electron-dense granules is not necessarily indicative of loss of hormone. Daniel and Lederis (1966) showed that extensive loss of electron-dense material from the infundibular process of rats could be achieved with little significant decrease in hormone content. This could be due to some change in the membrane or the enclosed granule rendering the material non-reactive to osmium tetroxide, and hence appearing electron-lucent (see review by Lederis, 1969). In this context note should be taken of the suggestion of Rodríguez (1971) that electron-dense and electron-lucent granules may each represent one of the two neurohypophysial hormones.

Apart from the 'typical' neurosecretory inclusions, some fibres in the mammalian neurohypophysis contain small electron-dense granules usually measuring about 100 nm in diameter or less (see p. 79). Morphologically these granules resemble the ones found in catecholamine-containing fibres. Dahlström and Fuxe (1966) and others have shown that fibres of the latter type do pass to the neurohypophysis, and recently Baumgarten *et al.* (1972) have shown that in the neural lobe of rats such fibres contain dense-cored vesicles measuring 50–120 nm in diameter.

The fourth commonly described inclusion in infundibular nerve fibres is the small electron-lucent vesicle which has often been likened to the synaptic vesicle (see p. 77). Collections of these are often found in the same fibres as neurosecretory granules, although profiles of some fibres may show the small vesicles only. These elements have been regarded by some as resembling true synaptic vesicles in function as well as in structure, being associated with acetylcholine which might play a part in the release of neurohypophysial hormones (see below). Such a view has long been questioned (e.g. Holmes and Knowles, 1960), and although acetylcholine does occur in the infundibular process and has been found in small vesicles (Lederis and Livingston, 1966) it has been localised to the perivascular regions and found to occur in nerve endings distinct from the neurosecretory ones (Livingston and Lederis, 1971).

It seems likely in the light of recent evidence that small vesicular elements are formed as a result of the passage of hormone-containing granules from the nerve fibres to the perivascular space. It has been clearly shown (Douglas, Nagasawa and Schultz, 1971; Krisch, Becker and Bargmann, 1972) that this is achieved by a process of exocytosis similar to that occurring in cells of the pars distalis. In this process, the membrane enclosing each individual granule fuses with the cell membrane; this breaks down over the granule which then lies outside the cell. The surplus membrane then forms small vesicular elements, the so-called synaptic vesicles (Douglas *et al.* 1971). Two alternative mechanisms for the disposal of the surplus membrane proposed by the latter authors are its incorporation in the cell membrane, or persistence as electron-lucent vesicles. It has been further suggested (Whitaker, LaBella and Sanwal, 1970) that lysosomes, which were demonstrated in nerve endings of the posterior pituitary, might be involved in digestion of membranes of the depleted neurosecretory granules or of the small vesicles.

The release of neurohypophysial hormones

In the intact animal, the release of ADH is brought about by a rise in the osmotic pressure of the blood passing through the internal carotid circulation (Verney, 1947), and suckling in lactating animals brings about release of oxytocin (see e.g. Cross, 1966); other stimuli are effective, and severe or prolonged stimuli will bring about the release of both hormones.

The synapses at the magnocellular hypothalamic neurons appear to be cholinergic. Pickford (1939, 1947) provided evidence for this based on the release of ADH by acetylcholine, and the neurons can be shown to contain a high concentration of cholinesterase (Holmes, 1961b). Neurosecretory neurons passing to the infundibular process transmit impulses in the same way as non-neurosecretory ones, and such impulses presumably bring about the release of hormones from the terminal parts of the fibres into the vessels of the process. Koelle and Geesey (1961) suggested that this terminal release might also be brought about by acetylcholine, but although cholinesterase can be demonstrated in the infundibular processes of some animals (Holmes, 1961b), it is not apparently present in appreciable quantities in all species.

The posterior lobe hormones can be released *in vitro* (Douglas, 1963; Daniel and Lederis, 1963; see Lederis and Jayasena, 1970, for later papers) by stimulation with K^+/Ca^{++}, without the need for transmitter substances. The probable mechanism is a depolarisation of the membrane of the neurohypophysial nerve fibres, followed by the passage of Ca^{++} into the fibres. The Ca^{++} may then reduce the binding of hormone to neurophysins, allowing the former to pass from the fibres into the blood.

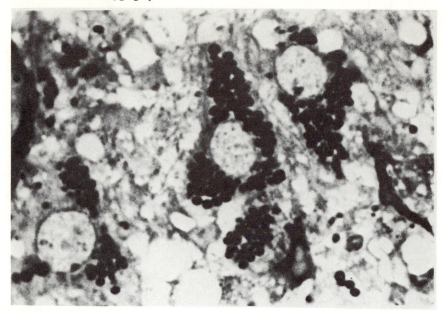

Fig. 5.9. Semi-thin section of the neurohypophysis of a rat dehydrated for 8 days. Pituicytes filled with round osmiophilic inclusions are present. Fixed in osmium tetroxide. Reproduced from Krsulovic and Brückner (1969), by permission of the authors and Springer-Verlag.

Pituicytes

The role of pituicytes in neurohypophysial activity is unknown. Essentially they appear to be modified glial cells, and electron microscopy shows that the nerve fibres are intimately associated with them. The early proposals that they were essentially the elements concerned in the elaboration of posterior lobe principles (Gersh, 1939) have long since been abandoned. They may act as sheath cells for the fibres in the same way as neuroglia in the central nervous system; there are, however, indications that they are not simply inert 'supporting elements'. Leveque and Small (1959) found that dehydration of rats was accompanied by increased mitotic activity of the pituicytes, and suggested that this might indicate a role in the separation of the posterior lobe hormones from carrier substances, or one involved in the actual release of hormone from nerve terminals. Rennels and Drager (1955) had earlier supported such a view. Later, Kurosumi *et al.* (1964) observed a considerable increase in lipid granules (which are a striking feature of the rat pituicyte) after increased release of posterior lobe hormones. These authors considered that the pituicyte lipid originated from the membrane bounding the hormone-containing neurosecretory vesicles which disintegrated during release of hormone. Sterba and Brückner (1969) provided evidence that

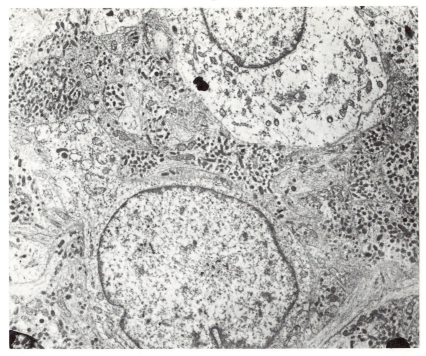

Fig. 5.10. Electron micrograph showing two types of pituicyte in the infundibular process of a hedgehog. The upper cell has abundant electron-lucent cytoplasm, the lower sparser and denser cytoplasm.

following transection of the stalk, pituicytes were able to phagocytose degenerating neuronal material. Later, Kruslovic and Brückner (1969) showed striking changes induced by dehydration in rats. They described a stage of hypertrophy of pituicytes from the third to the eighth days (fig. 5.9) followed by degeneration and reduced activity; and Whitaker, LaBella and Sanwal (1970) suggested that acid phosphatase-containing lysosomes in pituicytes might be concerned in the digestion of surplus membrane after liberation of secretory granules. Thus, there seem to be good grounds for assuming an active role for pituicytes in neurohypophysial activity.

It has been suggested that more than one type of pituicyte exists. Certainly they differ morphologically in both the same and different species (fig. 5.10); as noted, those of the rat are particularly rich in lipid. Kruslovic and Brückner (1969), and earlier authors, however, consider that morphological variations represent only different states of activity of a single cell type.

II. THE MEDIAN EMINENCE

It is now generally accepted that the more proximal parts of the neuro-hypophysis are essentially concerned with the transfer into the portal blood of the various releasing factors for adenohypophysial hormones, while neurosecretory fibres passing to the infundibular process traverse this region on the way. As already discussed (pp. 20–1), the form of the neurohypophysis varies considerably between species. Commonly, however, the infundibulum (median eminence) has the form of a distorted funnel, continuous above with the tuberal part of the hypothalamus and passing below, or posteriorly, into the infundibular stem, when this is well developed (Harris (1955) includes the stem in the infundibulum). Hence, the walls of the funnel surrounding the infundibular recess of the third ventricle, must be traversed by any neural elements linking the hypothalamus with more distal parts of the neurohypophysis.

The infundibulum, although in continuity with the tuber cinereum of the hypothalamus, can be distinguished from it. A boundary between the two can be defined, which may take the form of a groove, visible on surface examination, as in the cat (Martinez, 1960). This has been called the sulcus tuberis infundibularis by Spatz, Diepen and Gaupp (1948). As already considered, however (p. 9), the infundibulum is more clearly characterised by its particular vascular pattern, namely the primary capillary plexus of the portal vessels, which is supplied from a source (superior hypophysial vessels) distinct from that of the capillaries of the infundibular process (inferior hypophysial vessels). Such a demarcation on the grounds of the origin of the blood supply cannot be made in all species, for in some (notably man) capillary formations in the infundibular stem are also supplied from inferior hypophysial sources. Furthermore, an infundibular stem is not always present. On these grounds Green (1951) proposed to use only the terms 'median eminence' and 'neural lobe' to designate anatomically the two divisions of the neurohypophysis.

In 1960 Martinez published a detailed study of the structure of the neurohypophysis of the cat, based on cell and fibre stains. Prior to this, although the infundibular process had been extensively studied, relatively little attention had been paid to the more proximal part of the system.

Typically, the mammalian median eminence consists of three layers (fig. 5.11). Innermost is a layer of ependyma continuous with that extending throughout the third ventricle. Immediately external to this is the layer containing the fibres of the supraoptico-hypophysial tract, made up of fibres of supraoptic and paraventricular neurons passing to the infundibular process. The outermost zone is a neurovascular layer in which fine neuronal processes enter into relationship with the capillary formations of the primary plexus of the portal system. The three layers have been designated as zona ependymalis (inner), zona fibrillaris (middle) and zona

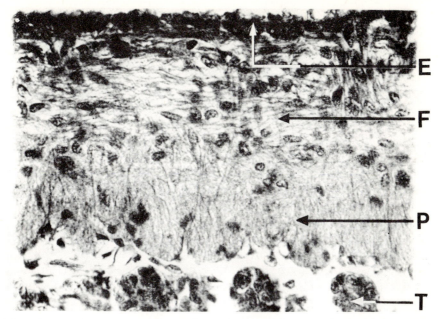

Fig. 5.11. The three layers of the median eminence of the cat, stained with haematoxylin. E, ependymal layer; F, fibrillary layer containing supraoptico-neurohypophysial fibres; P, palisade layer, the zone of neurovascular contact; T, pars tuberalis. Reproduced by permission from Martinez (1960).

palisadica (neurovascular outer zone). The surface of the eminence is clothed with a layer of cells of the pars tuberalis, but this may extend beyond the eminence itself, particularly rostrally, where, as in the ferret, it may reach the optic chiasma.

The layers are readily distinguishable by optical microscopy, their appearance naturally depending on the stains used. Bearing in mind the funnel-like form of the infundibulum, it can be understood that the three layers may extend to surround the infundibular recess, and once the infundibulum lies free from the tuber dorsal, ventral and lateral walls are present. In a typical horizontally-lying neurohypophysis, the ventral wall is more extensive than the dorsal, and commonly forms the largest part of the eminence. The thickness of the walls and also of the individual layers varies in different parts, and the lateral walls are generally much thinner than the others.

The inner ependymal zone is not simply a single layer of cells covering a plane surface; in many regions there is more than one layer of nuclei, while in others the lining may appear deficient. Clumps of cells also extend into the surrounding neural layer. Another feature is that the processes of the ependymal cells extend throughout the whole thickness of the median eminence (see pp. 92ff) and end either as branches around the sheaths of the capillary formations of the primary plexus, or at the basement membrane forming the outer limit of the neural tissue. These fibres cross the neural processes of the supraoptico-hypophysial tract at right angles.

The zona fibrillaris, as already noted, consists largely of neurosecretory fibres passing to the infundibular process. These are generally oriented in a sagittal plane, and pass into the infundibular stem. Usually in mammals the amount of NSM along the course of the tract itself is not great, and scattered beaded fibres and occasional Herring bodies only can be stained, compared with the denser staining of the infundibular process itself.

The outermost layer, the zona palisadica, is the destination of nerve fibres passing to the infundibulum from various hypothalamic nuclei. These fibres, which are designated as 'tubero-hypophysial', arise from neurons in the tuber and probably more widely in the hypothalamus; they enter the palisade zone and eventually end about the capillary formations of the primary plexus which penetrate the neural tissue (fig. 5.12) (see pp. 109ff). In their course some of the fibres decussate, and as in some areas of the tuber they lie internal to fibres of the supraoptico-hypophysial tract, these must also cross this tract to achieve their final external position. The vascular formations present in this external zone are discussed elsewhere (pp. 103ff) but essentially they consist of 'long' and 'short' loops. The latter lie entirely within the zona palisadica; while the former may extend beyond it and penetrate the zona fibrillaris, even reaching as far as the ependymal layer.

Optical microscopy reveals only some of the features of the neuro-vascular zones in the median eminence (see, e.g., Green, 1948). The blood vessels themselves can be readily stained to show endothelium and associated cells, probably smooth muscle, at any rate in the larger vessels. The vessels are surrounded by a 'sheath' which can be shown to contain nerve fibres in a kind of 'matrix' of poorly staining material, some of which is glial.

Studies with the electron microscope have added considerably to knowledge of the fine organisation of the median eminence. The cells lining the recessus infundibularis show typical microvilli, and as elsewhere in ependyma, zonulae adherens and zonulae occludens occur (Rinne, 1966). Processes of these cells can be traced to pericapillary zones.

The nerve fibres of the region can be classified into various categories, chiefly by their diameter and the type of inclusion they contain (see review by Kobayashi, Matsui and Ishii, 1970, and papers in Knigge, Scott and Weindl, 1972). In general fibres of the supraoptico-hypophysial tract lie in the zona fibrillaris external to the ependymal layer. This is made up largely of unmyelinated fibres, and although some myelinated ones are present (Rinne, 1966) many apparently lose their myelin sheath before leaving the median eminence. Some authors refer to these as type A

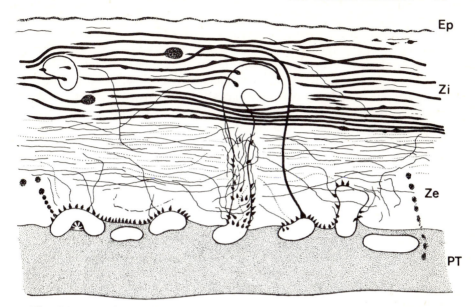

Fig. 5.12. Drawing to show the ultrastructural organisation of the mammalian median eminence. Ep, ependymal layer; Zi, the intermediate or fibrillary layer; Ze, the external layer; PT, pars tuberalis. Capillaries of the primary plexus can be seen lying at the interface between the pars tuberalis and the zona externa or penetrating more deeply; numerous neural swellings make contact with these vessels. From Barry (1961).

fibres, following the classification of Knowles (1965). This, originally introduced with reference to the pituitary of the dogfish, distinguishes two categories of fibre, type A containing large electron-dense vesicles with a mean diameter of 150 nm, which stain with CAH, and type B fibres which contain smaller electron-dense vesicles (60 nm), do not stain with CAH, and by contrast with type A are now known to be aminergic. A two-fibre classification, however, proved inadequate, since although it is difficult on present evidence to be sure how many types of fibre there may be, both in structural and functional terms, in the median eminence, there are certainly more than two. A third type (C) contains only clear vesicles; and Ishii (1972) for example, who applied a statistical method to a study of the median eminence of the horse, described five groups of fibres, which he called A_1, A_2, B_1, B_2 and C, with the possibility of further subgroups. In his classification, however, C refers to the fibres with the largest inclusions and A to those with the smallest.

Variations in the number of types of fibres described by different authors may be due to several factors, such as different technical methods, notably fixation; species differences, differences in the area sampled; in the physiological state of the animals used, and of course subjective errors. Furthermore, so many substances are present in the median eminence that it is not yet possible to correlate the complexity of its morphology with that of its function. Not only does the nervous tissue contain the two neurohypophysial hormones, but also the various releasing factors (see pp. 126ff), as well as acetylcholine, catecholamines and serotonin. The latter two substances have been extensively studied in recent years by the fluorescence techniques first introduced by Falck (1962). It has been clearly shown that there is an extensive system of catecholamine-containing neurons in the hypothalamus, and that groups of these extend processes into the median eminence. The amount of demonstrable fluorescent material varies both in different physiological states and also in response to drug and hormone treatment. Hökfelt and Fuxe (1972) suggest that the noradrenaline-containing part of this system may be concerned in the induction of a pattern of hormonal secretion by the pituitary, and many authors have postulated the involvement of monoaminergic neurons in the control of various adenohypophysial activities. These ideas have been discussed in a number of papers (see, for example, Bargmann and Scharrer, 1970; Knigge, Scott and Weindl, 1972).

At any rate some of the granular material demonstrable in nerve fibres of the median eminence seems to represent releasing factors. The granular content of certain fibres varies in different physiological and experimental states, although not in parallel with the changes in fluorescent material. Harris and Campbell (1966), for example, found changes in the ultrastructure of the median eminence of the rabbit occurring within 30 minutes of mating, an act which brings about the release of LRF into the portal vessels and LH from the pituitary. Changes of a comparable kind have been described associated with secretion of other tropic hormones. Another type of study is of the ontogeny of the median eminence. Monroe, Newman and Shapiro (1972) compared the ultrastructure of this region in neonatal and adult rats, and concluded that although in the neonatal period the eminence was not fully developed morphologically (and therefore presumably functionally), neurohaemal contact – a necessary prerequisite for the passage of transmitter substances into the portal blood – was present at the surface zone of the eminence. Clementi *et al.* (1970) have suggested, on the basis of ultrastructural studies, that each factor concerned in the release of tropic hormones may be stored in a different type of nerve ending, and that at least two such factors are associated with endings containing dopamine.

Tanycytes

Recently considerable interest has been directed to a possible non-neural transport system associated with (among other sites) the median eminence and pars tuberalis. In 1954 Horstmann described, in selachian brain, cells

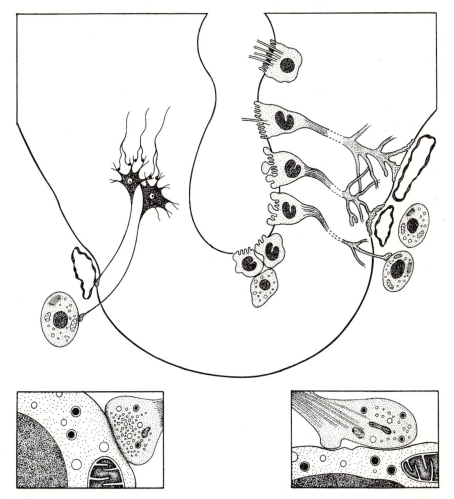

Fig. 5.13. Diagram of tanycytes in the hypothalamus of the monkey. On the left two neurons are seen with processes passing to a cell and a capillary; on the right tanycytes lying in the ependyma extend to the surface of the median eminence where they are closely associated with capillaries or cells of the pars tuberalis. The left inset shows the contact between a neurosecretory nerve fibre and a cell of the pars tuberalis, and the right inset contact between a tanycyte and a cell of the pars tuberalis. Reproduced from Knowles and Anand Kumar (1969), by permission of the authors and the Royal Society.

called tanycytes, which appeared to be essentially a modified type of ependymal cells. These have since been described by various authors both in mammalian and non-mammalian species; see for example Leonhardt, 1966 (rabbit), and Millhouse, 1971 (rat and mouse).

Although these tanycytes are by no means confined to the basal part of the hypothalamus, they appear to be particularly numerous and well developed in that region (fig. 5.13). Millhouse (1971), who used a rapid Golgi method to demonstrate these cells, describes them as consisting of a somatic part lying within the ependymal lining; a neck region deep to this, and a long process which passes through the thickness of the neural wall, ending in swelling either at the pial surface, or in close association with capillaries. The neck region bears processes which contact a vessel. Electron microscopy (Leonhardt, 1966) suggests that the cells might transport some material; and clearly from their situation it would be possible (fig. 5.13) for material to pass from the ventricular cerebrospinal fluid from adjacent neuronal elements in the wall of the ventricle or from subependymal capillaries to the blood passing through the capillaries about which the processes of the tanycytes end: in the median eminence the latter is part of the primary plexus of the portal vessels.

In an earlier study of this infundibular region Löfgren (1961) also put forward the idea that 'glial' elements might act as a transport system between hypothalamus and portal vascular system. This author considered indeed that capillary loops in the median eminence develop by a process of 'vacuolisation and canalisation' in part of this glial system – a possible but unusual mechanism underlying the intimate cell–capillary relationships clearly demonstrated by electron microscopy.

6

THE BASIS FOR NEURAL CONTROL
OF THE PARS DISTALIS

I. THE PROBLEM OF INNERVATION

The relationship of the pituitary gland to the nervous system must necessarily differ according to the origin of its major subdivisions. The neurohypophysis, formed as an outgrowth of the neural tube, is made up largely of nervous tissue. The adenohypophysis, however, being an epithelial derivative, must acquire any innervation by a secondary ingrowth of neuronal elements. Although it is now generally accepted that a direct innervation does not play any major part in the control of the secretory activity of the mammalian pars distalis, the gradual and sometimes reluctant acceptance of this view is of considerable historical interest.

Relatively little has changed in our understanding of all aspects of the innervation of the mammalian pars distalis since the topic was reviewed by Holmes and Zuckerman in 1962. The decline of the idea of a direct nervous control of the pars distalis was largely due to two factors – the demonstration that many of the techniques used to reveal nerve fibres (notably metallic impregnation methods) also demonstrate collagenous fibres, which are often not clearly distinguishable from nerves; and the emergence of the hypothalamo-hypophysial portal system as the major link between the central nervous system and the pars distalis. But even while fully accepting the predominant importance of this vascular system, it might be unwise, when dealing with so complex a structure as the pituitary, to discount entirely any possible role of a direct innervation, however scanty; nerves certainly are of considerable importance for the functioning of the mammalian pars intermedia, and some kind of vaso-motor control could possibly modify the activity of the rest of the adenohypophysis. Hence, although a detailed review would be out of place, a brief consideration of the development of ideas may serve to put our present views in their proper perspective.

Possible sources of nerves

The general anatomy of the pituitary region indicates the possible sources of innervating fibres, as well as routes over which they might reach the

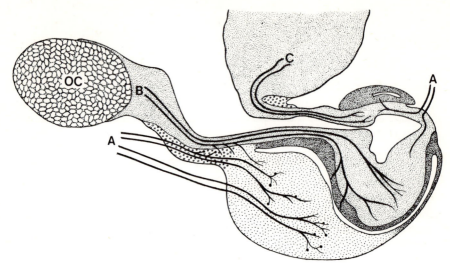

Fig. 6.1. Possible routes from nerve fibres to the pituitary gland. (A) by direct branches from nerves or blood vessels, or via the pars tuberalis; (B) and (C) via the stalk. OC, optic chiasma. From Hair (1938).

gland. The obvious sources are the central nervous system, particularly the hypothalamus; adjacent cranial nerves; and the perivascular plexuses on the vessels lying adjacent to, or passing to supply the gland. Nerve fibres from these sources might reach the pars distalis by several routes; directly from the hypothalamus, infundibular stem or infundibular process; along vessels entering the gland; or as direct branches from adjacent nerves or perivascular plexuses. Fibres passing from the neurohypophysis would be likely to travel through some other part of the gland, the pars tuberalis or the pars intermedia, according to the point at which they left the neurohypophysis (see fig. 6.1).

The earliest reports described filaments, presumed to be of a nervous nature, which passed to the gland from neighbouring structures, notably the internal carotid arteries. Bock (1817) seems to have been the first to describe such a feature, and traced a fine bundle of fibres which left the carotid artery as it passed through the cavernous sinus and ran with a branch of the vessel to enter the hypophysis. Others, such as Hirzel (1824), published similar findings, but it cannot be assumed that such filaments as were found were in fact neural, since no differentiation between nervous and connective tissue fibres was attempted until later. In 1860 Luschka made such an attempt, treating fibres with acetic acid and examining them by microscopy, and described, in the human, nerve fibres passing to the anterior pituitary from the carotid plexus.

None of the earlier investigators considered what happened to the nerve fibres once they had reached the gland. Berkley, however, in 1894, published a description of bundles of small nerve fibres following the course of arteries which gave off branches to the glandular elements of the pituitary. He described these as passing through the glandular substance and noted 'ball-shaped endings' within this. In common with many others, Berkley used silver techniques to demonstrate the intraglandular fibres. Later, methylene blue, a dye with a high specificity for staining nerve fibres, was used by Dandy, who described (1913) in cats and dogs nerves passing from the carotid plexus to the anterior lobe of the pituitary via arterial branches. He did not observe any intraglandular distribution, and indeed staining of nerve fibres within dense parenchymal tissue is often not reliable with this method.

Over the years the glands of many different species have been studied, silver techniques being the most favoured. Only a few publications will be mentioned, to give some idea of the often conflicting findings reported. Thus, a moderately rich or abundant innervation of the pars distalis was described by Tello (1912) in man, Pines (1926) in the dog, Hair (1938) in the cat, Drager (1947) in the armadillo, while Croll (1928) observed a patchy innervation in the rabbit, which she thought might be due to a faulty impregnation. More recently, Metuzals (1956) described an exceedingly rich innervation in the duck. Other papers described a somewhat sparse innervation (Gemelli, 1906, dog, horse and ox; Brooks and Gersh, 1941, rat and rabbit; Truscott, 1944, rat; Ribas-Mujal, 1958, ox; Kása, 1963, rodents).

Authors have described nerve endings of various forms, such as endbulbs; some observed pericellular baskets or networks; while others considered the glandular tissue to be permeated by a plexus of nervous filaments. Metuzals, in particular, described both a compact nervous end plexus with which each glandular cell came into contact, and an extensive sympathetic ground plexus, such as that which Boeke (1940) believed to represent the terminal part of the sympathetic nervous system. Hagen (1954) postulated a rich afferent innervation in man, macaque monkey and dog. The nerve fibres were ascribed to various sources and some of the authors attempted to determine their origin experimentally; thus Brooks and Gersh (1940) removed the superior cervical ganglia, but noted no apparent change in the richness of innervation. The other obvious experimental procedure, that of dividing the pituitary stalk, was also tried, but gave no very conclusive results.

Although many authors believed that the pars distalis had a more or less rich innervation, others disagreed. Inconsistency of observations was common, and Drager (1945), who observed nerve fibres in the armadillo, failed to find a comparable innervation in the chicken. The numerous positive reports were strongly criticised by Green, who in 1951 reported that the pars distalis of the cat, armadillo and rat was devoid of nerve fibres, although the techniques he used did reveal some in the other parts of the adenohypophysis – an indication that failure to reveal nerve fibres in the pars distalis was probably not due to faulty impregnation. This paper was followed by one in 1952 in which Green described the arrangement of connective tissue around both blood vessels and groups of cells of the pars distalis, and published photomicrographs showing the appearance of collagenous fibres which had not been fully impregnated by the silver, and certainly could be mistaken for nerve fibres. Green was firmly of the opinion that the pars distalis received no innervation, and that all reports to the contrary were based on the observation of connective tissue elements.

The possibility of such confusion between nervous and non-nervous elements probably did not occur to many of those who described in earlier papers a rich innervation. Latterly, however, anyone examining the possibility that the pars distalis might be directly innervated should have been clearly aware of the danger of confusion between the two types of tissue. Smith (1956) paid particular attention to distinguishing between nerve fibres and reticulin, and concluded that in the ferret some, although relatively few, nerve fibres were distributed throughout the pars distalis. Metuzals was also aware of the problem, and made the point that connective tissue was either not impregnated in his specimens or that a comparison of the argyrophilic connective tissue in the pars distalis with nervous structures revealed clear and recognisable differences in morphology.

It must be accepted that there are problems of distinguishing between the two kinds of tissue using the techniques of optical microscopy, and it is difficult for anyone who relies on a published report without being able to examine the material on which it is based to form an adequate opinion. Criticism is made more difficult by the fact that the majority of papers dealing with this problem are illustrated by drawings rather than photomicrographs. With the electron microscope, however, it is relatively simple to distinguish nervous and connective tissue. Hence it is significant that although the ultrastructure of the pars distalis has been extensively studied by electron microscopy, there have been few reports or published photographs showing nerve fibres in that part of the gland. Théret and Tamboise claimed to do so in a paper published in 1963. Rats were treated with chlorpromazine to induce hypertrophy of the somatotropic cells and dilatation of 'nerve terminals' which they describe as associated with such cells. The authors described in the pituitaries of such animals non-myelinated nerve fibres lying alongside capillaries, dilated nerve terminals, and 'pseudo-synaptic' contacts between nerve elements and secretory cells, with appearances suggesting the passage of secretion from 'cell to fibre'. Their micrographs, however, are not sufficiently convincing to support their claim without further evidence. A more recent study by

Unsicker (1971) gave negative results. He examined, with the electron microscope, a total of 2000 grid squares of pars distalis of mouse, rat, hamster, cat and pig, but failed to find a single axon profile; nerves were, however, observed in pars tuberalis.

In summary, it seems that there is clear evidence that nerves are associated with the vessels lying in relation to the pituitary gland; and despite the fact that usually there is no *direct* arterial blood supply to the pars distalis (see p. 105) a functional innervation of such vessels could perhaps exert some influence over the activity of the gland (see p. 113). As regards the pars distalis itself, it does not seem that there is sufficient evidence to assume that it has any considerable innervation, although nerve fibres may lie within it, having entered with vessels or passed in from some part of the neurohypophysis. But while there seem to be no grounds at present for assuming that such nerves play a part in the economy of this part of the mammalian pituitary gland, it may be premature, particularly in view of the situation in some non-mammalian vertebrates (see p. 113), to dismiss entirely the possibility that nerves might be able to exert some influence on secretory activity.

II. THE PORTAL SYSTEM:
THE NEUROVASCULAR LINK

The important – indeed dominant – role played by the vascular system in the control of adenohypophysial activity has already been referred to in chapter 1. A hypophysial portal system of vessels is found in mammals, birds, reptiles, amphibians and at any rate some fishes. We now appreciate that this system serves a dual purpose, namely to supply the metabolic requirements of the greater part of the adenohypophysis, and to transport releasing factors from neurons of the hypothalamus to the secretory cells of the pars distalis, whose activity they control. The realisation that the portal blood supply embodies these two functions came only as a result of numerous experimental studies, extending in effect over some thirty years from the first description of the portal system in the early 1930s and the later demonstration that the flow in these vessels was from hypothalamus to pituitary. The importance of the pituitary portal vascular system in the life of the higher vertebrates is so great that the development of our understanding of its significance warrants a brief outline.

The actual portal vessels had been described before 1930, but the earlier observations were mostly concerned with the source of the blood to the region (see Morato, 1939). It was generally appreciated that there was a difference in the blood supply to the anterior and posterior lobes, and a few papers suggested, at least to anyone reading them in the context of our present knowledge, that the main blood supply to the anterior pituitary followed a descending pathway. Thaon (1907) considered that the blood supply to the anterior lobe came mainly from above and Paulesco (1907) also noted that most of the vessels supplying the gland penetrated at the level of the stalk; but the fact that the venules lying along the stalk were portal in nature, namely that they connected two capillary nets, hypothalamic and hypophysial, was not appreciated until Popa and Fielding (1930) and Pietsch (1930) published their work. Even then, since no observations had been made on the living animals, it was concluded that blood passed upwards from the pituitary to the 'secondary distributing net' in the hypothalamus.

Clearly dynamic studies of this vascular system were not possible in the human, and even in animals the exposure of the pituitary to enable observation during life is not always easy. In 1935, however, Houssay, Biasotti and Sammartino observed the infundibular region of the living toad, and found that the flow of blood was from the hypothalamus to the pituitary. They noted also that a lesion of the 'lobus infundibularis' – presumably in the region of the median eminence – was followed by necrosis in the central region of the 'principle' lobe of the pituitary, and thus provided confirmatory evidence for the direction of the flow of blood. Wislocki and King (1936) studied the hypophysial vascular system in the rabbit, cat and monkey and concluded on histological grounds that blood flowed down the portal vessels to reach the anterior pituitary, having first passed through a rich capillary plexus situated between the pars tuberalis and the stalk or through vessels which penetrated the stalk. A point which these authors made, and one which Wislocki was to emphasise again in later papers, is a lack of any appreciable anastomosis between the vascular systems of the pituitary and of the hypothalamus beyond the limits of the tuber cinereum. Anastomoses with the neurohypophysis were also considered to be so slight as to be functionally negligible, although, as will be seen later, this point of view is not tenable.

In 1937 Popa still maintained that the flow of blood was from pituitary to hypothalamus. One of his pieces of evidence was an experiment in which the pituitary stalk of a live rabbit was constricted for two minutes, the region then flooded with formalin and later examined microscopically. The portal vessels were distended below the site of compression, a finding which could indicate an upward flow. In the light of later evidence, however, it seems likely that Popa had failed to take account of blood entering the portal vessels from the inferior hypophysial arteries, passing via anastomotic channels from the neuro- to the adenohypophysis and filling the lower part of the portal vessels by retrograde flow.

Morato (1939), after a critical review of earlier studies, went on to describe the results of injecting fat intravascularly in cats to produce emboli. Both living and dead animals were used, and he injected either a single dyed fat, or two fats, each dyed a different colour, successively. This procedure resulted in numerous emboli in the neurohypophysis, including the walls of the infundibulum, but very few in the pars distalis, a finding which seemed to indicate that most of the blood reaching the pars distalis had already passed through a capillary bed, namely that in the infundibulum, which had prevented the further progress of the emboli. The author came out strongly in favour of a downward portal flow, although he admitted the existence of anastomoses between the different vascular territories of the pituitary complex.

Further indirect evidence was presented by Green (1948), who showed that the superior capillary bed (the one often designated as the primary plexus) is fed by arterioles and drained by venules, suggesting a downward (arterio-venous) flow. Other suggestive evidence came from the examination of injected specimens. In the following year Green and Harris (1949) published the results of studies on the hypophysio-portal vessels of living rats, in which they had been able to observe directly the blood flowing from the median eminence to the pars distalis. It was thereby shown conclusively that the mammals resembled anuran amphibians in this respect.

THE ANATOMY OF THE HYPOPHYSIAL VASCULAR SYSTEM

The hypothalamo-hypophysial vascular system has reached its greatest complexity in the higher mammals, notably in man and the primates, but many features are common to a wide variety of species. The morphology inevitably varies considerably with that of the pituitary gland, notably with its orientation, degree of differentiation and the closeness of the association between its neural and epithelial components. A few general principles, applicable particularly to the system in mammals, are set out below.

1. The arterial supply is derived from the internal carotid arteries, which give off superior and inferior hypophysial branches. Branches of the superior hypophysial arteries enter the upper region of the neurohypophysis, the median eminence and infundibular stem (fig. 6.2); while the inferior hypophysial arteries supply the lower part of the neurohypophysis, namely the infundibular process itself.

2. The vessels entering the infundibulum supply a variety of specialised formations. These may take the form either of simple capillary loops which penetrate the neural tissue for a greater or lesser distance and return to the surface to empty into the portal venules, or of larger and more complex vascular formations which penetrate deeper into the tissue (figs. 6.5 to 6.8). The latter have been given different names by various authors, such as vascular spikes, tufted vessels, 'gomitoli' and 'Spezial-gefässe'. The largest and most complex of these have so far been found in man and monkeys, in which they consist of a central arteriole feeding a number of

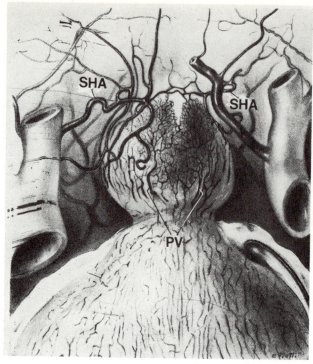

Fig. 6.2. Drawing of the vessels reaching the tuber cinereum of the monkey. SHA, superior hypophysial arteries; PV, portal venules. From Wislocki (1938*b*).

capillaries, which in turn empty into a venule which runs towards the surface and leads into the portal vessels. The capillaries may form a 'sheath' enclosing the main central vessels (fig. 6.3).

3. The adenohypophysis commonly receives the whole of its blood via the portal vessels, and thus is supplied largely by the superior hypophysial arteries. The distal neurohypophysis is supplied largely by inferior hypophysial arteries.

4. In most (but not all) mammalian species so far studied the pars distalis receives no significant direct arterial blood supply, but is entirely dependent on portal blood.

5. According to some authors, there is no significant anastomosis between various vascular territories in the complex, that is between the median eminence and the hypothalamus proper, or between the infundibular process and the adenohypophysis (see, however, p. 112).

6. The venous drainage from the pituitary passes into the neighbouring intracranial venous sinuses and thus enters the general systemic circulation.

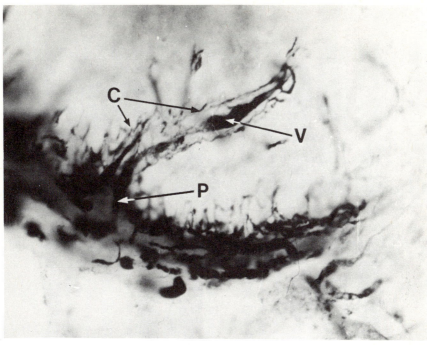

Fig. 6.3. Thick section through the median eminence of a monkey with blood vessels injected with Indian ink. Many of the capillary formations penetrating the nervous tissue are out of focus; one large complex, however, shows partially filled capillaries (C) surrounding a central venule (V) which runs directly into a portal venule (P).

THE PITUITARY VASCULAR SYSTEM IN MAMMALS

Primates

The arrangement of the blood vessels associated with the human pituitary is of particular interest in relation both to surgery of the region and to certain pathological conditions of the gland which particularly involve its vessels.

The disposition of the vessels supplying the human pituitary gland (see Xuereb, Prichard and Daniel, 1954a, b) in general conforms with the plan outlined above (fig. 6.4). Thus, the superior hypophysial arteries give rise to smaller vessels, which form a vascular collar around the upper stalk within the subarachnoid space; from here short stalk arteries penetrate the upper stalk and median eminence. Before the superior hypophysial vessels divide, however, each gives off a 'loral' artery which descends to the superior surface of the anterior pituitary; these penetrate the substance of the lobe and then pass towards the intraglandular stalk, lying in fibrous tissue of the 'loral septum'. On reaching the stalk each artery

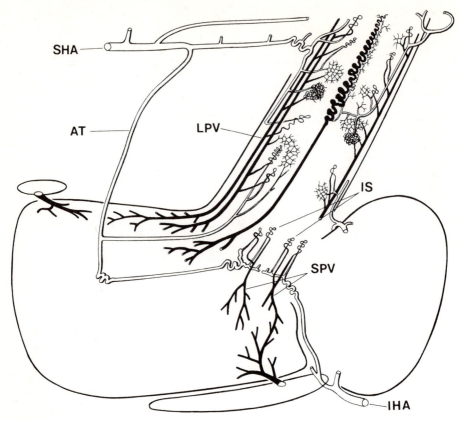

Fig. 6.4. Diagram of the vascular system of the human anterior pituitary. The superior hypophysial arteries (SHA) supply capillary spikes in the upper stalk which are drained via long portal veins (LPV) to the pars distalis. A branch of the superior hypophysial artery, the artery of the trabecula (AT, loral artery), enters the gland and supplies blood to spikes in the lower stalk. Some spikes (IS) in the intraglandular stalk receive blood from the inferior hypophysial arteries (IHA) and drain via short portal veins (SPV) to the posterior part of the pars distalis. From Xuereb, Prichard and Daniel (1954*a*).

divides into several branches, which pass upwards in a septum of fibrous tissue which lies between the stalk and the adenohypophysis. These vessels, which usually receive anastomoses from the superior hypophysial system, are called long stalk arteries. Both long and short stalk arteries supply blood to the special vascular formations lying within the neural tissue of the median eminence and stalk.

The inferior hypophysial arteries arise on each side from the internal carotid artery in the cavernous sinus and give off branches which directly penetrate and supply the infundibular process, as well as small capsular branches. They also give off large interlobar arteries which pass between the neural and adenohypophysial parts of the gland; these anastomose with each other and give rise to several small vessels which Stanfield (1960) called 'genual arteries'. A branch from each interlobar artery or from the genual arteries ('communicating artery', Stanfield) passes into the fibrous core which runs through the pars distalis and here anastomoses with either the loral artery or with a branch of that vessel supplying the fibrous core. Other anastomoses between the superior and inferior hypophysial systems occur between branches of the genual arteries (the parallel vessels) and the long stalk vessels.

Published accounts differ somewhat in the importance attributed to anastomoses between superior and inferior vessels; no doubt this difference of opinion is in part due to the fact that the size of the anastomoses varies in different specimens. Clearly the size of any anastomosis, however, could be of considerable importance in the event of interruption of one or other set of vessels.

The bulk of the blood passing into the arterial vessels of the stalk is destined for the capillary complexes which constitute the 'primary plexus' of the portal system, which in the human pituitary is not confined to the median eminence but extends into virtually the whole of the infundibular stem, both extraglandular and intraglandular parts (fig. 6.4). Large 'gomitoli' or vascular spikes occur, particularly in the upper part of the neurohypophysis, and simpler capillary formations in other parts. The final pathway draining the blood to the pars distalis can be described as having two components, 'long' portal veins draining the median eminence–upper stem region, and 'short' portal veins draining the lower, intraglandular stem.

McConnell (1953) made the point that there is no anatomical reason why either an ascending or descending flow of blood should not occur in the stalk, although he noted that the only vascular communications between the stalk and hypothalamus are of capillary size. Some earlier authors (for example Spanner, 1952) considered that blood from the proximal parts of the 'spike' portal veins could pass into the basilar veins as well as in the opposite direction.

A point of some importance on which the descriptions of the human pituitary vascular system disagree is whether or not there is any direct arterial supply to the parenchymal tissue. McConnell considered that there is such a contribution from the artery of the fibrous core, and from the capsular vessels; Xuereb *et al.* (1954*a*, *b*), however, denied that there is a direct arterial supply. Stanfield (1960) maintained that there is a direct supply from three main sources – the artery of the fibrous core, which arises on each side from the loral artery within the anterior lobe; from interlobar branches of the inferior hypophysial artery, via the communicating artery already described which runs forwards into the upper half of the anterior lobe and anastomoses with the loral system; and a

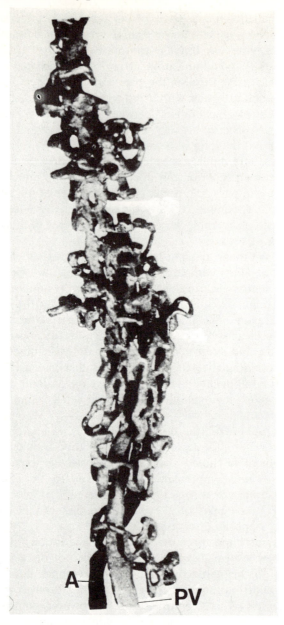

Fig. 6.5. Reconstruction of a spike ('gomitolo'). A, arteriole; PV, portal venule. From Fumagalli (1942).

small contribution from branches of the inferior capsular artery. Here again, of course, variation in the size of any such direct arterial contributions can be expected in different specimens. It must follow, however, that if the direct contribution is of any significant size, then arrest of the portal circulation alone, even if the supply passing via the short portal veins were included, would not produce a total necrosis of the pars distalis, although changes resulting from the lack of hypothalamic releasing factors might well result in cellular atrophy.

The complexity of the vascular spikes can be seen from the photographs of latex casts of the vessels (fig. 6.6). In 1942 Fumagalli published a detailed description of these 'gomitoli'. He described the larger ones disposed around the infundibular recess of the third ventricle, as being formed of a mass of sinusoidal capillaries fed by a terminal arterial branch and running into a 'rete mirabile' which in turn communicates with a portal venule, and observed that peripheral gomitoli were more numerous and smaller. Wax reconstructions or casts of these vascular formations give an excellent idea of their structure (figs. 6.5, 6.6). McConnell (1953) described three different types of capillary formation in different parts of the stalk and suggested that there might be corresponding differences in their function.

The vascularisation of the hypophysial region has been studied in few species of primates apart from man. In the monkey (*Macacus rhesus*) vascular tufts of varying complexity are located in the upper part of the neurohypophysis (Wislocki and King, 1936; Wislocki, 1938*b*; Engelhardt, 1956; Holmes, 1967). The larger formations are fed by arterial afferents and drained by venules as in man. Wislocki also suggested that the 'sinusoids' of the anterior pituitary are fed not only by portal venules but by arterioles, derived from the superior hypophysial arteries. In view of the findings that in most species there is no direct arterial supply to the epithelial tissue of the pars distalis, the possibility that such arterioles in fact supply capillary complexes in the lower stalk, so that their blood reaches the glandular tissue only via the portal venules, should be considered.

Five different types of vascular formation occur in the upper neurohypophysis of the rhesus monkey, of varying complexity correlated with their position. The largest and most complex seem comparable to those found in man, and consist of a spike or loop of many capillaries supplied by an arteriole and draining into a vein, which lies at the centre of the complex and runs to the portal vessels. Other vascular formations are less complex in structure. Loops made up of a number of capillaries, or shorter single-channelled ones, penetrate into the neural tissue from the interface between pars tuberalis and the median eminence, and in the caudal zone of the eminence long, straight and generally single capillary loops penetrate the nervous tissue.

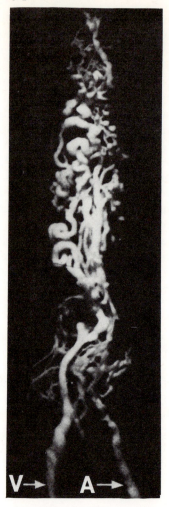

Fig. 6.6. Latex injection of a vascular spike in the human. A, artery; V, portal vein. Reproduced from Daniel, *Br. med. Bull.* **22**, 202–208 (1966).

Non-primates

The vascular architecture of the median eminence has been studied in a number of subprimate mammals, particularly in readily available laboratory or domestic animals. Enemar (1961) listed according to species numerous descriptions published up to that date. As the detailed anatomy of the region varies considerably from one species to another, so inevitably does the vascular pattern. Nevertheless, the same general plan seems to apply widely, namely the penetration of the nervous tissue of the median eminence by vascular loops arising from vessels at the interface between adeno- and neurohypophysis.

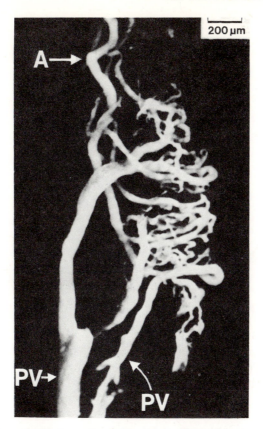

Fig. 6.7. Complex vascular formation in the sheep. PV, portal vein; A, artery. From Daniel and Prichard (1957).

Although comparable vascular formations occur in other mammals, such as the sheep (fig. 6.7), the penetrating vessels do not always form such complex arrangements as in the primates. The median eminence, particularly in smaller mammals, is often relatively thin so that there is simply not enough neural tissue available to contain complex formations. In such species the pattern is essentially one of loops of capillaries, which often penetrate through the greater part of the median eminence, rather than of complexes fed by a specific arteriole and drained by a venule. Not all the penetrating vessels are single loops, however, and even in small mammals there may be also tufts of capillaries (fig. 6.8).

The primary plexus
Descriptions of hypophysial vasculature commonly make use of the term 'primary plexus'; Harris, in his monograph on the pituitary (1955),

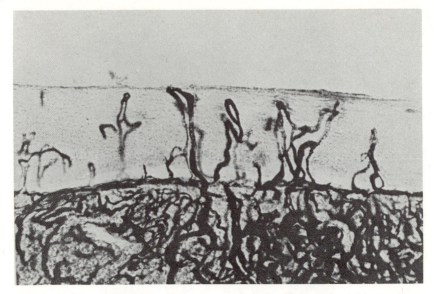

Fig. 6.8. Typical pattern of capillary loops in the infundibular floor in the rat. From Landsmeer (1963).

defined this as a collective name for the loops or tufts of capillaries which penetrate the median eminence, and which arise from 'a rich vascular plexus, situated in the pars tuberalis of the pituitary gland' (p. 25). Unless the various loops and tufts are interconnected both basally and at their apices, it would seem inappropriate to designate the whole complex as a plexus – and although some apical interconnections between the formations in the median eminence as well as connections with the capillaries of the surrounding nervous tissue do occur, these are by no means sufficiently abundant to merit such a term. Nevertheless, examination of injected specimens in section usually gives the impression that the dense layer of vessels lying in the junctional zone between the pars tuberalis and the median eminence may indeed be plexiform. But if this is so, and the penetrating loops and tufts arise from a vascular network, then it seems unlikely that the haemodynamic characteristics of the complex would be appropriate for what we now know is the purpose of the arrangement, namely the close association of capillary loops and nerve terminals in the median eminence and transfer of the various hypothalamic releasing factors. The situation would be even more difficult to appreciate if the portal venules themselves took origin from this same plexus, as they sometimes appear to do. Furthermore, as Landsmeer (1963) noted, if the capillary loops themselves form part of the plexus, originating from it and draining to it, then the two sides of the loop should be functionally identical. If, on the other hand, the loops have

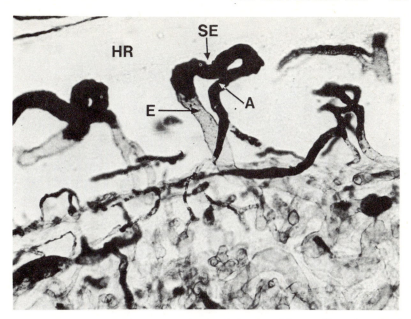

Fig. 6.9. Sagittal section of the hypophysis of the dog. The capillary loop in the centre penetrating the neural tissue below the hypophysial recess (HR) shows a narrow afferent branch (A), a thicker efferent one (E) and an apical region (SE) lying just deep to the ependyma. Reproduced by permission from Duvernoy (1972).

arterial and venous segments some morphological difference should be detectable. Even if the 'arterial' end arose from a plexus of vessels, the 'venous' end should conduct blood to the adenohypophysis, via the portal vessels.

It is often not possible to be certain of the precise mode of termination of many of the loops. Landsmeer (1963) considered that in the rat the capillary loops form a system of interconnected capillaries, and noted that 'only rarely' does a loop lead directly into a portal 'sinus'. This author did, however, publish figures of loops in the infundibular floor in the cat, in which thin (ascending) and thick (descending) limbs can be clearly distinguished and some of the latter can be seen to continue into vessels lying within the pars distalis (fig. 6.8). The appearance is indeed very similar to that found in the monkey (Holmes, 1967). Daniel and Prichard (1957a) also showed in the sheep a cast of an afferent artery supplying capillary loops which drain directly in a portal vein (fig. 6.7). In other mammals, also, clearly arterial and venous limbs of loops have been observed (fig. 6.9).

A feature described in several species (see for example Duvernoy, 1972) is the penetration of capillary loops so far into the nervous tissue that they become closely associated with the ependymal lining of the infundibular

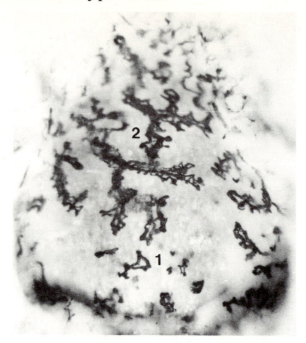

Fig. 6.10. View of the infundibular recess in a rabbit from the ependymal aspect, to show the subependymal network of capillaries (2). 1, tops of capillary loops. Reproduced by permission from Duvernoy (1972).

recess (fig. 6.10). This clearly raises the possibility of passage of substances from the cerebrospinal fluid to the portal blood.

CONTRIBUTIONS OF BLOOD FROM THE INFUNDIBULAR STEM AND PROCESS

It has already been seen that, in primates, an appreciable part of the blood passing to the pars distalis reaches it from inferior hypophysial vessels via capillaries in the lower infundibular stem and the short portal vessels. Veins of the latter type originating in the lower stem are also found in the non-primate mammals, for example the rat, where portal veins emerge from the rostral pole of the infundibular process and from the adjacent part of the infundibular stem, as well as from the more lateral regions of the capillary network which surround the stalk. A further possible source of blood for the adenohypophysis is the infundibular process itself. Where a well-developed cleft remains between the pars intermedia and pars distalis, as in the cat, direct vessels are not likely to run across it; but there remains the possibility of vessels tracking through the peripheral zones of continuity between the pars distalis and pars intermedia. If there is such cleft, however, the contiguity of the various parts of the gland might serve as a bed for anastomotic vessels. In the rat Daniel and Prichard (1956) noted that in addition to portal vessels draining capillary beds in the stem, the neural lobe (infundibular process) drains partly to the pars distalis, and partly into systemic veins. The latter drainage is from the deeper part of the lobe, the more superficial capillaries draining via portal vessels, which are found only on the dorsal and caudal aspects of the gland and do not pass through the pars intermedia or traverse the intraglandular cleft. Similar anastomoses occur between the vascular beds of the anterior and posterior lobes via the pars intermedia in the guinea-pig, rabbit, rat and cat (Duvernoy, 1958) as well as in the rhesus monkey (Holmes and Zuckerman, 1959). Connections such as these do not necessarily constitute portal vessels, although if the blood flows from neural to glandular divisions of the gland, then they could theoretically serve a similar function.

As already discussed, there is some uncertainty whether in man there is any direct supply to adenohypophysial tissue of blood that has not first passed through capillaries and portal vessels. In some species there is such a supply, notably the rabbit (Harris, 1947), but in none does it replace the typical portal supply.

In summary, blood may reach the pars distalis of the mammalian pituitary gland after having first passed through either the median eminence, the upper or lower infundibular stem or infundibular process, and (rarely) by direct arterial branches. One or more of these routes may be utilised, according to the species. An extreme example is provided by the Cetacea, in which the adenohypophysis is almost completely separated from the infundibular process by a septum of connective tissue, so that there can be no direct passage of vessels from most of the neurohypophysis to the adenohypophysis. The pars tuberalis, however, extends upwards to make contact with the upper stalk–median eminence, and provides the basis for a vascular link between the median eminence and adenohypophysis via a system of portal vessels (Harris, 1950).

A recurrent question is whether or not there is any significant anastomosis between the vessels of the hypophysial complex and the hypothalamus beyond the median eminence. There is no doubt that capillary anastomoses do occur, both in the macaque and other species (e g. Holmes, 1967), but it is far from clear what possible significance such anastomoses might have in the functioning of the pituitary.

Functional considerations

Worthington (1960) studied the hypophysial vascular system in living mice, and found that although the arterial vessels supplying the primary plexus were highly contractile, the actual portal venules were not so under any circumstances. Worthington's observations of the effects of various drugs and stresses in modifying the flow through the whole system suggested at any rate the possibility that such changes might influence the secretory activity of the gland. Regional variations in the blood supply to the stalk (Worthington, 1963) might also provide a mechanism for such control, in which event a vasomotor innervation of the vessels carrying blood to the pituitary complex should assume a new importance. Some support for such a view came from a report by Fendler and Endroczi (1965) that bilateral cervical sympathectomy resulted in inhibition of compensatory adrenal hypersecretion, which suggested that the blood supply to the pituitary might be under sympathetic control. Goldman (1968), however, failed to detect any change in the pituitary blood flow following cervical sympathectomy, and concluded that following this operation some vasomotor mechanism continues to control the flow of blood to the gland. But in any event we cannot yet dismiss the possible influences of vasomotor nerve fibres on pituitary activity.

The primary role of the portal vessels in the supply of oxygen and essential metabolites to the pars distalis is clearly shown by the effects of interrupting the vessels, either by division of the pituitary stalk or by direct cautery of the vessels. Since these vessels appear to have the ability to regenerate rapidly, however, it is necessary, if the long-term effects of such lesions are to be studied, to ensure that such regeneration does not occur. This can be done by the insertion of a thin lamina of some impermeable material (waxed paper, polythene or foil) between the divided ends of the stalk at operation. Such lesions have been made in a number of different mammalian species (rat: Daniel and Prichard, 1956; sheep: Daniel and Prichard, 1957*b*; goat: Daniel and Prichard, 1958: rhesus monkey: Holmes, Hughes and Zuckerman, 1959; ferret: Holmes, 1961*a*). Furthermore, observations have been made on human pituitary glands in which the stalk had been divided, either surgically for therapeutic reasons (Adams, Daniel, Prichard and Schurr, 1963; Daniel, Prichard and Schurr, 1958) or following head injury (Russell, 1956).

It is clear that, provided the vascular patterns of the pituitary conform to the long and short portal vein patterns, division of the extraglandular stalk would be expected to deprive a considerable part of the pars distalis of its blood supply. Furthermore, the region so deprived would lie anteriorly within the gland (see fig. 6.11) and its size would be greater the lower the site of transection. Sparing of the short portal venule system would allow a continued supply of blood from the inferior hypophysial arteries to that zone of the pars distalis lying close to the lower stem and infundibular process.

The various published data accord well with these expectations (see Adams, Daniel and Prichard, 1966). Interruption of the long portal vessels is followed by a large infarct (area of necrosis) in the pars distalis,

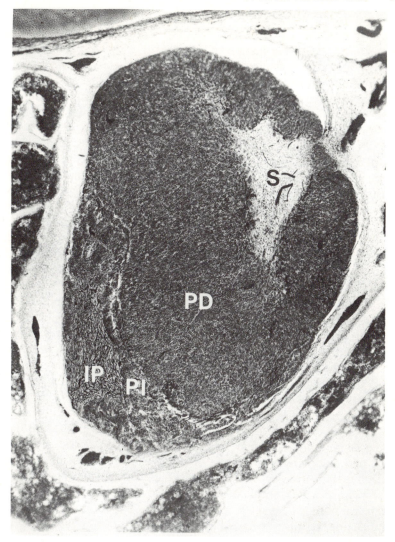

Fig. 6.11. Sagittal section through the pituitary gland of a rhesus monkey in which the pituitary stalk had been divided some months previously. The infundibular process (IP) has atrophied and a large scar of fibrous tissue (S) is present in the upper anterior part of the pars distalis (PD). PI, pars intermedia. From Holmes and Zuckerman (1959).

involving the greater part of the glandular tissue. A zone of the pars distalis which derives its supply from short portal vessels (lying dorsally and caudally) is spared, together with a rather thin rim of tissue along the ventral and lateral borders, which presumably can derive some blood by venous reflux or from arterial vessels supplying the surrounding connective tissue. Incomplete interruption of the long portal vessels, either by partial transection of the stalk, selective cautery or pressure from a malpositioned barrier (Daniel and Prichard, 1956, 1957) results in a smaller zone of necrosis limited to the side of the stalk lesion.

Following the acute necrotic phase the dead tissue becomes organised into a fibrous scar (fig. 6.11) which over weeks and months contracts, so that ultimately it is much smaller than the initial lesion (Adams, Daniel and Prichard, 1963). The surviving glandular tissue also contracts, the individual cells becoming smaller, and losing at any rate some of their typical chromophil characteristics, a finding reminiscent of pituitary glands transplanted to a site remote from the median eminence. This is not surprising, since even if the supply of blood to the surviving paren- chymal zone is sufficient to keep these cells alive, a transection of the stalk which interrupts the blood vessels must also interrupt the nerve fibres passing down the stalk to end about the capillaries of the primary capillary bed of the short portal venules. Hence the blood passing through these vessels, although entirely adequate to supply the basic metabolic needs of pituitary cells, will lack the hypothalamic releasing factors (see pp. 126ff) which normally control the activity of the adenohypophysial cells.

An important lesion of the human anterior pituitary involves its vascular supply (Sheehan, 1954). This is post-partum necrosis. In its extreme form, often associated with severe blood loss or shock at the time of delivery, the patient develops gross hypopituitarism, and may pass into coma. The glands of patients dying from this condition in the early post-partum period show extensive necrosis of the pars distalis, the necrotic zone being replaced by fibrous scar tissue progressively with increasing time of survival. Lesser degrees of scarring may be associated with less marked hypopituitarism, and small scars have been found in patients dying, perhaps many years later, of other causes. The primary lesion underlying such necrosis was at first thought to be thrombosis of the portal vessels. Later Sheehan and Stanfield (1961) suggested that the primary cause may be a spasm of the arteries supplying the gland, which, if long lasting, results in necrosis and secondary thrombosis in the portal system.

III. THE HYPOTHALAMUS

It is now generally accepted that control of the secretory activity of the adenohypophysis is largely, if not entirely, vested in the hypothalamus, and that the essential link between the nervous and endocrine system in this respect is the portal vascular system. The gradual realisation of the importance of the latter for full secretory activity of the pars distalis, and the equally slow acceptance of the relative unimportance of a direct innervation of the glandular cells, eventually led to the present concept of control by blood-borne hypothalamic factors (see review by Harris, 1972).

The study of the role of the portal blood as a carrier of factors controlling pituitary activity was made difficult by the dependence of the pars distalis on portal blood for its basic metabolic requirements. As already discussed, interruption of this supply, as by dividing the pituitary stalk, is followed by necrosis of secretory tissue of the pars distalis. Gradually, however, it became clear that the portal blood also serves another function, and the late G. W. Harris proposed that in this vascular system lay the key to the control of the anterior pituitary. It followed that, if this system was indeed the link via which neural control of the gland was mediated, then it was also the link which indirectly brought the activity of the adrenal cortex, thyroid and gonads under the control of the central nervous system.

A number of reports published before 1950 had indicated that a pituitary gland transplanted to a site remote from its normal one commonly showed little evidence of functional activity, even though the transplant acquired an apparently adequate blood supply (see for example Westman and Jacobsohn, 1940). It must be admitted, however, that authors were not always in agreement with this observation, although in some instances where active hormone secretion from a transplanted gland was described, the completeness of the removal of glandular tissue from the sella turcica had not always been verified (see Harris, 1955).

Harris and Jacobsohn in 1952 published the results of experiments which strongly indicated that a close association with the hypothalamus was important for pituitary function. Using rats, they removed the pituitary gland from its normal position in the sella turcica, and implanted it either under the temporal lobe of the brain, within the pituitary capsule, or under the median eminence. In each site the transplant acquired a new blood supply from neighbouring vessels. Only those glands placed under the median eminence, however, which regained a blood supply from the site of the primary plexus of the portal vessels, showed anything more than a minimum of function. Female rats with glands replaced in this site underwent normal oestrous cycles, became pregnant after mating and carried young to term. Lactation occurred, although normal suckling was not possible owing to lack of oxytocin.

Five years later Nikitovitch-Winer and Everett (1957, 1958) published the results of a series of experiments which provided evidence strongly in favour of the probability that some hypothalamic neurohumoral mechanism controlled pituitary activity. The authors had made use of the structural and functional regression of pituitary tissue transplanted away from its usual site in a two-phase experiment. The glands of female rats were transplanted to the capsule of the kidney, a site which enabled them to become well vascularised. Nevertheless, as expected, oestrous cycles ceased and ovarian follicles were not maintained. The grafts were re-transplanted after 3–4 weeks, in one group of animals to a site beneath

5

the median eminence, in another group to the under-surface of the temporal lobe; in a third group they were left on the kidney. Only in those animals in which the grafts were replaced beneath the median eminence did gonadotropic activity return, in the form of oestrous cycles and, in some animals, pregnancy after mating.

A survey of the whole range of experiments involving assessment of the activity of the pituitary gland separated from its usual blood supply, whether this be by transplantation or by division of the stalk, certainly shows no unanimity in the results reported (for references see Thomson and Zuckerman, 1954; Harris, 1955). In a number of reports there is a lack of conclusive evidence that all the glandular tissue had been removed from the sella, and it is known that pituitary-dependent endocrine glands can be sustained by a relatively small amount of secretory tissue remaining in its normal situation (Smith, 1932). Experiments involving transection of the pituitary stalk, which was assumed to separate the pituitary effectively from the hypothalamus, also gave varied results in terms of function since it was not realised by earlier investigators that unless an impermeable barrier is placed between the cut ends of the stalk rapid restoration of the portal vascular link often occurs. Hence, experiments such as those described by Dempsey (1939) in which division of the stalk had either no effect on oestrous cycles, or was followed by irregular cycles, or by their cessation, can be ascribed to varying degrees of vascular regeneration.

Nevertheless, some anomalies remain. Notable are the findings of Thomson and Zuckerman (1954), who found that two out of seventeen ferrets in which the stalk had been divided and the cut ends separated by a barrier came into oestrus after operation in response to photoperiodic stimulation. If, as the authors claimed, no vascular connections between the median eminence and the pituitary gland either remained or regenerated, then clearly the portal system as such is not essential for the mediation of nervous control over the adenohypophysis. Donovan and Harris (1954) repeated these experiments using what they considered a better surgical approach to the stalk, and were unable to confirm Thomson and Zuckerman's findings, which remain unexplained.

Other anomalous results not in keeping with the assertion that the hypophysio-portal vascular link is essential for the continued secretion of pituitary tropic hormones have also been reported. Firstly, an exception must be made for the lactotropic hormone, LTH, whose secretion actually increases when the gland is separated from its portal supply (see p. 128), and it is now accepted that the hypothalamus normally exerts an inhibitory influence over its secretion. Other observations are more difficult to explain. For example Martinovitch and his colleagues grafted pituitary glands of infantile rats into the anterior chamber of the eye of hypophysectomised hosts (Martinovitch and Pavić, 1960). Their results were not consistent, but nevertheless an appreciable proportion of their grafted animals showed restoration of pituitary activity as evidenced by testicular weight, reproductive activity and adrenal weight. It must be noted, however, that multiple grafts were used (three or so at a time) and if a response was not obtained, the procedure was repeated, if necessary more than once. The authors considered the age of the donors to be important, better results following grafting of glands from 19 to 22-day-old rats than from adults. Better results also followed grafting immediately after hypophysectomy than if the procedure was delayed; good vascularisation of the graft and health of the host were also of importance. Removal of the grafts in responsive animals was followed by regression of testicular weight.

Other authors have produced evidence of slight tropic hormone secretion in hypophysectomised animals bearing grafts. Goldberg and Knobil (1957), for example, using 21-day fetal pituitaries considered that the grafts secreted STH, TSH, ACTH, and in some instances FSH and LH, all at a low level. Hertz (1959) published evidence for some production of ACTH by pituitary tissue transplanted to the kidney capsule, and Knigge (1961) for some TSH production by anterior chamber grafts. Many other reports for and against some secretion of tropic hormones by pituitary tissue transplanted away from direct portal vascular influence have appeared.

The bulk of pituitary tissue grafted is perhaps an important factor in determining whether secretory activity of grafts is detectable or not. Even if the substances necessary for the secretion of tropic hormones (pp. 126ff) are released directly only into the blood passing through the capillary formations of the median eminence (and stalk) this blood does enter the general circulation, so that such substances may circulate widely, albeit in extremely low concentrations, and hence they may be able to exert some effect on ectopic adenohypophysial tissue. They will normally of course be present in highest concentration in portal blood (see p. 128) and the evidence in favour of the portal vascular link playing an over-riding role in neural control of the adenohypophysis is now overwhelming.

Lesions of the nervous system and pituitary function

Among the techniques used to elucidate the precise relationship between the nervous system and the pituitary gland has been the placing of lesions in various parts of the brain, notably, at any rate in the earlier studies, in the hypothalamus. Aschner in 1912 reported atrophy of the gonads following hypothalamic lesions, and since this early paper, many reports of similar observations have been published. These have described the effect of hypothalamic lesions not only on the weight and histological structure of endocrine glands, but on their function as shown by oestrous cycles and mating behaviour, response to stress and so on. Typical examples of such studies are those reported by Dey and his colleagues (see Dey, 1943), in which lesions were made in the hypothalamus of female guinea-pigs. It was found that large bilateral lesions at the caudal end of the optic chiasma resulted in persistent hypertrophy of the ovaries and reproductive tract, an observation interpreted as indicating lack of secretion of LH; destruction of a large part of the median eminence was associated with loss of cyclical oestrous activity. Hillarp (1949) found that in rats lesions immediately lateral to the wall of the third ventricle below or just caudal to the paraventricular nuclei were associated with ovaries containing large and small follicles but no corpora lutea, and with persistent oestrus. He found that in the zone between the paraventricular nuclei and the stalk very limited lesions could have such effects, provided they were bilaterally symmetrical, and suggested that the lesions damaged a system of fibres passing from the anterior hypothalamic area towards the stalk. In some studies other criteria of alteration in the function of the 'gonadotropic system' of the pituitary have been used. Werff ten Bosch and Donovan (1957), for example, found that lesions in the anterior hypothalamus in infantile rats induced the appearance of puberty (as indicated by opening of the vagina) earlier than usual and early onset of oestrous cycles. The authors considered that this was due to injury to a hypothalamic centre inhibiting the release of FSH in early life.

Many studies of non-gonadal effects of hypothalamic lesions have also been published, such as those of Ganong, Frederickson and Hume (1955), who found that in the dog lesions at the anterior end of the median eminence and extending upwards from there resulted in a depression of thyroid function not necessarily linked to effects on other tropic hormones. The extensive studies of the effect of lesions of the central nervous system are reviewed in the monograph of Szentágothai *et al.* (1968).

Assessment of the full significance of the results of many experiments of this nature is difficult. There is no doubt that lesions of the hypothalamus do affect the secretion of tropic hormones of the pars distalis; and there is good evidence that an element of localisation is present, so that lesions in, for example, the anterior hypothalamus may exert a certain effect not obtained with lesions placed more superiorly or caudally. Problems of interpretation may, however, arise on several grounds, such as:

1. It is difficult to achieve really accurate bilateral placement of lesions, particularly small ones; similarly, it is difficult, if not practically impossible, to reproduce *precisely* the location of lesions. Authors have attempted to overcome objections to interpretations of results arising from such technical problems by plotting the extent of a number of lesions

found to be associated with a given effect, delimiting an area common to all such lesions and ascribing the effects to destruction of this circumscribed area. Similarly, see the figure from Halász and Pupp, fig. 6.12.

2. Even with circumscribed lesions, it is difficult to be certain just what is being destroyed. The microscopic structure of the hypothalamus of the commoner species of animal used in experimental studies is well known as far as nuclear (neuronal) pattern is concerned, but far less so in respect of the dendritic and axonal pattern of the neuropil. Furthermore, it is difficult to assess with any degree of precision the true extent of lesions. This problem is likely to be greater when small animals, such as rats, are used, in which within a single millimetre a variety of neurons and processes are likely to be included.

3. Many authors have not assessed the effects of lesions on more than one or two parameters. This is certainly understandable, for the labour involved in making anything like full assessments can be enormous. Nevertheless, attention confined to the effect of a lesion on gonadotropic activity might overlook effects on other endocrine systems.

4. Lesions in the region of the median eminence and origin of the pituitary stalk may exert an effect in three ways: by destroying 'centres of activity'; by damaging pathways from other parts of the hypothalamus to the region of the primary plexus of the portal vessels; or by direct damage to the portal system.

Bearing in mind these points, it must be said that lesioning experiments have, within their limitations, added considerably to our knowledge of the relationship between the hypothalamus and pituitary, and have formed a basis for other kinds of approach such as the placing of hormonal implants into the hypothalamus, and electrical stimulation. A few examples of such studies must suffice.

It was shown by Fee and Parkes (1929) that ovulation in the rabbit (an induced ovulator, in which ovulation occurs about ten hours after copulation) was prevented by hypophysectomy within an hour of mating, but not if the removal of the gland was delayed for longer than this. Harris in 1937 showed that ovulation could be achieved by electrical stimulation (in anaesthetised rabbits) of the tuber cinereum, posterior hypothalamus or the pituitary gland. Later work indicated that the essential stimulus was one affecting the hypothalamus (tuber cinereum) rather than the pituitary gland itself (Markee, Sawyer and Hollinshead, 1946) and Harris (1948) later found that a brief stimulation of the tuberal region lasting only a few minutes, in the conscious animal, was sufficient to produce ovulation. Stimulation of various parts of the pituitary gland itself, however, even for periods of up to $7\frac{1}{2}$ hours, did not result in ovulation.

Other species have been similarly studied; ovulation was obtained following stimulation (at certain times of the menstrual cycle) by electrodes implanted into the median eminence of monkeys, while stimulation of other parts of the central nervous system did not produce such an effect (Anand, Malkani and Dua, 1957). Using rabbits, Kurachi and Suchowsky (1958) reported the induction of ovulation in a third of their animals in which the ventromedial hypothalamic nucleus was stimulated.

A different approach to the study of the part played by the hypothalamus in the control of pituitary activity makes use of the feedback mechanisms which play a major part in the control of secretion. For example, under the stimulation of GtH during the pre-oestrous period or the first part of the menstrual cycle, the ovaries increasingly secrete oestrogen; by the negative feedback effect this hormone decreases the secretion of FSH, largely or entirely by acting on the hypothalamus. Sawyer (1959) showed that lesions in the region of the posterior median eminence prevented the usual response, in the rabbit, of ovulation following copulation, and in some instances also produced ovarian atrophy. Later Davidson and Sawyer (1961) implanted small amounts (*c.* 0.2 μg) of oestradiol benzoate into various regions of the forebrain and pituitary gland of female rabbits; they found that implants in the region of the posterior median eminence resulted in ovarian atrophy, and that these animals also developed failure to ovulate after copulation, although they did ovulate after mating a week after the implant. Failure of induced ovulation might indicate a suppression of the secretion of LH, or of FSH, when the result could be due to the inability of inadequately mature ovarian follicles to respond to the ovulatory surge of LH. A dual effect, the oestrogen suppressing both hormones, might also have occurred. Suppression of ovulation did not occur when oestrogen was implanted elsewhere in the forebrain, or in the pituitary gland itself.

In any event, despite the inevitable trauma associated with the implantation of the hormone and the examination of the ovaries by laparotomy, the results support, when the null effects in controls are taken into account, the assumption that the oestrogen was acting directly on cells in the region of the posterior median eminence and probably, in the light of current ideas, suppressing the release of FSH–RF into the portal blood.

Other observers have used similar kinds of approach. Yamada (1959) examined the effect of repeated intrahypothalamic injections of thyroxine into rats with propylthiouracil(PTU)-induced goitres. PTU, in common with some other thiocarbamide derivates, prevents the iodination of tyrosine by the thyroid and blocks the formation of thyroxine. This disturbs the negative feedback effect of thyroxine on the hypothalamo-pituitary system and as a result large amounts of TSH are secreted, bringing about hypertrophy of the thyroid. Yamada found that injections of thyroxine, in amounts which had no effect when given systemically, inhibited the development of goitre in animals treated with PTU, but only

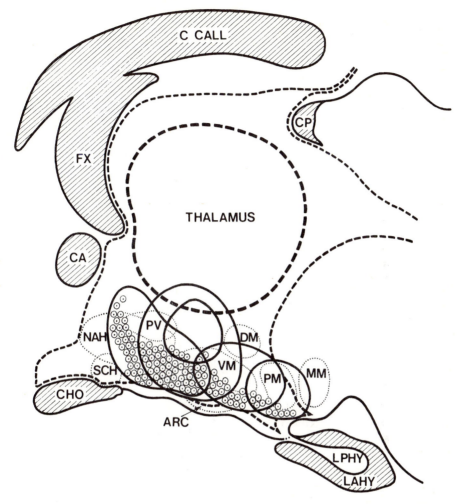

Fig. 6.12. Figure to show the hypophysiotropic area of the hypothalamus; circles with dots denote areas where PAS+ basophils were maintained in the implanted graft. CHO, optic chiasma; LPHY and LAHY, posterior and anterior lobes of the pituitary. Lettered areas within the hypothalamus indicate various hypothalamic nuclei. From Halász and Pupp (1962).

when the injection was made into an area of the anterior hypothalamus; the author mapped out a 'thyrotropic area' in this region.

A variation of the technique of injecting or implanting hormone into the hypothalamus is to implant tissue actively secreting a hormone which will act locally on the nervous tissue. An example of this type of approach is the work of Flerkó and Szentágothai (1957) who implanted small pieces of ovarian tissue (autografts) into the hypothalamus or pituitary gland of adult female rats. They found that implants into the hypothalamus in the region of the paraventricular nuclei were followed by significant decreases in uterine weight while implants into the pituitary, or implants of a non-endocrine tissue (liver) did not have this effect. The authors concluded that the observed results demonstrated the negative feedback of oestrogen, inhibiting the gonadotropic secretion (FSH) of the pituitary via the hypothalamus.

The technique of implantation of tissue into the hypothalamus was later used to demarcate the 'hypophysiotropic' area, that is, a zone which is immediately involved in the production of substances able to maintain structural and functional activity of the cells of the adenohypophysis. Halász, Pupp and Uhlarik (1962) used the criterion of the presence of PAS+ cells in grafts of pituitary tissue to define this hypophysial area, which they located in the medio-basal region of the hypothalamus (fig. 7.1). The zone extended no further than 0.5–1.0 mm from the midline; grafts extending or lying more laterally showed no appreciable content of PAS+ cells. In a sagittal plane the zone extended from above the posterior part of the optic chiasma (superiorly up to the paraventricular nuclei) in a ventral direction to the region of the anterior mammillary plane – here being limited to a narrow zone around the inframammillary recess. Hypophysectomy of grafted animals produced variable effects on the target organs. In some animals these were maintained in a near-normal state, but in others marked atrophy occurred. Histological assessment of the graft with the techniques used by Halász and his colleagues could not, however, differentiate between thyrotropic and the two types of gonadotropic-secreting cells. Also, the effect of an implant on target organs could presumably depend to some extent at any rate on the degree of vascularisation and the availability of an adequate route for the tropic hormones to pass into the systemic circulation.

Confirmation of the presence of a hypophysiotropic zone came from the work by Flament-Durand (1965) who found that basophils in the grafts were particularly numerous in the region of the arcuate nuclei, and that in this zone castration cells developed after hypophysectomy or castration. Few hypophysectomised female rats of this series showed cyclical ovarian activity. Later it was shown by combined hypophysectomy and intrahypothalamic grafting of pituitary tissue, followed by the placing of lesions in the hypothalamus, that lesions which disrupt oestrous cycles in normal animals have the same effect in those bearing functional grafts, as manifested by the reappearance of oestrous cycles (Halász et al. 1965).

The general conclusions from experiments involving intrahypothalamic grafts in relation to secretion of tropic hormones, up to the late 1960s, is well summarised in Szentágothai et al. (1968). The evidence suggests that the 'hypophysiotropic area' is concerned with the control of secretion by cells of the pars distalis of FSH, LH, TSH, ACTH and STH. There is also evidence, however, that not all parts of this area are equivalent in functional terms. Reference has already been made to the findings of Flament-Durand (1965) that gonadotropic effects were most marked in the region of the arcuate nuclei, although also detectable elsewhere. Halász *et al.* (1965) found that although compensatory hypertrophy of the remaining ovary after the removal of one occurred when a pituitary graft (in a hypophysectomised animal) lay within the hypophysiotropic area, adrenal hypertrophy after unilateral adrenalectomy only occurred if the graft was closely connected with the median eminence. In a somewhat similar way, a graft closely associated with the median eminence appeared to be essential for a marked increase in secretion of TSH following treatment with thiouracil to block the synthesis of thyroxine.

These and many other similar experiments have provided strong evidence that a particular region of the hypothalamus does have a special relationship with the pituitary, and that this hypophysiotropic area is necessary for full pituitary function. Problems of localisation of control mechanisms for individual tropic hormones within this whole region remain, although there are indications that such subdivisions are present. A further problem is that of the status of this zone of the hypothalamus in relation to the rest of the central nervous system. It is well known that a variety of stimuli involving the central nervous system can modify pituitary activity, ultimately through the portal blood. How does the hypophysiotropic area fit into this scheme – particularly, has it a degree of action completely independent of the rest of the nervous system, or does it serve only as part of the 'final common path' between the nervous system and the adenohypophysis?

This problem has been studied by experiments involving the destruction of all neural connections between the basal hypothalamus and the rest of the central nervous system, leaving a basal hypothalamic-pituitary unit. Halász and Pupp (1965), using a specially designed knife, carried out this operation in rats – and produced either a complete separation dividing all neural connections, or various partial ones, by limiting the cuts to particular aspects of the basal hypothalamic tissue. The authors came to the conclusion that the hypophysiotropic area did not act simply as part of the 'final common path' between the rest of the central nervous system and the pituitary gland, but itself played a role in the regulation of adenohypophysial activity. Thus, despite the severance of all neural connections between the basal hypothalamus and the rest of the nervous system, the weight and histological structure of the testes were not markedly changed in the three weeks after operation. In female rats, ovarian weight did not diminish, although there seemed to be a considerable disruption of the normal cyclical release of gonadotropic hormones necessary for oestrous cycles.

Halász and his colleagues also found (1967) that complete separation of the medial basal hypothalamus, as above (the operation was called 'deafferentation') was not followed by a decrease in the basal secretion of ACTH. Furthermore, in animals with such lesions an increase in the secretion of ACTH could be obtained as a response to stress. There were indications that the secretion of TSH and STH was slightly reduced after deafferentation, but nevertheless considerable secretion persisted.

Releasing factors

At the time when it was becoming apparent that the portal system played an important regulatory role, there was, however, no precise evidence as to the way in which this was achieved. Proof of the hypothesis that portal blood contained substances capable of acting specifically on cells of the pars distalis to bring about release of tropic factors required the isolation of such substances, their purification, analysis and ultimately their synthesis.

It was of course already known at the time when ideas of 'releasing factors' were being formulated that at least two active hormones were produced, stored and released in the hypothalamo-neurohypophysial system, namely the neurohypophysial hormones oxytocin and vaso-pressin (ADH). Understandably attention was directed to these as possible releasing factors for anterior pituitary tropic hormones (e.g. see Martini and De Poli, 1956). The demonstration that the administration of a given substance results in an increase in the amount of a hormone in the blood (or urine) does not of course necessarily indicate that the substance either normally acts as a releasing factor, or that if it does, it is the only one to do so. Consider the hypothesis that the release of, for example, ACTH from cells of the pars distalis is brought about by a specific factor elaborated in the hypothalamus, which reaches the secretory cells via the portal system, and an observation that injections of an extract of posterior lobe rich in ADH are followed by a raised plasma level of ACTH. A number of mechanisms might be involved in this. The ADH or perhaps a contaminant of the preparation might indeed have acted as a specific releasing factor. On the other hand it might have acted in a non-specific way, only one of a number of effects being observed. It might have acted at the level of the hypothalamus or of the pituitary; it might have acted on the adrenal cortex, evoking a change in the output of adrenocortical hormones and thus modifying the feedback effect on the pituitary; it might have effected the release of a specific CRF through a change in blood pressure or in response to stress induced by the substance injected or to the physical handling of the animal.

The administration of vasopressin is certainly followed by the release of ACTH (McDonald and Weise, 1956); but the dose required for this effect is greater when animals are under the influence of stress-reducing drugs such as morphine (Briggs and Munson, 1955). These and other observations (see Guillemin, 1964) indicate that although ADH can act as releasing factor for ACTH, so may other substances which can be extracted from posterior pituitary tissues; but a specific corticotropin-releasing factor (CRF) distinct from these is apparently secreted by the hypothalamus, and lesions placed bilaterally at the junction of the stalk and median eminence block its release (Porter, Dhariwal and McCann, 1967).

Specific releasing factors for other adenohypophysial hormones have been found. In 1962 Guillemin and his colleagues reported the isolation from hypothalamic tissue of a substance with thyrotropin-releasing activity. Since that time thyrotropin-releasing factor (TRF) has been extracted from hypothalamic tissue of several species, including man (see McCann and Porter (1969) for references).

As regards the gonadotropins, infusion of extracts of hypothalamic tissues were shown to be capable of producing ovulation both in rats (Nikitovitch-Winer, 1962) and rabbits (Campbell, Feuer and Harris, 1964). McCann (1962) showed that hypothalamic extracts raised plasma LH in normal female rates, and it seems that in the rat at any rate the anterior half of the hypothalamus from the region of the optic chiasma to the median eminence is particularly concerned with LH-releasing factor (LRF). This area has been localised both by assay of extracts of different zones of the hypothalamus (McCann, 1962), and also by a technique of implanting pituitary tissue into the hypothalamus of hypophysectomised rats. Implants into the anterior basal area, but not elsewhere, showed differentiation of basophil (LH-secreting) cells and maintenance of gonadotropic activity (Flament-Durand, 1965). Lesions of the supra-chiasmatic region of the hypothalamus (Crighton and Schneider, 1969) resulted in reduced LRF activity on later assay of the stalk–median eminence tissue. Activity was not abolished, however, despite the lesions, so presumably LRF is secreted by neurons lying more caudally than the suprachiasmatic region.

If the secretion of LRF is a major factor in the control of variation in the plasma levels of LH during the phases of the oestrous cycle, it would be anticipated that some evidence of varying rates of secretion of this factor would occur at different times of the cycle. The pre-ovulatory surge of LH, responsible for ovulation, has been associated with a diminution of the LRF content of the hypothalamus during pro-oestrus (Ramirez and Sawyer, 1965), an observation which might indicate increased release of LRF at this time. Hypothalamic extracts have also been shown to exercise a releasing effect on FSH, and the factor (FRF) has been extracted from hypothalami of several species of mammals including man (Schally *et al.* 1970). There is still some doubt, however, as to whether LRF and FRF are distinct compounds (Matsuo, Arimura, Nair and Schally, 1971).

It has already been noted that although secretory activity of the cell of the pars distalis is in general considerably reduced or almost absent in tissue removed from its normal relationship to the median eminence, one hormone, LTH (prolactin), is secreted in amounts greater than usual, and acidophils thought to be concerned with the secretion of this hormone are the only chromophils to retain their granulation and normal staining properties in ectopic grafts. The phenomenon of enhanced secretion of LTH has also been noted when the gland is cultivated *in vitro*. In 1961 Pasteels reported that the addition of hypothalamic extract to cultured pituitary tissue resulted in a reduction of the amount of prolactin in the medium. Later an inhibiting factor was purified, although Dhariwal *et al.* (1968) were unable to achieve its complete separation from LRF. The factor has been called prolactin-inhibiting factor, or PIF.

The sixth tropic hormone secreted by the pars distalis is STH or growth hormone. In this context there is again evidence that a releasing factor (GRF) can be extracted from hypothalamic tissue of a number of species. Another factor influencing the release of STH from pituitary cells has also been found and appears to constitute an antagonistic growth inhibiting factor (GIH) (Dhariwal, Krulich and McCann, 1969). A potent inhibitory factor for the release of MSH has also been isolated from hypothalamic tissue (Nair, Kastin and Schally, 1971).

Methods for the extraction of peptides have been used to obtain pure preparations of releasing factors, and determination of chemical structure of these is now well advanced (see Harris, 1972). Synthesis of LRF, for example, has already been reported (Matsuo *et al.* 1971), and the structure of others (TRF, GRF, MIF) is known, and they have been synthesised.

Further proof of the involvement of the portal vascular system in the control of the adenohypophysis has come with the demonstration that releasing factors occur in portal blood in a greater concentration than in systemic blood. For example the amount of portal LRF has been shown to vary with the phase of the oestrous cycle (Fink and Harris, 1970) and can be increased by electrical stimulation of the hypothalamus (Harris and Ruf, 1970). Similar studies have been directed towards other releasing factors.

7

THE PITUITARY GLAND IN AGNATHANS

The term 'fishes' covers several groups of vertebrates that differ fundamentally from each other. The most primitive living vertebrates – the lampreys and hagfishes – are superficially fishes; but in fact they represent a stage in vertebrate evolution before the development of jaws and paired limbs, and are placed by taxonomists in their own superclass, the Agnatha (jawless fish). All other living vertebrates have jaws, and occupy the superclass Gnathostomata (fig. 7.1). Living agnathans differ greatly from their primitive fossil ancestors, being modified in many ways for a scavenging or semi-parasitic mode of life, and because of this, and with reference to their round suctorial mouths, they are placed in the class Cyclostomata. Living cyclostomes are of two kinds, the lampreys (petromyzontids) and the hagfishes (myxinoids), and in these survivors of the earliest vertebrate stock we find the most primitive pituitary gland.

The cyclostome pituitary has a much simpler structure than that of gnathostomes. Both neural and glandular components can be recognised, but nervous or vascular communications between the two are limited and peculiar. Many of the adenohypophysial cells, especially in young animals, are chromophobic, and this has hampered histophysiological investigations. Another difficulty is that the primitive evolutionary position of these animals makes it hazardous to assume that their pituitary secretes the full complement of hormones known for gnathostomes. In fact, evidence for the secretion of hormones other than gonadotropin, MSH and arginine vasotocin (AVT) is very uncertain (see Ball and Baker, 1969; Perks, 1969; Larsen, 1969).

MYXINOIDS

The myxinoid pituitary appears to be more primitive than that of lampreys, although it is impossible to know to what extent its peculiarities are functional specialisations.

ADENOHYPOPHYSIS

The adenohypophysis consists of clusters and follicles of cells, embedded in the thick connective tissue below the diencephalon (fig. 7.2). The

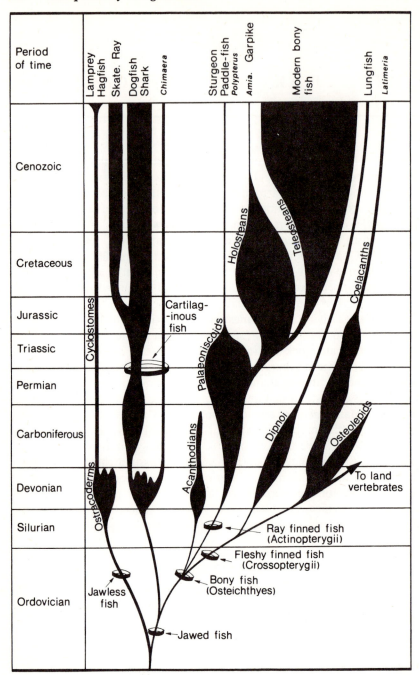

Fig. 7.1. Evolutionary relationships of fishes. Modified from A. S. Romer (1968), *The procession of life*, courtesy Weidenfeld and Nicolson.

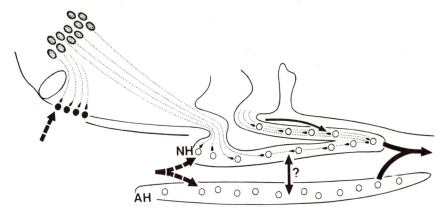

Fig. 7.2. Myxinoid pituitary, diagrammatic sagittal section, to show hypothalamo-hypophysial vascular and neurosecretory links. Question mark indicates unsettled direction of blood in the vertical vessels between neurohypophysis (NH) and adenohypophysis (AH). Dotted circles, neurosecretory cells of the preoptic nucleus; dotted lines, neurosecretory axons, with axon terminals marked at their endings; filled circles, prehypophysial plexus; empty circles, intrahypophysial capillaries; interrupted arrows, arteries; solid arrows, veins; thin arrows, possible portal veins. From Jasinski (1969).

follicles may contain colloid (PAS+, AF+, AB+, aniline blue+), but most cells lie in solid clusters. Vascularisation is poor, with no capillaries within the cell clusters and only a few in the thick connective tissue separating the cells from the overlying neurohypophysis (Olsson, 1959; Wingstrand, 1966a; Fernholm and Olsson, 1969; Fernholm, 1972a). There is no differentiation into pars distalis and pars intermedia. In large animals, several workers have described a posterior area of contact between adenohypophysial tissue and neurohypophysis, the cell clusters in this area being disorganised, small, and with irregular nuclei (Ball and Baker, 1969; Fernholm and Olsson, 1969). Other workers have denied the existence of this, the only area of direct adeno-neurohypophysial contact, but it is possible that they were dealing with juvenile animals and that the zone of contact develops with age (see Ball and Baker, 1969) and may vary in extent with species (Honma, 1969).

The adenohypophysis in cyclostomes is related in development to the median nasopharyngeal duct, a structure probably also present in extinct agnathans and seemingly representing an enormously expanded olfactory pit. It opens on the snout and runs backwards beneath the brain, giving rise to the olfactory organ close to the tip of the brain. The adeno-hypophysial anlage buds from the dorsal wall of the nasopharyngeal duct just below the diencephalon. Unfortunately, the details of pituitary embryology are not known in great detail. Attempts have been made to equate the posterior part of the nasopharyngeal duct, which may open into the pharynx (myxinoids) or end blindly (lampreys), with part of Rathke's pouch; this homology is not now generally accepted, and it is more likely, considering its embryological development, that the duct represents simply a backward extension of the nasal pit (Wingstrand, 1966a). Rathke's pouch is probably expressed in epithelial cell cords which in young *Myxine* connect the roof of the nasopharyngeal duct with the overlying adenohypophysial cell clusters, the cords being composed apparently of adenohypophysial basophils (Fernholm and Olsson, 1969).

The adenohypophysial cell clusters seem able to function as separate units, but nevertheless there is some evidence of regional concentration of different cell-types. Earlier work (reviewed by Ball and Baker, 1969) had identified some functional cell-types, but more recent investigations have cast doubt on the earlier conclusions (Fernholm and Olsson, 1969). This recent work identifies basophils (PAS+, AF+) of various types, two erythrosinophils, one with coarse and one with fine granules, and several types of chromophobes. The only positive functional identification achieved by exhaustive experimental investigations was of the finely-granulated erythrosinophil as the corticotrope, on the basis of its responses to adrenocortical blocking agents and general morphology (Fernholm and Olsson, 1969). This accords with earlier demonstrations of ACTH activity in the myxinoid gland (Chester Jones *et al.* 1969). Gonadotropes and thyrotropes could not be identified by appropriate experimental procedures, nor could Fernholm and Olsson support their earlier identification of the coarsely-granulated erythrosinophil as a lactotrope; LTH activity could not be detected in the myxinoid pituitary either by bioassay (Sage and Bern, 1972) or by immunochemical methods (Aler, Båge and Fernholm, 1971).

In a recent EM study of the adenohypophysis of *Myxine*, Fernholm (1972a) identified two cell-types which appear to secrete simple protein hormones. Type 1, with secretory granules of mean diameter 88 nm, probably secretes a hormone similar to ACTH/MSH, and type 2, with granules of mean diameter 176 nm, is probably the source of a hormone similar to STH/LTH. The type 1 cell is presumed to correspond to the corticotrope identified earlier with the light microscope (Fernholm and Olsson, 1969). In interpreting his findings, Fernholm (1972a) favoured the concept that each cell-type produces a molecule resembling the ancestral or 'parent' molecule of one of the two protidic hormone families (ACTH–MSH–lipotropin, and STH–LTH) rather than making the assumption that each cell-type secretes two different hormones. The basophilic (PAS+) cells could not be separated into different types with the EM. These cells are associated with cysts containing a PAS+ colloid, and because their ultrastructure is different from that of the thyrotropes and gonadotropes of other vertebrates, and because there is evidence that neither thyrotropin nor gonadotropin occurs in hagfishes, Fernholm does not regard these as endocrine cells. Instead he points to their marked ultrastructural resemblance to the mucous cells of the hagfish skin, and concludes that they are simply mucus-secreting cells incorporated into the pituitary but not transformed into endocrine cells. This interesting interpretation contains the implication that the myxinoid pituitary is genuinely primitive, representing an evolutionary stage before the development of thyrotropes and gonadotropes, and before the differentiation of ACTH from MSH and of LTH from STH.

In view of the poor vascularisation of the adenohypophysial region, it is not obvious how hormones produced in the cell clusters can reach the bloodstream. The cells are embedded in connective tissue, and since connective tissue transports NSM and other substances in insects, Fernholm and Olsson (1969) suggest that the myxinoid adenohypophysial hormones probably pass slowly through the connective tissue to blood vessels. In addition, 'ependymal' cells have been found, with the perikarya in the middle of the cell clusters and with long processes reaching the connective tissue at the periphery of the clusters. These cells, which contain many microtubules, may be homologous with the stellate cells of the gnathostome adenohypophysis, and may be concerned with transport to and from the adenohypophysial cells in myxinoids (Fernholm and Olsson, 1969). There are no nerve fibres in the adenohypophysis (Olsson, 1969; Fernholm, 1972a).

NEUROHYPOPHYSIS AND BLOOD SUPPLY

The myxinoid neurohypophysis is a dorso-ventrally flattened hollow sac, lying above the adenohypophysis. The cavity of the sac communicates with the third ventricle only by a narrow aperture (fig. 7.2). In the hypothalamus, the ill-defined preoptic nucleus (PON) lies far anterior to the pituitary, and some of its neurons contain an atypical NSM, AF − and CAH −, but stainable with Astra blue (Perks, 1969). In contrast to the hypothalamic nuclei of other vertebrates, these neurons do not appear to bear processes projecting into the third ventricle. The PON is found in all fishes and amphibians, and is regarded as the homologue of the supraoptic and paraventricular nuclei of amniotes. There are two pathways for NSM from the myxinoid PON. The first is probably unique: PON axons terminate ventrally behind the optic chiasma on the capillaries of a *prehypophysial plexus* from which portal vessels drain into the dorsal part of the neurohypophysis (fig. 7.2; Ball and Baker, 1969; Jasinski, 1969). The ultrastructure of the neurohaemal contact area in the plexus is very like that of the tetrapod median eminence (Gorbman, Kobayashi and Uemura, 1963; Nishioka and Bern, 1966). The second route from the PON is the more orthodox PON–neurohypophysial tract, formed of neurosecretory fibres. A few fibres terminate on blood capillaries in the anterior face of the neurohypophysis, but most end on the dorsal wall of the neurohypophysis, which probably represents the neural lobe of gnathostomes. In this region, a rich accumulation of AF+ NSM lies in a dense vascular bed draining into the general circulation. The EM shows axonal terminations on capillaries, the endings containing secretory granules of various sizes. Some fibres contain larger granules (100–400 nm diameter), and may correspond to the type A fibres (peptidergic and AF+) of the gnathostome hypothalamic neurosecretory system. Other fibres with smaller granules (65, 80 and 110 nm) may represent three kinds of type B fibres (aminergic AF−) such as are found in gnathostomes (Nishioka and Bern, 1966; Kobayashi and Uemura, 1972). This myxinoid arrangement seems adapted to deliver into the general circulation the NSM from the PON and perhaps from other hypothalamic nuclei, via the neurohaemal contacts in the dorsal neurohypophysis ('neural lobe') or less directly via the hypothalamo-neurohypophysial portal vessels. There is some evidence, though scant, for the production of neuro-hypophysial hormone(s) in myxinoids (Perks, 1969).

The ventral floor of the neurohypophysis, immediately above the adenohypophysis, may be a primitive median eminence. Kobayashi and Uemura (1972) report that this area in *Eptatretus burgeri* has an ultrastructure similar to the tetrapod median eminence. Axons in this region are type B (with secretory granules 65, 80 or 110 nm in diameter, and also 'synaptic' vesicles) and type C (containing only 'synaptic' vesicles). The type B axons have endings, often synaptoid, on ependymal cell processes lying against the connective tissue that separates neurohypophysis and adenohypophysis. The ependymal cells appear to secrete into the infundibular cavity, and they also contain vesicles and colloid droplets which seem to be extruded into the connective tissue. Few or no putative portal vessels traverse this connective tissue in *Polistotrema* and *Myxine* (Jasinski, 1969; Fernholm 1972*b*), but *Eptatretus* displays about 20 small vessels running from the 'median eminence' to the adenohypophysis (Kobayashi and Uemura, 1972). Thus in *Eptatretus*, it is possible, though not certain, that neurohormones from the axons of the 'median eminence' could travel in these putative portal vessels, entering them from connective tissues spaces continuous with pericapillary spaces. However, capillaries are rare in the 'median eminence', and the direction of blood flow in the vessels is not known. There is also the possibility that neurohormones could reach the adenohypophysis by transport through the connective tissue itself. Though unusual in structure, this newly-discovered 'median eminence' offers a route by which the myxinoid hypothalamus could influence adenohypophysial activity (Kobayashi and Uemura, 1972).

Blood reaches the neurohypophysis and adenohypophysis by separate branches of the carotid artery (Ball and Baker, 1969; fig. 7.2). In addition, the 'neural lobe' receives blood in the portal vessels from the prehypophysial plexus. Hypophysial veins drain the two components separately (fig. 7.2).

The myxinoid pituitary may well be degenerate. Hagfishes such as *Polistotrema* and *Myxine* live in a nearly uniform cold dark environment in deep seas, and they are scavengers so that even their food is constantly available. It follows that they must encounter few sensory clues of the kind that in higher vertebrates are translated (often by way of the pituitary) into cyclical physiological activity; for example, these animals exhibit no seasonal cycle in the gonads (Gorbman, Kobayashi and Uemura, 1963; Fernholm, 1972*b*). A constant environment, also, will not present the animal with sudden changes (stress) requiring rapid endocrine adjustments, and certainly would appear to exert the least possible selection pressure for the development (or maintenance) of the typical hypothalamo-hypophysial controlling system. It is interesting therefore that *Polistotrema stouti* has very few putative portal vessels, and that the adenohypophysis of *Myxine* can be cultured *in vitro* for as long as two weeks with no signs of changes in the secretory activity of its cells, indicating greater functional autonomy than in gnathostomes (Fernholm, 1972*b*). On the other hand, it may be significant that *Eptatretus burgeri*, with its 'median eminence' and up to twenty putative portal vessels, moves into shallow waters for part of the year and appears to have a seasonal gonadal cycle (Kobayashi and Uemura, 1972).

PETROMYZONTIDS

In lampreys the pituitary is organised in a more orthodox way than in myxinids, and has been investigated extensively. Earlier work is summarised by Ball and Baker (1969) and Perks (1969).

ADENOHYPOPHYSIS

The adenohypophysis is a compact structure, obviously divided into an anterior pars distalis, separated by connective tissue from the overlying infundibular floor, and a posterior pars intermedia, with a connective tissue septum between the two. The intermedia is virtually fused with the overlying neural lobe, the two being separated only by a thin septum containing a rich capillary plexus, the plexus intermedius. On the basis of its constituent cell-types, the pars distalis is further divided into rostral and proximal zones (fig. 7.3).

The rostral pars distalis is shown by its development to be homologous with the rostral pars distalis of gnathostome fishes (Wingstrand, 1966*a*). During the spawning migration of adult *Lampetra fluviatilis* from sea to river, empty cysts develop in this region, and open via a ciliated canal into the nasopharyngeal duct (Rühle and Sterba, 1966), recalling the organ-

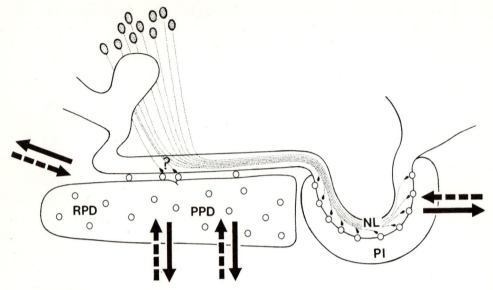

Fig. 7.3. Lamprey pituitary, diagrammatic sagittal section, to show hypothalamo-hypophysial vascular and neurosecretory links. Question mark indicates possible contacts between neurosecretory axons and capillaries of the pars distalis, in the putative median eminence. RPD, rostral pars distalis; PPD, proximal pars distalis; NL, neural lobe; PI, pars intermedia; dotted circles, neurosecretory cells of the PON; dotted lines, neurosecretory axons with axon terminals marked at their endings; empty circles, intrahypophysial capillaries; interrupted arrows, arteries; solid arrows, veins. From Jasinski (1969).

isation of the rostral pars distalis in certain primitive fishes (chapter 9). Otherwise, the lamprey rostral pars distalis, like the rest of the gland, consists of solid convoluted cell cords, divided into lobules by vertical connective tissue septa containing capillaries. The cells in the rostral region are either chromophobes, or the predominant PAS+ and AF+ basophils, divisible with the EM into two or three types on the basis of the size of their secretory granules (Larsen and Rothwell, 1972). In various lampreys the rostral basophils increase in number and staining affinities at metamorphosis of the ammocoete larva into the adult, and the entire pars distalis may then enlarge; this activation of rostral basophils at metamorphosis has been taken to mean that they are thyrotropes, by analogy with amphibian metamorphosis, although in fact there is no evidence that lamprey metamorphosis is thyroid-dependent (Pickering, 1972). In the adult, rostral basophils (possibly a second category) exhibit changes which are suggestive of a gonadotropic function (Ball and Baker, 1969).

The proximal pars distalis exhibits both acidophils and basophils, arranged in vertical cell cords (Honma, 1969). Older workers described two types of acidophils, but it now seems that these are amphiphils, since recent work on *Lampetra* showed them to stain violet after Aliz BT (Aler, Båge and Fernholm, 1971). Two undoubted acidophil types, erythrosinophilic after Aliz BT, have been described in *Lampetra*, but neither secretes LTH judging from the negative results of immunochemical studies (Aler *et al.* 1971). In another species, the Transylvanian lamprey *Eudontomyzon*, one of the proximal acidophils has been studied in some detail. It is carminophilic after Azan, weakly Aliz B+, and strongly PbH+. Treatment with the adrenocortical antagonist aldactone produced degranulation and vacuolation in these cells, responses which, like their staining properties, suggest that they are corticotropes (Molnár and Szabó, 1968). Basophils are scarce in the proximal pars distalis, and are all PAS+ and AF+. They become most active during metamorphosis, and relatively inactive in the adult after spawning. During gonadal maturation, these basophils degranulate, a change prevented by gonadectomy. These cells, together with some of the rostral basophils, would thus appear to be gonadotropes. Partial hypophysectomy has indicated that gonadotropic function is located in the proximal pars distalis, either totally (Evennett, 1963) or mainly, with some gonadotropin produced by the rostral pars distalis (Larsen, 1965).

Since thyroid activity in the adult river lamprey is not affected by hypophysectomy, TSH or thyroxine (Larsen and Rosenkilde, 1971; Pickering, 1972) it is uncertain that the pituitary secretes TSH (Larsen and Rothwell, 1972). Nor is the endostyle of the ammocoete larva altered by hypophysectomy, although this structure, which changes into the thyroid gland at metamorphosis, is responsive in its handling of iodine and in its histology to injections of mammalian TSH (Pickering, 1972). It may be that TSH control of the adult thyroid is established during the ectoparasitic marine phase of the life history, and that TSH cells will be identified in the pituitary only when marine lampreys are investigated.

The proximal pars distalis also contains chromophobes, said to be most active at metamorphosis or during the upstream river migration to the spawning beds and suggested to be somatotropes (Sterba, 1969). The EM differentiates two or three types of granulated cells in this region, as well as chromophobes and stellate cells (see Ball and Baker, 1969; Larsen and Rothwell, 1972).

The large pars intermedia has been shown by experiments to secrete MSH (see van Oordt, 1968; Ball and Baker, 1969; Larsen and Rothwell, 1972). It is separated from the neural lobe by the connective tissue septum containing the plexus intermedius, a system of capillaries found in this position in most vertebrates, and is not penetrated to any extent by neurohypophysial processes (fig. 7.3). Many of the intermedia cells are chromophobic, but some workers have described a single chromophilic type, carminophilic, PAS+ or PAS− according to species, and PbH+

in *Lampetra fluviatilis* (van Oordt, 1968). With the EM, four kinds of cell can be differentiated, but probably all represent stages in the cycle of a single cell-type (Larsen and Rothwell, 1972). Other workers have differentiated two chromophilic types, one AF+ and PAS−, situated ventrally with processes extending to the neuro-intermedia septum, the other AF+ and PAS+, and situated close to the plexus intermedius. Various cytological changes have been described in the pars intermedia, related to illumination, metamorphosis, migration and spawning, but the functional significance of these changes remains unknown (van Oordt, 1968; Ball and Baker, 1969). Following the usual vertebrate pattern, neurosecretory fibres have been observed with the EM, terminating singly on the pars intermedia cells (Sterba, 1969).

NEUROHYPOPHYSIS AND BLOOD SUPPLY

The lamprey neurohypophysis, simpler than that of myxinoids, is merely a slight thickening of the floor of the diencephalon, with little sign of an infundibular stem. In the ammocoete larva the region is even less differentiated, but at metamorphosis a slight evagination is produced which may represent the delayed formation of the saccus infundibuli (Wingstrand, 1966a). The thickened floor of this evagination forms the neural lobe, in contact with the pars intermedia. Despite its poor demarcation this neural lobe has a typical construction, with a dorsal ependymal layer, a fibre layer and a ventral palisade layer containing AF+ NSM and apposed to the neuro-intermedia septum (Wingstrand, 1966a). The PON is well-developed, elongated from the optic chiasma to the posterior end of the diencephalon, and rather poorly vascularised. Its neurons secrete AF+ CAH+ NSM, even in the youngest larva, and they bear short dendrites projecting between the adjacent ependymal cells into the cerebrospinal fluid, a characteristic feature of hypothalamic neurosecretory centres in higher vertebrates. There is no sign of the curious prehypophysial plexus with its portal vessels seen in myxinoids (Perks, 1969). Some workers have described some PON fibres terminating on capillaries in the connective tissue lamina between the hypothalamic floor and the rostral pars distalis (fig. 7.3), but most of the PON fibres run in a well-defined PON-neurohypophysial tract in the hypothalamic floor, laden with NSM, and pass backwards to terminate in the neural lobe. A few fibres end on the ependymal cells of the shallow infundibular recess, but most terminate on the blood vessels of the plexus intermedius, there being no capillaries within the neural lobe itself (Rodríguez, 1971). The nerve endings often contain Herring bodies, and with the EM can be seen to terminate not directly on perivascular spaces, but on processes from the ependymal cells, which pass downwards through the neural tissue as a complicated network between the nerve fibres, and end as expanded end feet against the perivascular membrane of the plexus intermedius. These end feet make a nearly complete barrier between the neurosecretory endings on their dorsal surfaces and the perivascular membrane ventrally. Occasional fibres pass between the ependymal end feet and make direct perivascular contacts, but in the case of most fibres the ependymal processes must transmit the NSM in some way to the perivascular space. This pattern is common in higher vertebrates, and not unlike the architecture of the 'median eminence' in myxinoids. Rodríguez (1971) found that most fibre endings in the lamprey neural lobe were type A, with granules 150–180 nm in diameter, some elongated up to 300–500 nm. A possible second type A fibre was rare and had paler granules of the same size. The predominant type A fibre presumably carries arginine vasotocin (AVT), the only neurohypophysial factor so far detected in lampreys (Perks, 1969). In addition, Rodríguez (1971) found numerous type B fibres, with granules smaller than 100 nm, and many type C fibres, containing only 'synaptic' vesicles, and possibly cholinergic. A neurosecretory hypothalamic nucleus posterior to the infundibular recess has been described as the origin of some fibres to the neural lobe (Perks, 1969). At present, the origin of the type B and type C fibres is unknown. The neurosecretory fibres found in the pars intermedia (Sterba, 1969) presumably travel via the neural lobe.

The amount of NSM in the neural lobe has been described as changing in relation to alterations in illumination, metamorphosis and sexual maturation (Ball and Baker, 1969). Unlike myxinoids, adult lampreys lead active predatory lives, in many species involving migrations between rivers and sea, and these animals face the necessity of making rapid adjustments to environmental changes such as myxinoids never encounter. The changes observed in the NSM of the neural lobe, though not fully understood, do at least suggest some adaptive physiological role for the lamprey hypothalamo-neurohypophysial system.

Whether lampreys possess a median eminence and portal system is uncertain. We have seen that a few PON fibres terminate in the vascular connective tissue sheet between the hypothalamus and rostral pars distalis, which is the region where the median eminence differentiates in higher vertebrates. A few blood vessels have been traced from this 'contact area' into the rostral pars distalis (fig. 7.3; Jasinski, 1969). The blood capillaries within the pars distalis itself ascend between the cell cords and descend as wider sinusoids; where the vessels loop over dorsally, they are very close to the 'contact area', and could conceivably receive PON fibre endings (Gorbman, 1965). In the absence of a detailed EM study of this area, it seems possible that apart from the relatively few AF+ fibre endings, there may be numerous type B (AF−) endings, as in the median eminence of gnathostomes; and it is also possible that, as in myxinoids, NSM could pass through the connective tissue lamina as well as by way of capillaries from the 'contact area'. No alternative route of hypothalamic control of the pars distalis is known, although there have been claims that a few PON fibres terminate directly on pars distalis cells (Perks, 1969; Jasinski, 1969). However, there is in fact little evidence that the pars distalis is under hypothalamic control, since ectopic pars distalis auto-transplants can induce complete gonadal maturation in male lampreys (Larsen, 1969). It seems fairly certain that MSH secretion is inhibited by the hypothalamus, presumably by way of the direct innervation of the pars intermedia (Larsen and Rothwell, 1972).

The pars distalis is supplied with blood mainly from several small branches of the internal carotid artery, and is drained by several venules. This supply is independent of the neuro-intermediate lobe, which has its own branch from the internal carotid to the plexus intermedius, with drainage into an independent hypophysial vein (Gorbman, 1965).

8

THE PITUITARY GLAND
IN ELASMOBRANCHS

Living elasmobranchs (class Elasmobranchii or Chondrichthyes) fall into two groups, unequal in numbers of species and individuals. On the one hand the subclass Selachii includes the familiar sharks and dogfishes (Pleurotremata, about 250 species) and the skates and rays (Hypotremata, about 350 species); on the other hand, the subclass Bradyodonti includes the little-known oceanic chimaeroids (Holocephali), about 25 species known as rat-fishes or rabbit fishes. The fossil record shows that elasmobranchs diverged from the ancestral gnathostome stock very early, and pursued their own evolution independently of all other fish groups. They are themselves specialised in many ways, notably in having a completely cartilaginous skeleton, and are in no sense ancestral to 'higher' fishes; but they are, nevertheless, the most primitive living gnathostomes.

Nearly all information about the elasmobranch pituitary comes from work on selachians. The holocephalian gland has been studied only to a limited extent, but it does appear to resemble the selachian pituitary in most respects. The following account applies to selachians, except where holocephalians are specifically mentioned.

THE ADENOHYPOPHYSIS

At first sight, the adenohypophysis is very unlike that in other fishes (figs. 8.1, 8.2, 8.3). There is a very large posterior pars intermedia, elaborately invaded by the neurohypophysis to form a *neuro-intermediate lobe*; an elongated pars distalis, divided into a *dorsal lobe* which includes a narrow rostral part (head) and a wider caudal part (tail of the dorsal lobe) and extending forwards beneath the infundibular floor; and a *ventral lobe*, attached to the tail of the dorsal lobe by an epithelial stalk which is hollow in the embryo (Alluchon-Gérard, 1971). The ventral lobe is closely associated with the cranial floor. Elasmobranchs are the only fishes to have a hollow Rathke's pouch during development, but it is so complicated that in the past the interpretation of the homologies of its various derivatives has given rise to controversy. It now seems reasonably certain that the head of the dorsal lobe is formed from the anterior process, and the tail of the dorsal lobe from part of the aboral process of

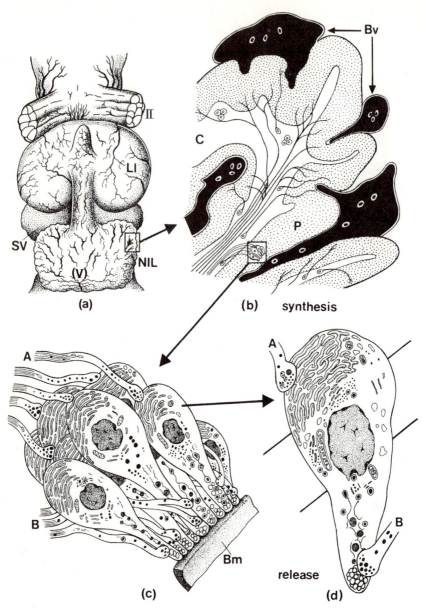

Fig. 8.1. The distribution of intrinsic cells and neurosecretory fibres in the neuro-intermediate lobe of the pituitary of *Scyliorhinus stellaris*.

(*a*) Ventral view of the pituitary and associated structures. II, the base of the optic nerve; LI, inferior lobe of hypothalamus, pituitary dorsal lobe in midline; SV, saccus vasculosus; NIL, neuro-intermediate lobe; (V), position of attachment of ventral lobe.

(*b*) Diagram of a small portion of the neuro-intermediate lobe, showing the

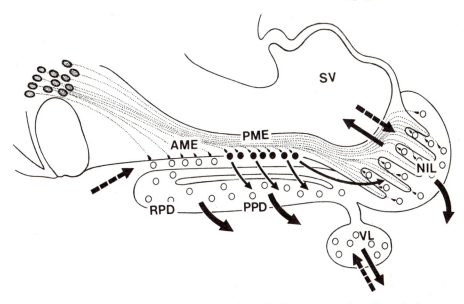

Fig. 8.2. Selachian pituitary, diagrammatic sagittal section to show hypothalamo-hypophysial vascular and neurosecretory links. RPD, rostral pars distalis (=head of dorsal lobe); PPD, proximal pars distalis (=tail of dorsal lobe); VL, ventral lobe; NIL, neuro-intermediate lobe; SV, saccus vasculosus; AME, anterior median eminence; PME, posterior median eminence. Dotted circles, neurosecretory cells of the PON; dotted lines, neurosecretory axons, with axon terminals marked; filled circles, primary portal capillaries; empty circles, secondary portal capillaries and other intrahypophysial capillaries; interrupted arrows, arteries; solid arrows, veins; thin arrows, portal veins. From Jasinski (1969).

Rathke's pouch, so that the two regions correspond respectively to the cephalic and caudal lobes of the avian pars distalis. The pars intermedia is orthodox, in developing from the region of the aboral process that contacts the infundibulum (Wingstrand, 1966a). The ventral lobe appears totally anomalous in its adult condition; but in embryology it arises from the paired lateral lobes which uniquely bend downwards and fuse beneath the main gland. Thus the ventral lobe seems to be homologous with the tetrapod pars tuberalis (Wingstrand, 1966a; Alluchon-Gérard, 1971),

relationships of blood vessels (Bv), endocrine cells of the peripheral layer (P) and nervous and other elements in the central region (C).

(c) A few peripheral cells and their innervation by type A and type B neuro-secretory fibres. Bm, basement membrane.

(d) A single peripheral endocrine cell of the intermedia, showing the distinct regions of hormone synthesis, hormone assemblage, and hormone storage and release. This and the preceding figures are semi-diagrammatic, and the relative sizes of some of the cell components have been altered slightly for the sake of clarity. From Knowles (1965).

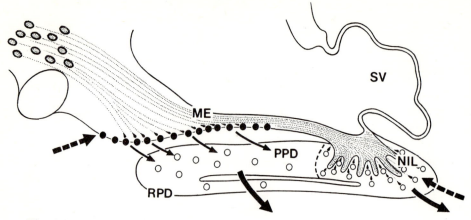

Fig. 8.3. Holocephalian pituitary, diagrammatic sagittal section to show hypo-thalamo-hypophysial vascular and neurosecretory links. Abbreviations and symbols as in fig. 8.2. From Jasinski (1969).

despite some dissenting opinions (Gorbman and Bern, 1962). In adult holocephalians the structure of the gland is similar, but the dorsal lobe is not clearly divisible into head and tail, and instead of a ventral lobe these fishes have a follicular glandular structure, the *Rachendachhypophyse*, lying far ahead of the main gland outside the cranium in the roof of the mouth. This is usually regarded as homologous with the selachian ventral lobe, although its embryology is hardly known (Sathyanesan, 1965; Wingstrand, 1966a). However, unlike the ventral lobe, the Rachendach-hypophyse in young *Chimaera monstrosa* is connected to the *head* of the dorsal lobe (not to the tail) by an epithelial cord (Honma, 1969), and in *Hydrolagus colliei* it develops as an evagination from the oral part of Rathke's pouch, not from the lateral processes which give rise to the ventral lobe and pars tuberalis; at first the epithelial stalk of Rathke's pouch connects the Rachendachhypophyse anlage to the head of the dorsal lobe, as in young *Chimaera*, but this stalk gradually disappears and cartilage grows to separate the Rachendachhypophyse from the rest of the gland (Honma, 1969). Thus, the Rachendachhypophyse is not embryologically comparable with the selachian ventral lobe, and its development suggests instead a tentative homology with the buccal part of the pituitary of the coelacanth, *Latimeria* (chapter 11); both structures may simply represent a detached piece of the rostral tip of the pars distalis.

Two conditions of the selachian adenohypophysis are recognisable. In the *squaloid type*, found in sharks, dogfishes, and certain shark-like rays, the entire pars distalis is hollow, the head of the dorsal lobe containing vesicles or tubules communicating with an extension of the hypophysial cavity, and the tail of the dorsal lobe consisting simply of folds of epithelial tissue around a voluminous hypophysial cavity. In the *batoid type*, found in typical skates and rays, the hypophysial cavity is small or obliterated, and the entire dorsal lobe is a mass of compact cords and clusters of cells (Wingstrand, 1966*a*). The holocephalian dorsal lobe is always hollow. The selachian ventral lobe is hollow, often vesicular (Ball and Baker, 1969), while the follicular structure of the Rachendach-hypophyse in holocephalians was mentioned earlier. All these spaces and vesicles appear to represent a persistent hypophysial cleft (i.e. the cavity of Rathke's pouch; Alluchon-Gérard, 1971), and they often contain a colloid, PAS+, AF+ and AB+. It has been thought that this colloid might represent a stored form of gonadotropin and thyrotropin (see Ball and Baker, 1969), but more recent work indicates that it is secreted by non-endocrine cells which line the walls of the various cavities. These 'pericavity cells' are chromophobic and linked to each other by desmosomes, and in their structure and their secretion of a glycoproteinaceous colloid they resemble the mucus-secreting stomodeal epithelial cells from which they ultimately derive (Mellinger, 1969; Alluchon-Gérard, 1971). The suggestion was recently made that they are homologous with the stellate cells found in the adenohypophysis in most vertebrates (Vila-Porcile, 1972), an idea returned to in chapter 15. Again, one is reminded of the follicles of the rostral pars distalis in primitive actinopterygian fishes which frequently are filled with a PAS+ colloid, and of the chromophobes lining the hypophysial canal in palaeoniscoid fishes, which apparently secrete a PAS+ material into the canal (chapter 9).

Giant cells, varying in number with endocrine condition, appear in the walls of the selachian cavities, and may resorb the colloid (Mellinger, 1969).

Experiments involving bioassay (Scanes *et al.* 1972), total or partial hypophysectomy, and replacement treatment with mammalian hormones have suggested that the ventral lobe secretes gonadotropin, and bioassay of different parts of the gland also locates TSH secretion in the ventral lobe (see Ball and Baker, 1969; Mellinger, 1972). ACTH has been located in the head of the dorsal lobe by bioassay (deRoos and deRoos, 1967), and in corroboration the cells of this region are activated by chemical or surgical adrenalectomy (Mellinger, 1969, 1972). The head of the dorsal lobe also secretes LTH, detectable by bioassay (Sage and Bern, 1972). Thus the head of the dorsal lobe and the ventral lobe taken together account for four of the five functions found in the teleost pars distalis. The rostral location of the sources of ACTH and LTH accords with the location of these functions in teleosts (chapter 10), and the head of the dorsal lobe may be truly homologous with the teleostean rostral pars distalis. In secreting TSH and gonadotropin, the ventral lobe resembles somewhat the teleostean proximal pars distalis (chapter 10); it may be that the missing hormone, STH, is secreted by the tail of the dorsal lobe, but we have no evidence for this at present, although certainly the selachian pituitary appears from limited data to be essential for growth (see Ball, 1969). The dilemma here is that the ventral lobe and the tail of the dorsal lobe together are apparently functionally equivalent to the proximal pars distalis of teleosts, and yet on embryological grounds the ventral lobe seems to be homologous with the tetrapod pars tuberalis, which is not represented as far as we know in teleost fishes. It is true that the mammalian pars tuberalis probably secretes some gonadotropin (see Legait, 1969; Pickford and Atz, 1957), and that the amphibian tuberalis has some unspecified endocrine function(s) (chapter 12), so that it would be wrong to regard the pars tuberalis as a non-functional lobe. But it is surprising to say the least to find that its probable homologue in elasmobranchs seems to be the sole source of gonadotropin and TSH.

The limited information we have about the histology of the elasmobranch adenohypophysis is sometimes contradictory, and cannot be related satisfactorily to the location of functions within the various regions of the gland. The head of the dorsal lobe, which apparently secretes ACTH and LTH, seems to contain only one cell-type which is quite unlike the corticotropes and lactotropes of teleosts. This cell is strongly PAS+, and OG+, AF− and AB−; thus it reacts as an amphiphilic cell-type (Ball and Baker, 1969; Alluchon-Gérard, 1971), not unlike the corticotropes of amphibians (chapter 12) and reptiles (chapter 13). The tail of the dorsal lobe, of uncertain endocrine function, contains acidophils, PAS+ to a varying extent though PAS− in the young post-embryonic dogfish *Scyllium canicula* (Alluchon-Gérard, 1971). The ventral lobe contains large basophils, PAS+, AF+ and AB+, which may represent two categories, possibly thyrotropes and gonadotropes (Ball and Baker, 1969).

In holocephalians, the dorsal lobe contains basophils, acidophils and chromophobes, while the Rachendachhypophyse contains two kinds of basophils, both PAS+, but one AF+, the other AF− (Ball and Baker, 1969).

Mellinger (1960b) has described neural ganglion cells, accompanied by glial elements, in the middle of the tail of the dorsal lobe of *Scyliorhinus caniculus*. The significance of this curious arrangement is quite unknown.

The *pars intermedia* lies below the neural lobe, with which it is intimately fused to form a composite neuro-intermedia. The degree of intermingling of the two components varies, but the intermedia cell cords are always penetrated to some extent by neural tissue. This region has been shown to secrete MSH in selachians (see Ball and Baker, 1969), and the intermedia cells, as in other vertebrates, contain large acidophilic and osmiophilic globules, variously interpreted as products of cellular degeneration or as hormone stores (see Ball and Baker, 1969). The intermedia cells may be arranged in distinct lobules separated by highly vascular connective tissue, or (fig. 8.1) the cell cords may fuse to form a parenchymatous mass penetrated by an irregular blood plexus (Meurling, 1962). The penetration of this lobe by neurohypophysial fibres may be slight, as in the sharks *Squalus* and *Etmopterus* (Meurling, 1962, 1963) or very extensive as in the dogfish *Scyliorhinus* (fig. 8.1) and the rays *Torpedo* and *Raia* (Della Corte and Chieffi, 1962; Knowles, 1965; Chevins, 1968). Most workers agree that only a single amphiphilic cell-type occurs in the pars intermedia cords, weakly PAS+ and staining with OG, azocarmine, etc. (Ball and Baker, 1969). Knowles (1965) differentiated peripheral and central cells in the intermedia cords of *Scyliorhinus stellaris*, on the basis of shape, position and ultrastructure, and suggested that they both probably secrete MSH but that the peripheral cells, closer to the blood vessels, might specialise in storage and sudden release of the hormone, while the central cells, which do not appear to store much MSH, might release the hormone slowly and maintain a steady background level of MSH as a 'tonic' stimulus to the melanophores. In the peripheral cells, Knowles (1965) distinguished a synthetic apical region from a basal hormone release region (fig. 8.1). In his original (1965) account, Knowles described type A neurosecretory fibres from the PON as terminating on the synthetic pole, and type B fibres, possibly from the NLT (Mellinger, 1962) as terminating on the release pole, and interpreted these observations as indicating that synthesis and release are under independent neurosecretory control. More recently, Knowles, Weatherhead and Martin (1970) have indicated that the synthetic pole in *S. stellaris* is innervated by both type A and type B fibres, and the same is true of both poles of the cells in the skate *Raja* (= *Raia*) *radiata* (Meurling and Björklund, 1970), which complicates the original hypothesis. No doubt there are species differences in the details of the innervation of the pars intermedia cells, and generalisations at this stage would be inadvisable. However, there can be no doubt that type A fibres do penetrate the pars intermedia in all selachians investigated to date, and that these fibres terminate on the MSH cells and, according to some reports, on the neuro-intermedia blood vessels as well (see Ball and Baker, 1969; Perks, 1969; Chevins and Dodd, 1970; Meurling and Björklund, 1970). Type B fibres have been recorded in this region less often, though it is impossible to be sure that this might not be due to the greater technical difficulty of identifying these fibres; for example, Mellinger (1962, 1963, 1964) described only type A fibres in the neuro-intermediate lobe of *Scyliorhinus caniculus*, although type B fibres must surely be present in view of Knowles' (1965) finding them in *S. stellaris*.

Mellinger (1962, 1963, 1964) showed that destruction of the PON-neurohypophysial tract in *S. caniculus* led to ultrastructural signs of hyperactivity in the intermedia cells and to continuous release of MSH, suggesting that the lesion had removed inhibitory control of both synthesis and release of MSH. In the embryo of *Squalus acanthias* with its distinct neural lobe and pars intermedia, Meurling (1972) has found evidence that hypothalamic inhibitory control of MSH secretion, which involves catecholamines in the intermedia, may be mediated by a combination of neuroglandular and neurovascular mechanisms. Chevins and Dodd (1970) working on *Raia* spp. found that not only tract section and ectopic transplantation of the neuro-intermediate lobe, but also destruction of the PON itself, led to excessive MSH secretion, which suggests either a single inhibitory control of both synthesis and release (contrary to Knowles' hypothesis) or a common origin for both type A and type B fibres in the PON. However, work on *Raia radiata* has shown that in the pituitary stem type A fibres travel medially while aminergic type B fibres travel laterally, making it possible to section either fibre tract independently (Meurling, Fremberg and Björklund, 1969; Meurling and Björklund, 1970); section of the type A fibres had little effect on MSH secretion, but reserpine treatment, or sectioning the type B tracts, led to sustained MSH secretion. Thus, type B aminergic fibres inhibit both synthesis and release of MSH in *R. radiata*, and the type A fibres seem not to be involved in pars intermedia control. Nevertheless, in *Raia* spp. (including *R. radiata*) both type A and type B fibres make synaptoid contacts with pars inter-media cells and with pituicytes, and some type B fibres also make non-synaptoid contacts with neuro-intermediate capillaries (Chevins, 1972). To reconcile all these findings, one must postulate either marked species variation, even within the same genus, in the role played by type A and type B fibres, or else suppose that the inhibitory type B fibres in the species studied by Chevins and Dodd (1970) originate in the PON rather than in the NLT. The matter clearly requires further investigations, although the salient feature of a hypothalamic inhibitory control of MSH secretion is firmly established.

THE NEUROHYPOPHYSIS AND BLOOD SUPPLY

The neurohypophysis can be divided into the *neural lobe*, derived from the ventral wall of the saccus infundibuli and in contact with the pars inter-media, the *infundibular stem*, and the *median eminence*. The dorsal wall of the saccus infundibuli gives rise to the *saccus vasculosus*, an enigmatic structure found in many fishes and always close to the neural lobe (figs. 8.1, 8.2, 8.4). In the hypothalamus, two neurosecretory centres are known. The *nucleus lateralis tuberis* (NLT) was first described in 1962 (Mellinger, 1962). It lies just beneath the ependymal lining of the infundibular recess, above the median eminence (fig. 8.4), and its cells do not contain classical NSM, but secrete AF− type B granules, 80 nm in diameter. Fibres from

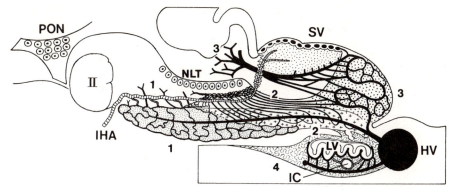

Fig. 8.4. *Scyliorhinus caniculus*. Diagrammatic sagittal section of the pituitary region, to show the blood supply. PON, preoptic nucleus; NLT, nucleus lateralis tuberis; II, optic nerve; IHA, inferior hypothalamic artery; SV, saccus vasculosus; LV, ventral lobe; HV, hypophysial vein; IC, anastomosis of internal carotid arteries; 1, head of the dorsal lobe, and the corresponding primary portal capillaries in the anterior median eminence; 2, tail of the dorsal lobe, and its portal vessels issuing from the glomeruloid capillaries of the posterior median eminence; 3, neuro-intermediate lobe, and its special venous supply; 4, ventral lobe, with its blood supply from the carotid system. From Follénius (1965).

the NLT seem to pass into the neuro-intermedia and to the median eminence. The cells of the NLT contain monamine oxidase, an indication that they secrete monoamines (Urano, 1971*a*). The *preoptic nucleus* (PON) is better known, lying close to the ependyma of the third ventricle (fig. 8.4), further anterior in sharks than in rays. Its cells contain AF + NSM, and this material can be seen in their dendritic projections into the third ventricle. Most PON fibres pass into the PON-neurohypophysial tract, running backwards in midline in the infundibular floor above the median eminence. Some fibres terminate in the median eminence, on the primary portal capillaries (Perks, 1969), and Mellinger (1964) has proposed that the PON elaborates two kinds of NSM corresponding to (i) granules 180 nm in diameter, which are distributed mainly to the neuro-intermedia (type A1 fibres), and (ii) granules 130 nm in diameter, which pass in type A2 fibres mainly to the median eminence.

The majority of PON fibres continue along the infundibular stem, perhaps generally confined to the median region as in *Raia radiata* (Meurling, Fremberg and Björklund, 1969). On entering the neuro-intermedia the PON fibres lie close to the ependymal lining of the infundibular recess, and ependymal processes project ventrally and mingle with the neurosecretory fibres. Some ependymal cells are enclosed within the tract itself, as pituicytes (Perks, 1969).

The architecture of the neuro-intermediate lobe varies from the perhaps primitive condition in the shark *Squalus*, in which a well-defined neural

6

lobe lies above the intermedia and sends nerve fibres down between the intermedia cords, to probably the most advanced condition, seen in skates and rays, and in the holocephalian *Hydrolagus* (Sathyanesan, 1965), in which there is total fusion of neural and intermedia tissue, with no sign of a discrete neural lobe (Perks, 1969). In the latter condition, the pars intermedia cords are elaborately penetrated by blood vessels and both type A and type B fibres. Where a discrete neural lobe occurs, it shows the usual three-layered arrangement, a dorsal ependyma overlying a middle fibre layer, poor in AF + NSM, and a ventral palisade layer, rich in NSM and in contact with a neuro-intermediate septum containing the plexus intermedius. The blood vessels of the pars intermedia derive from the plexus intermedius, and nerve fibres terminate on the plexus as well as passing beyond it to terminate on the intermedia cells. Thus the plexus intermedius with its capillary projections into the intermedia may form part of a neurovascular link for control of MSH secretion (Perks, 1969). In older specimens of *Squalus*, and in various primitive sharks, diverticuli of the infundibular recess penetrate into the pars intermedia, lined with ependymal cells and accompanied by nerve fibres (Ball and Baker, 1969; Perks, 1969), an arrangement strikingly like that found in the eel (chapter 10) and in ganoid fishes (chapter 9). In the advanced state of complete neuro-intermedia fusion there is no distinct neural lobe, and no trace of a neuro-intermedia septum and plexus intermedius; the compound tissue contains its own intrinsic capillary plexus, with abundant NSM, and type A and type B fibres. Transitional conditions between the two extremes have been found (Perks, 1969).

Type A neurosecretory terminations in the neuro-intermedia vary, and include direct contacts with the endocrine cells, endings on the plexus intermedius when it is present, on blood vessels within the intermingled gland of skates, and on pituicytes (Perks, 1969; Ball and Baker, 1969; Chevins and Dodd, 1970; Meurling and Björklund, 1970). In addition, type B fibres, some at least coming from the NLT (Mellinger, 1962*a*), have been found in the neuro-intermedia, and have been traced in various species to endings on the MSH cells (Perks, 1969; Ball and Baker, 1969; Meurling and Björklund, 1970; Chevins, 1972), and to endings near blood vessels in the compound neuro-intermedia (Ball and Baker, 1969; Meurling and Björklund, 1970; Chevins, 1972). Strong monoamine oxidase activity around the neuro-intermediate blood vessels of the dogfish *Triakis* is indicative of type B fibre terminations (Urano, 1971*a*).

It seems possible that there may be two categories of type A fibres in the neuro-intermedia, the one involved in control of the pars intermedia, and the other conveying neurohypophysial octapeptides (Acher, Chauvet and Chauvet, 1972) to be released into the blood vessels of the neuro-intermedia and thence into the general circulation. Mellinger (1962) distinguished type A1 fibres (granule diameter 180 nm) from type A2 fibres (granule diameter 130 nm), both occurring in the dogfish neuro-intermedia and both deriving from the PON.

The *median eminence* is elongated and lies in the infundibular floor above the dorsal lobe (figs. 8.2, 8.3, 8.4). It is separated from the dorsal lobe only by a connective tissue sheet that may be missing in places (Mellinger, 1966). In selachians, the median eminence is divisible into anterior and posterior regions, corresponding roughly to the division between head and tail of the adenohypophysial dorsal lobe (fig. 8.4). As in other fishes, branches from the inferior hypothalamic artery supply the primary capillary plexus (Mellinger, 1964; Follénius, 1965; Jasinski, 1969). The outer layer of the median eminence has the typical palisade structure. In the anterior region the primary capillaries are superficial, but in the posterior region in dogfish, though not in skates, they form two longitudinal groups of glomerular vessels, the glomerular loops pene-trating upwards into the palisade layer (fig. 8.4). In the anterior region, the primary capillaries are directly continuous with the capillaries of the head of the adenohypophysial dorsal lobe, with no formation of inter-vening portal vessels; however, in the posterior median eminence the glomeruloid capillary complex gives rise to distinct portal veins which run across the intervening space to supply the capillaries of the tail of the dorsal lobe (fig. 8.4). Type A2 fibres from the PON (secretory granules 130 nm in diameter) and type B fibres from the NLT (granules 80 nm in diameter) terminate on the anterior primary capillaries, usually in folds of the palisade layer which project downwards into the adenohypophysial tissue. Both types of fibres also end on the perivascular spaces of the glomeruloid capillaries in the palisade layer of the posterior median eminence (Mellinger, 1960a, 1962, 1964, 1966; Mellinger, Follénius and Porte, 1962; Follénius, 1965; Chevins, 1968). In the dogfish *Triakis*, monoamine oxidase activity, presumably in the type B fibre endings, is distributed throughout the median eminence and is particularly strong in the posterior region (Urano, 1972). The holocephalian median eminence is also elongated, but unlike the selachian structure it shows no division into anterior and posterior regions (Jasinski and Gorbman, 1966).

Blood from the primary portal vessels passes into both regions of the dorsal lobe, and in addition the posterior glomeruloid capillaries give rise to portal vessels which supply the neuro-intermedia in several selachians (Mellinger, 1960c; Follénius, 1965; Meurling, 1967a; Chevins, 1968), although the importance of these vessels varies with species and they are missing altogether in the dogfishes *Squalus* and *Etmopterus* (Meurling, 1967a). All parts of the selachian pituitary receive arterial blood from the carotid system, in addition to the portal supply (Mellinger, 1964; Follénius, 1965; Meurling, 1967a); the ventral lobe is generally described as receiving no portal blood at all (see Ball and Baker, 1969), but in *Raia* spp. it probably receives some, via the dorsal lobe vessels (Chevins, 1968). The relative importance of portal and arterial blood in the tail of the dorsal lobe varies with species; very little portal blood supplies this region in *Squalus* and *Etmopterus*, whereas in *Scyliorhinus* and *Pristiurus* nearly all its supply is portal (Meurling, 1967a). On first sight, the absence or insignificance of a portal supply to the ventral lobe is puzzling, since this region, secreting gonadotropin and TSH, would seem to be a likely target for hypothalamic NSM. However, although seasonal cycles in gonadotropic function certainly occur (Jørgensen, 1968), there is no evidence that they are in fact under hypothalamic control, since gonado-tropin secretion continues in *Scyliorhinus caniculus* after sectioning the PON-neurohypophysial tract and after lesioning the median eminence (Mellinger, 1964).

A specialisation in some selachians is that the neuro-intermediate lobe receives some blood from a pair of large lateral veins (fig. 8.4; Follénius, 1965). All parts of the pituitary drain into a posterior hypophysial vein.

In the holocephalians, the dorsal lobe receives only portal blood, and there is no portal supply to the neuro-intermedia (Jasinski and Gorbman, 1966; Meurling, 1967b).

All descriptions agree on the absence of direct neurosecretory inner-vation of the dorsal and ventral lobes, in contract to the pars distalis in teleosts (chapter 10), so that the portal system seems to be the only route for hypothalamic control. The presence in some selachians of a portal supply to the neuro-intermediate lobe is puzzling, in view of the rich neurosecretory innervation of this region. It recalls the prehypophysial–neurohypophysial portal system of myxinoids (chapter 7), but its func-tional significance in elasmobranchs remains unknown. The well-developed median eminence, with its glomeruloid capillaries and type A and type B terminations, is clearly similar to that in ganoid fishes, and its marked development is to be correlated with the absence of direct innervation of the pars distalis.

9

THE PITUITARY GLAND IN PRIMITIVE ACTINOPTERYGIAN FISHES

At the same time as elasmobranchs were evolving away from the original gnathostome stock, another group of fishes was pursuing an evolutionary destiny which was eventually to lead to the teleosts, the dominant fishes alive today. With a few exceptions, these fishes retained the ancestral bony skeleton, and because of the structure of their paired fins they are classified together with teleosts as the class Actinopterygii, the ray-finned fishes (fig. 7.1).

Still alive today are some non-teleostean actinopterygians, collectively termed the 'ganoid' fishes in reference to the ganoid-type scales some of them possess. These are descendants of ancient fishes which included the ancestors of the teleosts, and which were perhaps not very far from the main line of vertebrate evolution. There are two groups, the more primitive super-order Chondrostei (including the orders Palaeoniscoidei and Acipenseroidei), and the more recent super-order Holostei. The few living survivors of these once-numerous groups have something of the status of 'living fossils', and their pituitary gland is obviously of great potential interest in helping to clarify the evolutionary developments which led to the highly specialised gland of the teleosts.

SUPER-ORDER CHONDROSTEI

ORDER PALAEONISCOIDEI (=BRACHIOPTERYGII, POLYPTERIFORMES)

Two palaeoniscoid genera survive, *Polypterus* and *Calamoichthys*, living in African rivers and lakes. They are primitive in many respects, and their pituitary is not well-known. General accounts of the gland have been given by Dodd and Kerr (1963) and Wingstrand (1966a), Kerr (1968) has made a detailed histological study, and Lagios (1968) has made important ultrastructural observations on the median eminence, portal system and neurohypophysis.

The pituitary is apparently similar in both genera. Its most remarkable feature is the persistence in the adult of part of the ventral region of the solid Rathke's pouch, as the hypophysial (orohypophysial, buccohypophysial) duct or canal, opening ventrally into the roof of the mouth and

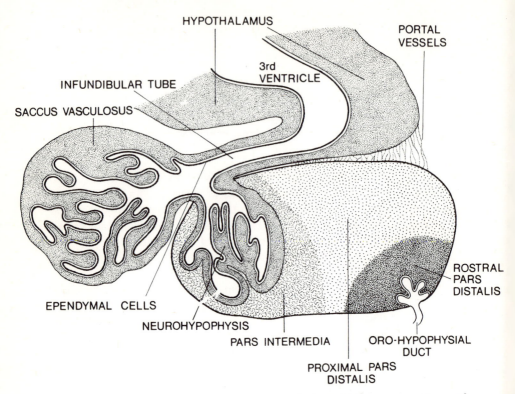

Fig. 9.1. Diagrammatic sagittal section of the pituitary and saccus vasculosus of *Polypterus ornatipinnis*, anterior to right. Note the continuation of the third ventricle (infundibular tube or recess) into the neurohypophysis and saccus vasculosus, and the close relationship between these two structures. From Marquet *et al.* (1972).

dorsally into an expanded space in the antero-ventral region of the pars distalis (fig. 9.1). Short diverticuli from this space penetrate the pars distalis, looking like vesicles when seen in cross section. This antero-ventral part of the gland, related to the hypophysial duct, is probably the homologue of the teleostean rostral pars distalis (Kerr, 1968; Lagios, 1968; Marquet *et al.* 1972). The hypophysial duct and its diverticuli are lined by columnar mucinous cells, regarded as mucus-secreting and non-endocrine by Lagios (1968), and certainly changing along the course of the duct to become indistinguishable from the mucous cells of the buccal epithelium, in shape as well as staining reactions (Kerr, 1968). Kerr described these duct cells as elongated adenohypophysial chromo-phobes, with a small mass of PAS+, AB+ secretion at their outer ends. In other ganoid fishes, and in primitive teleosts, the follicles of the rostral pars distalis, remnants of the hypophysial duct system (Kerr, 1968; Ball and Baker, 1969) are lined by acidophils (the lactotropes in teleosts), and

Kerr (1968) speculated that the duct cells changed function in the course of evolution, altering their staining reactions in the process. However fluorescent antibody to ovine LTH is bound by cells scattered throughout the pars distalis in both *Polypterus* and *Calamoichthys*, and not by the duct cells (Aler, 1971*b*); thus cells other than the duct cells are probably lactotropes in these fishes, and the duct cells are not likely to have given rise to lactotropes in evolution, contrary to the hypothesis advanced by Olsson (1967). It should be noted that the follicles of the teleostean rostral pars distalis, like the elasmobranch hypophysial cavities, frequently contain PAS+, AB+ colloid, which resembles the secretion of the palaeoniscoid duct cells, and which may be secreted by elements of the stellate cell system (chapters 8 and 15).

Apart from the duct cells, the rostral pars distalis consists of one (Kerr, 1968) or two (Lagios, 1968) types of basophils, PAS+, AB+, but AF−, which are intercalated between the bases of the duct cells, and also form cell cords between the adenohypophysial capillaries. According to Kerr (1968), his single (*type 3*) rostral basophil occurs also in the dorsal region (proximal pars distalis); as he points out, some teleosts also have a basophil cell type that occurs in both rostral and proximal regions, in some cases the gonadotrope, in others the thyrotrope (chapter 10).

The proximal pars distalis, which in fact lies dorsal to the rostral zone (fig. 9.1) contains a small scattered acidophil, and two further types of basophil, Kerr's *type 1* (AF−) and *type 2* (AF+). Type 1 is strongly PAS+, type 2 only weakly PAS+. It seems likely that type 1 is the small polygonal PAS+ cell of Lagios (1968), which with the EM is seen to have a convoluted nucleus and small tubular cisternae in the RER. The type 2 basophil may be the large amphiphil of Lagios (1968), which in his investigation was absent in young male *Polypterus* but abundant in mature female *Calamoichthys*. It displays ultrastructural similarities to teleost gonadotropes, including dilated RER cisternae, and it may well be the palaeoniscoid gonadotrope. Fluorescent antibody to ovine LTH located rather sparsely in cells scattered throughout the pars distalis, which may correspond to Kerr's scattered acidophil (Aler, 1971*b*). *Polypterus* pituitary contains an STH, which is immunochemically and biologically similar to rat STH (Hayashida, 1971), but its cellular source is unknown.

The pars intermedia is penetrated by neurohypophysial processes, and contains only one cell-type, PAS+ and (unusually) PbH− (Kerr, 1968; Lagios, 1968; Ball and Baker, 1969), arranged radially around the neurohypophysial projections. The intermedia cells are separated from the neural tissue by a double basement membrane, enclosing an extra-vascular space which contains strong inosine phosphatase activity (Marquet *et al.* 1972).

No NLT has been described in the hypothalamus, although type B

fibres are present in the median eminence. There is an elongated AF +
PON, indistinctly differentiated into magnocellular and parvocellular
regions, and this is a source of type A fibres, and possibly of type B fibres
also. An AF + PON-neurohypophysial tract runs via the internal layer
of the median eminence to the neural lobe (Kerr, 1968; Lagios, 1968;
Perks, 1969). No neurohypophysial processes or nerve fibres penetrate
the pars distalis, which in this respect is primitive and unlike the teleostean gland. Extensive and complicated processes of the neural lobe
penetrate the pars intermedia; these are hollow tubes containing diverticuli of the deep infundibular recess, as in primitive teleosts such as
Anguilla, and they are lined by an epithelium strikingly like that of the
saccus vasculosus (Marquet *et al.* 1972). As fig. 9.1 shows, the saccus
vasculosus and hollow neural lobe are closely linked in *Polypterus*,
which bears on discussions about the relationship between these two
structures. The lining of the neural lobe and its hollow processes contains
crown cells, which are generally regarded as confined to the saccus
vasculosus. These are secretory, and extrude material by apocrine secretion
into the infundibular recess (Marquet *et al.* 1972). There are also ependymal cells, and neurons with ciliated swollen ends which project into the
infundibular recess; these 'liquor-contacting neurons' have been described
in the walls of the third ventricle of all vertebrate classes, and they
probably release neurosecretory vesicles into the cerebrospinal fluid
(Marquet *et al.* 1972). Especially in possessing crown cells, probably
secreting a mucopolysaccharide or sugar and hitherto considered unique
to the saccus vasculosus, the lining of the neural lobe and its processes in
Polypterus furnishes independent evidence of the close affinity in fishes
of the saccus vasculosus and neural lobe, additional to the fact that both
structures derive embryologically from the saccus infundibuli (Wingstrand, 1966a).

Distally, the lumina of the neurohypophysial tubes become occluded,
but solid strands of ependymal cells continue together with neurosecretory
fibres deep into the cords of intermedia cells. The main PON-neurohypophysial tract ends in the neural lobe, which contains typical AF +
NSM. The fibres in the neural lobe contain type A granules, rather
electron-lucent and 106–167 nm in diameter, and these fibres have
synaptic endings on glial processes which surround the collagen-filled
perivascular space of the neural lobe capillaries (Lagios, 1968). These
terminations may well be the site of release of neurohypophysial hormones
into the bloodstream; typical octapeptides (arginine vasotocin and
isotocin) occur in these fishes (Perks, 1969; Sawyer, 1969). In addition,
type A fibres with larger secretory granules (120–229 nm in diameter)
innervate the pars intermedia, with synaptic endings on the very narrow
extravascular space that separates intermedia cells from the neural
processes (Lagios, 1968; Marquet *et al.* 1972). This second class of type A

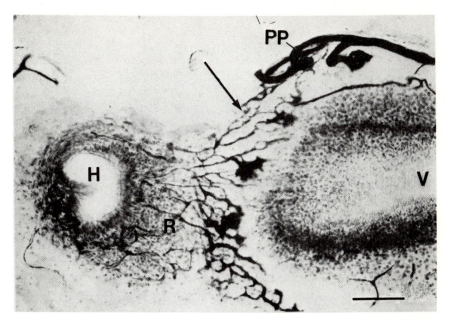

Fig. 9.2. *Calamoichthys calabaricus.* Coronal section through median eminence and rostral pars distalis (R) of specimen injected with Indian ink. H, hypophysial duct; V, third ventricle; PP, convoluted pre-portal arteriole. Arrow indicates primary capillaries in the median eminence; the dark blotches overlying these vessels are melanophores in the meninges. 50 μm section, alum–carmine nuclear stain. Scale, 100 μm. From Lagios (1968).

fibres presumably forms the main route for hypothalamic control of the pars intermedia, although the region is also irrigated by portal blood via the pars distalis capillary system (Lagios, 1968).

Polypterus and *Calamoichthys* possess a typical median eminence and portal system, in sharp contrast to their remote and phylogenetically younger cousins the teleosts. The sole vascularisation of the entire pituitary is portal according to Lagios (1968), although Kerr (1968) thought that an independent arterial supply reaches the neural lobe from vessels in the wall of the brain, rather as in the trout (chapter 10). The median eminence lies just ahead of the pituitary in the infundibular floor (figs. 9.1, 9.2). It is supplied by a subsidiary nerve tract from the PON; if the absence of an NLT be eventually confirmed, the PON may prove to be the source of both type A and type B fibres in these animals. The primary capillary network of the median eminence derives from looped and twisted arterioles from the hypophysial artery (fig. 9.2); such tortuous pre-portal arterioles have been noticed in many vertebrates, and may retard blood flow in order to facilitate neurohaemal exchanges in the median eminence. The primary capillary bed anastomoses from side to

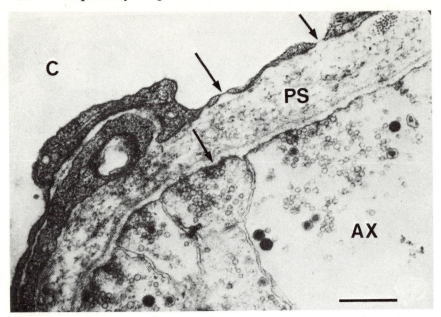

Fig. 9.3. *Calamoichthys calabaricus*. Electron micrograph of the median eminence neurohaemal contact area. AX, neurosecretory axon; PS, pericapillary space; C, capillary lumen. Arrows indicate fenestrations in the capillary endothelium, and synaptoid endings of the neurosecretory axons. Scale, 500 nm. From Lagios (1968).

side and lies within the median eminence palisade layers (fig. 9.2). From this plexus, portal vessels pass into the pars distalis (Lagios, 1968). The anterior vessels supply the rostral pars distalis, which lies ventrally (fig. 9.1), and these vessels are long and supported in connective tissue (Kerr, 1968). More posteriorly the primary capillaries lie so close to the proximal pars distalis that they tend to pass directly into the secondary capillaries of the glandular parenchyma without forming definite portal connections. The wide capillaries of the secondary plexus supply the pars distalis, pars intermedia and, in part, the neural lobe and saccus vasculosus, and the entire gland is drained by a pair of lateral hypophysial veins (Lagios, 1968; Kerr, 1968).

The detailed structure of the median eminence is remarkably like that of tetrapods. It is divided into two layers: below the ependyma, an inner layer contains the longitudinal AF+ PON-neurohypophysial tract, and below this an external thickened palisade layer displays little or no AF+ NSM, but contains many nerve fibres around the primary portal capillaries. These are nearly all type B fibres, with secretion granules 91–106 nm in diameter, very electron-dense, and containing also 'synaptic' vesicles. They make typical synaptic contacts with the basement membrane of the perivascular space around the primary portal capillaries; the capillary endothelium opposite these axonal terminations is occasionally fenestrated, and shows pinocytotic vesicles (fig. 9.3: Lagios, 1968). There can be no doubt that this arrangement, indistinguishable from the median eminence structure of many tetrapods, serves for the transfer of type B neurosecretory material into the portal blood and so to the adeno-hypophysis.

Points of particular interest in the brain–pituitary relationships of these primitive fishes are the presence of a definite median eminence and portal system; the absence of direct innervation of the pars distalis; the separation of type B fibres to supply the median eminence and type A fibres to supply the neural lobe and pars intermedia; and, though not established for certain, the possibility that both type A and type B fibres might originate in the PON.

ORDER ACIPENSEROIDEI (= ORDER CHONDROSTEI)

Of the two extant genera, the paddlefish (*Polyodon*) and sturgeon (*Acipenser*), the pituitary of sturgeons has been studied many times, particularly by Russian workers, but there is still little detailed information about its histophysiology, and very little is known about *Polyodon*.

The most notable anatomical feature is a large central hypophysial cavity within the adenohypophysis. This apparently represents the dorsal part of Řathke's pouch, although unlike the palaeoniscoids the sturgeons do not retain a hypophysial duct and the adenohypophysial anlage is in fact solid, the hypophysial cavity or cleft arising as a schizocoel, i.e. a split in the solid anlage (Kerr, 1949; Dodd and Kerr, 1963; Wingstrand, 1966a). The hypophysial cavity almost completely separates the posterior pars intermedia from the anterior pars distalis, and also largely splits the latter into dorsal and ventral zones (fig. 9.4). The cavity gives off numerous tubular extensions, mainly dorsally but also some running anteriorly and ventrally. In addition to these tubules there are in the anterior and ventral pars distalis numerous closed vesicles, not connected to the hypophysial cavity in the adult but probably derived from it during embryology (Kerr, 1949). These vesicles are presumably homologous with the follicles of the rostral pars distalis of holosteans and primitive teleosts. *Acipenser fluvescens* has acidophils oriented radially around the vesicles, often elongated like the LTH cells of primitive teleosts, and mixed with equally abundant basophils and chromophobes (Kerr, 1949). However, in the rostral region of *A. stellatus* Barannikova (1949) described strongly acidophilic cells together with amphiphils, and only a few basophils. In both species, the vesicles usually contain a basophilic colloid, similar to that in holostean and teleostean rostral zones. The rostral acidophils may secrete LTH, which has been detected in *Acipenser* pituitaries by bioassay (Sage and Bern, 1972).

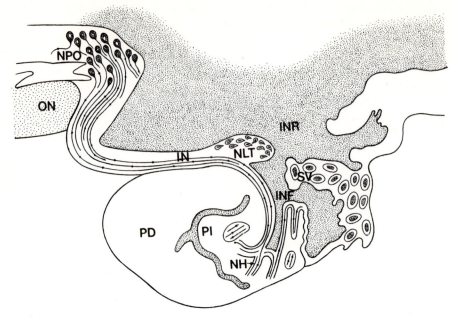

Fig. 9.4. *Acipenser fluvescens* (sturgeon). Diagrammatic sagittal representation of hypothalamic and pituitary structures, with lateral structures imposed. IN, infundibulum; INR, infundibular recess; NH, neurohypophysis (neural lobe); NLT, nucleus lateralis tuberis; NPO, nucleus preopticus (preoptic nucleus); ON, optic nerve; PD, pars distalis; PI, pars intermedia; SV, saccus vasculosus; INF, infundibular funnel. From Sathyanesan and Chavin (1967).

The ventral pars distalis, below the hypophysial cavity, was regarded by Kerr as an extension of the rostral zone, with the same cellular composition, but Barannikova separates this region from the rostral zone because its acidophils stain more weakly and it contains many more basophils and chromophobes. In the dorsal pars distalis Kerr (1949) described regular columns of cells, arranged around the tubular diverticuli of the central cavity and containing both basophils and acidophils. Barannikova (1949) states that this region contains the same cells as the ventral region (faint acidophils, basophils and chromophobes), together with strongly staining acidophils (the same as the rostral acidophil cell type?). Bioassay of dissected glands of *A. stellatus* located gonadotropin in the ventral and dorsal pars distalis (Barannikova, 1949); the basophils of these regions display secretory changes correlated with gonadal development, which identifies them as the gonadotropes (Barannikova, 1949, 1954). They display a marked development of acidophilic granules during their cycle of activity, similar to the lysosomal R granules of the gonadotropes in teleosts and amphibians (chapters 10 and 11). Since the gonadotropes are associated in both dorsal and ventral regions with a weakly-staining acidophil, it is reasonable to regard the two regions together as equivalent to the teleostean proximal pars distalis, the acidophil presumably being the source of the typical STH that has been detected by bioassay and radioimmunoassay in the acipenseroid pituitary (Hayashida and Lagios, 1969).

The pars intermedia is very large (fig. 9.4) and consists of cell cords almost entirely occupied by large basophils together with a few chromophobes and acidophils (Kerr, 1949). The neural lobe is hollow, and produces long hollow diverticuli lined with ependyma, which penetrate deeply among the pars intermedia cords. Neural and intermedia tissues are separated by a highly vascular double basement membrane. The relationships of the infundibular recess, saccus vasculosus, neural lobe diverticuli and pars intermedia are reminiscent of the palaeoniscoids (fig. 9.4). No neural processes or separate nerve fibres penetrate the pars distalis (Kerr, 1949; Sathyanesan and Chavin, 1967).

The hypothalamus contains an extensive PON, giving rise to the AF + PON-neurohypophysial tract which runs in the infundibular floor and extends to the neural lobe (Sathyanesan and Chavin, 1967; Perks, 1969). The cells of the PON and the NSM in the neural lobe show changes related to spawning and to osmotic stress (Polenov, Pavlovic and Garlov, 1972). The NLT lies in the usual position (fig. 9.4), with most of its cells AF − but a few AF +, and like the cells of the PON they have some dendrites projecting into the third ventricle (Sathyanesan and Chavin, 1967).

The neural lobe, mainly represented by hollow tubes between the pars intermedia cords, contains ependymal cells, a few pituicytes, and many type A and type B fibres, the latter containing catecholamines (Polenov, Garlov, Konstantinova and Belenky, 1972). The type A fibres (two categories, with secretory granules 140–180 nm and 100–140 nm in diameter) presumably originate in the PON, the type B (secretory granules 40–110 nm in diameter) in the NLT, but further studies are needed to confirm this distribution. Both types of fibres terminate on the basement membrane of the typical collagenous extravascular space separating the neural and intermedia elements, but no fibres have been found to penetrate beyond this boundary into the intermedia (Polenov, Garlov, Konstantinova and Belenky, 1972). The extravascular space contains large capillaries, and the entire arrangement is like that in the eel (chapter 10), some neurosecretory endings being related via the extravascular space to pars intermedia cells, and others to the capillaries. Some of the type B fibres contact ependymal cells in the neural lobe (Polenov, Garlov, Konstantinova and Belenky, 1972). Thus catecholamines from type B fibres may pass into capillaries, intermedia cells or ependymal cells, whereas the contents of type A fibres can reach only capillaries and intermedia cells. The type A fibres presumably secrete neurohypophysial

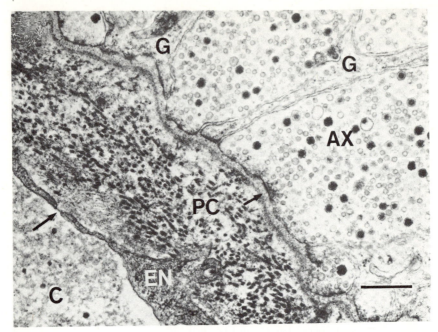

Fig. 9.5. *Acipenser transmontanus* (sturgeon). Electron micrograph of median eminence. Bulbous axons, AX, abut against basement membrane of pericapillary space, PC. The endothelium of the capillary, EN, is fenestrated (arrow). Other arrow indicates synaptoid region of neurosecretory axon termination. G, glial processes; C, capillary lumen. Scale, 500 nm. From Hayashida and Lagios (1969).

hormones into the capillaries, arginine vasotocin and a second principle being present in the sturgeon pituitary (Perks, 1969). Concerning the innervation of the pars intermedia, type A endings are more numerous than type B, but double innervation of the intermedia by both peptidergic (type A) and aminergic (type B) fibres is undoubtedly a feature of the sturgeon pituitary, as of the gland in other vertebrates (Polenov, Garlov, Konstantinova and Belenky, 1972). These workers emphasise that the amount of catecholamines in the sturgeon pituitary is greater than can be accounted for by the visible type B granules, and conclude that catecholamines in the gland need not always be present in granular form.

Predictably, the absence of direct innervation of the pars distalis is accompanied by a well-developed median eminence–portal system (Ball and Baker, 1969; Hayashida and Lagios, 1969). The dorsal surface of the pars distalis is closely applied to the anterior infundibular floor (fig. 9.4), the two structures being separated by a flat sheet of connective tissue. Blood vessels and nerve endings within this connective tissue form the median eminence, called the 'proximal contact area' by earlier workers (see Jasinski, 1969; Perks, 1969). The complex network of the primary capillaries receives endings of neurosecretory fibres (fig. 9.5), almost all type B; more dorsally, the PON-neurohypophysial tract passes backwards, containing mainly type A fibres, with secretory granules 130 nm or more in diameter (Hayashida and Lagios, 1969). In the neurohaemal contact region, numerous bulbous type B fibre endings, with 76–105 nm diameter secretory granules, mix with glial processes on the border of a very wide collagenous pericapillary space, the nerve endings being clearly synaptoid. The capillary endothelium opposite the fibre endings is characteristically fenestrated (fig. 9.5). The source of these median eminence type B fibres is uncertain; Sathyanesan and Chavin (1967) described a ventral branch of the PON-neurohypophysial tract, which may innervate the median eminence as in palaeoniscoids, but with the presence of an NLT now established (Sathyanesan and Chavin, 1967), the type B fibres are more likely to originate there. From the primary capillary plexus, short vessels pass into the underlying pars distalis. The acipenseroid median eminence–portal system is obviously comparable to that in tetrapods, particularly in the urodele amphibians (chapter 12), but in contrast to other ganoid fishes the neurohaemal contact zone lies outside the neural bulk of the median eminence, within a connective tissue lamina.

SUPER-ORDER HOLOSTEI

The holostean fishes evolved from the early chondrosteans, radiated widely, and were the dominant bony fishes during the Triassic, later being replaced by their descendants, the teleosts (fig. 7.1). Today there are only two living holosteans, inhabitants of freshwaters in North America, the bowfin *Amia* and the garpike, *Lepisosteus* (= *Lepidosteus*). As the closest living primitive relatives of the teleosts, the pituitary of these forms has some very interesting features. A general account of the holostean pituitary was given by Kerr (1949), and Ball and Baker (1969) have recently studied the gland with more modern and discriminating staining techniques. The hypothalamo-neurohypophysial system was described by Sathyanesan and Chavin (1967), and the median eminence–portal system by Lagios (1970).

The adenohypophysial anlage is solid, as in all actinopterygians, and the hypophysial cleft appears as a transitory schizocoel (Wingstrand, 1966a). Neither genus preserves a hypophysial cavity or hypophysial duct in the adult. The pituitary lies attached along most of its length to the infundibular floor, with vascular connective tissue in between. The pituitary of *Amia* is relatively shorter and deeper than that of *Lepisosteus*, and is rotated forwards to lie below the optic chiasma (fig. 9.6). A large and elaborate saccus vasculosus lies behind and close to the pituitary. In both genera, but more especially in *Lepisosteus*, the pars distalis resembles that of sturgeons in having mixtures of cell-types in broad transitional

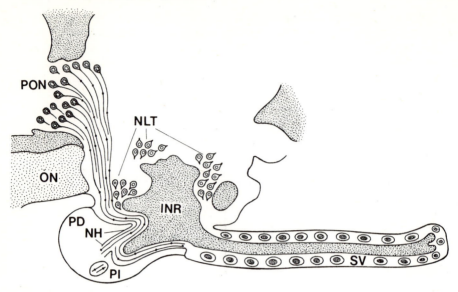

Fig. 9.6. *Amia calva*. Diagrammatic sagittal representation of hypothalamo-hypophysial interrelationships with lateral structures imposed. Note the division of the preoptic nucleus (PON) into dorsal pars magnocellularis and ventral pars parvocellularis. ON, optic nerve; PD, pars distalis; PI, pars intermedia; NH, neurohypophysis (neural lobe); NLT, nucleus lateralis tuberis; INR, infundibular recess; SV, saccus vasculosus. From Sathyanesan and Chavin (1967).

zones, but nevertheless it is more possible in these fish than in the other ganoids to distinguish rostral and proximal pars distalis, as in teleosts. *Amia* pituitary is the better-known, and the following account applies mainly to this genus, although *Lepisosteus* exhibits only minor differences (Kerr, 1949; Ball and Baker, 1969).

The rostral pars distalis contains the characteristic closed vesicles or follicles (fig. 9.7) also found in primitive teleosts (chapter 10). It is likely from embryological evidence that these follicles do indeed represent diverticuli from the hypophysial cleft (Kerr, 1949). They are lined by elongated acidophils, erythrosinophilic after Aliz BT, and very like the lactotropes of the eel; these *acidophils 1* are the probable source of LTH, which has been detected by bioassay in *Amia* pituitary at about the same concentration as in teleosts (Sage and Bern, 1972). Intercalated amongst these cells, but not usually reaching the follicular lumen, is a second cell-type, *acidophil 2*, erythrosinophilic but also taking alizarin blue, so that it generally stains a blue-red in contrast to the scarlet acidophil 1 after Aliz BT. Acidophil 2 is strongly PbH +, and in its staining properties it resembles the teleostean corticotrope. The follicular lumen usually contains a colloidal material, PAS+, AB+ and AF+, resembling the follicular colloid of the eel and salmon (chapter 10). A few cells of the

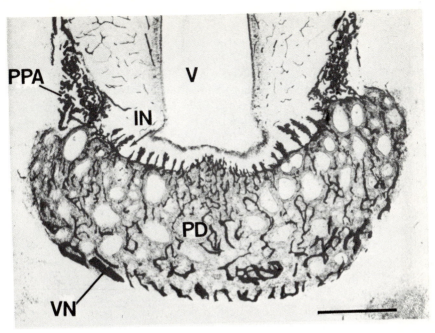

Fig. 9.7. *Amia calva*. Thick (50 μm) coronal section through median eminence and rostral pars distalis after vascular perfusion of Indian ink. PD, pars distalis, largely composed of rostral follicles at this level; V, third ventricle; IN, infundibulum; PPA, convoluted preportal arterioles; VN, venous network on surface of gland. Arrow indicates the capillary glomeruloids of the median eminence. Alum–carmine nuclear stain. Scale, 0.5 mm. From Lagios (1970).

proximal pars distalis may be mixed with the follicles, especially in the ventral region. Also ventrally, the follicles are joined by a very peculiar cell-type. This is strongly PAS+, AF+, AB+ and PbH+, and has therefore been called *basophil 1* (Ball and Baker, 1969). However, after Aliz BT, its coarse refractile granulation is brilliantly stained with erythrosin; the cell usually also contains a few large perinuclear aniline blue+ granules, which, together with the larger size of its erythrosinophilic granules and details of cell shape, allow an easy distinction between basophil 1 and the erythrosinophilic acidophil 1 after Aliz BT. It may be that basophil 1 should be called an amphiphil. A mantle of these cells extends laterally and ventrally round the gland, enclosing the proximal pars distalis and neuro-intermedia, and containing an admixture of acidophils 1 and 3. Although there is no experimental evidence, its staining properties and distribution suggest that basophil 1 may be a gonadotrope.

The proximal pars distalis is composed of vertical cell cords. Prominent in the cords is an *acidophil 3*, sharply distinguished from acidophils 1 and

2 by staining with OG after Aliz BT, and very possibly a somatotrope. Like the teleostean somatotrope, acidophil 3 has a slight PAS affinity. An STH, with considerable biological and immunochemical relatedness to mammalian STH, occurs in both *Amia* and *Lepisosteus* (Hayashida, 1971). The acidophil 3 is most numerous dorsally, close to the connective tissue interface with the median eminence and infundibular floor, but it occurs throughout the proximal pars distalis. Two kinds of basophils are present, although it is difficult to be certain that they do not represent two stages in the cycle of a single cell-type. *Basophil 2* is the smaller, with rounded contours, stains a clear blue in Aliz BT, is slate-blue after AB–PAS–OG and is AF+ and PbH+; this cell occurs mostly in the dorsal and central regions. *Basophil 3* is larger, with angular contours, and stains lavender in Aliz BT (it contains scattered red granules as well as dull blue granules), often with a few large clear blue granules close to the nucleus. It stains magenta with AB–PAS–OG, and is more strongly AF+ and PbH+ than basophil 2. It occurs mostly in the ventral and lateral regions. Basophils 2 and 3 probably correspond to the two basophils described by Kerr (1949), and one of them is presumably a thyrotrope. If the other is indeed a separate cell-type, its function is at present uncertain.

The pars intermedia is elaborately invaded by branching processes of the neural lobe, which are hollow proximally with a lining of ependymal cells. Two intermedia cell-types can be distinguished: a predominant PbH+ cell, with the club-shape often displayed by the similar cell of teleosts (chapter 10), its prolongation being in contact with the neuro-intermedia interface; and a rather scarce PAS+ cell, which is usually rounded. The PbH+ cell stains various shades of blue after Aliz BT, and with the same stain the PAS+ cell is variably amphiphilic, colouring red to mauve.

In the hypothalamus the PON is like that of teleosts, divisible into dorsal pars magnocellularis and ventral pars parvocellularis. The NLT is rather diffuse (fig. 9.6) and divisible into several regions (Sathyanesan and Chavin, 1967). The neural lobe is essentially the thin floor of the infundibulum which has folded down and penetrated the pars intermedia by a hollow projection, the infundibular funnel, its cavity continuous with the third ventricle. Branches of the funnel, hollow tubes lined by ependyma and neurosecretory fibres, penetrate between the pars inter-media cell cords, and distally these become solid processes with a central core of ependymal cells. The neural lobe is rich in NSM, AF+, AB+, PAS+, CAH+ and aniline blue+. Most of the neurosecretory fibres come from the PON, and some terminate on capillaries, but a few AF− fibres from the NLT also enter the neural lobe (Sathyanesan and Chavin, 1967). The pituitary has been shown to contain typical octapeptides (arginine vasotocin, isotocin), which may be released by the PON fibre endings on the capillaries of the plexus intermedius, in the boundary between neural and intermedia tissue (Perks, 1969); however, Lagios (1970) could find only occasional type A fibre perivascular endings on capillaries in his EM study.

In contrast to teleosts, no large neurohypophysial processes penetrate the pars distalis, and it used to be thought that there was no direct innervation of this region (see Ball and Baker, 1969; Perks, 1969). However, it now seems that small numbers of neural lobe processes, containing AB+ NSM, extend into and abut against the posterior cell cords of the proximal pars distalis, and in places these cords also border the main part of the neural lobe (Lagios, 1970). At such places the pars distalis cells are separated from neural tissue by a typical extravascular space, and on the neural border of this space can be found the endings of many type A fibres (granule size 124–201 nm), together with occasional type B fibres (granule size 74–120 nm) (fig. 9.8). We see here the beginnings, as it were, of the neurohypophysial 'invasion' of the pars distalis so characteristic of teleosts (Lagios, 1970).

Innervation of the pars intermedia is similar to that of other ganoids and primitive teleosts, with type A fibres making synaptoid contact on the basement membrane of the collagenous intervascular space separating the neural processes from the endocrine cells. This immensely sinuous intervascular division, extending around all the neural lobe diverticuli, represents the simple neuro-intermedia septum seen in cyclostomes and tetrapods, and the numerous capillaries within it represent the plexus intermedius. There are also rare examples (fig. 9.8) of type A fibres penetrating beyond this septum and making direct synaptoid contacts with intermedia cells (Lagios, 1970); these direct neuro-intermedia contacts, absent in other ganoids, are common in teleosts (chapter 10).

It is particularly interesting that together with the slight but phylogenetically novel direct innervation of the pars distalis, the modern holosteans preserve a well-developed median eminence, more highly developed indeed than the median eminence of the acipenseroids which show no hint of direct pars distalis innervation. The median eminence–portal system of *Amia*, very like that of tetrapods, but a primitive feature in the context of actinopterygian evolution, has been described in detail by Lagios (1970), and a light-microscope account was given earlier (Ball and Baker, 1969). Lying dorsal to the pars distalis, the median eminence occupies the entire width of the infundibular floor, the connective tissue between the infundibulum and the pituitary being here very thin (fig. 9.7). Blood reaches the median eminence from a branch of the hypothalamic artery. The vascular organisation is typical, with convoluted pre-portal arterioles, and an elaborate primary capillary bed consisting of many discrete groups (glomeruloids) of two or three capillary loops which anastomose between their afferent and efferent limbs deep within the median eminence itself (fig. 9.7). As Lagios (1970) points out,

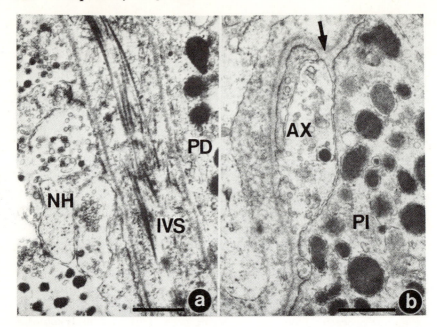

Fig. 9.8. (*a*) *Amia calva.* Electron micrograph of part of proximal pars distalis. Neurohypophysial process (NH) in relation to intervascular space (IVS) bordering a pars distalis (PD) cell. Note type B axon endings upper left, and a type A axon, lower left. Scale, 500 nm. From Lagios (1970).

(*b*) *Amia calva.* Electron micrograph of pars intermedia. Synaptoid contact of type A axon (AX) with pars intermedia cell (PI). Note axon lying within basement membrane of pars intermedia; arrow indicates the continuity of the basement membrane. Scale, 500 nm. From Lagios (1970).

these capillary loops are as well-developed as the glomeruloid complexes of the mammalian median eminence, and they also resemble the glomeruloids of the posterior median eminence in selachians (chapter 8). From the glomeruloids, short portal vessels pass directly into the pars distalis. Neurosecretory fibres end against the distal parts of the glomeruloids, and, especially anteriorly, contain NSM similar to that in the NLT (Ball and Baker, 1969). With the EM, each glomeruloid capillary is seen to be surrounded by a typical perivascular space, contacted by infrequent glial processes and by numerous synaptoid endings of type B fibres. The perivascular space commonly contains several overlapping strata of endothelial-cell processes among the more usual collagen fibres, and the endothelium itself is fenestrated (fig. 9.9; Lagios, 1970). The anterior short portal vessels enter the pars distalis and form a secondary perifollicular capillary plexus in the rostral pars distalis, which supplies the capillaries in the connective tissue between the cords of the proximal pars distalis. Portal vessels from the more posterior median eminence supply

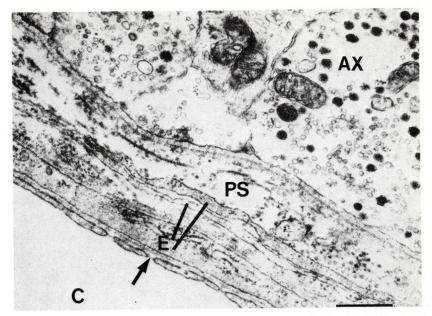

Fig. 9.9. *Amia calva.* Electron micrograph of the median eminence. Bulbous type B axonal ending (AX), with clear 'synaptic' vesicles and large dense-cored vesicles, abutting on perivascular space (PS) containing abundant collagen fibres and layered endothelial cell processes (E). C, capillary; arrow indicates fenestration in surface endothelium. Scale, 500 nm. From Lagios (1970).

the proximal pars distalis directly (cf. elasmobranchs, chapter 8). Capillaries from the pars distalis system supply the convoluted plexus intermedius. The portal system apparently supplies blood to the entire gland, with no separation of a posterior independent vascular bed such as occurs in some teleosts (chapter 10). As in teleosts, blood drains from the pituitary by a superficial venous plexus (fig. 9.7; Lagios, 1970).

We have seen in this chapter that all the primitive actinopterygians have a median eminence, sandwiched between the infundibular floor and the pars distalis. Its blood capillaries and portal vessels, like those in all vertebrates, can be regarded as specialisations of the generalised 'mantle plexus' of this region. It is easy to imagine the evolution of the teleostean condition, with its median eminence enclosed within the pars distalis, and with neurosecretory fibres reaching beyond the enclosed portal system to innervate the distalis cells directly. What the pituitary of *Amia* indicates is that innervation of the pars distalis started in evolution before any modification of the median eminence–portal system.

10

THE PITUITARY GLAND
IN TELEOST FISHES

After the chondrosteans and the holosteans, the actinopterygian stock gave rise to the teleosteans, which flourished exceedingly and now form the major component of the fish fauna in all habitats. With more than 20000 known living species, the super-order Teleostei includes animals which differ widely in biology; the group has radiated to occupy all possible aquatic ecological niches, and has even ventured with some success on to land. The pituitary gland in these animals is remarkably specialised in two fundamental ways: in the loss of the typical median eminence and portal system external to the pituitary; and in the direct innervation of the pars distalis by hypothalamic neurosecretory fibres. The two features are obviously interrelated, and presumably evolved together. Possibly related to the direct innervation of the cells is the fact that the various cell-types in the pars distalis are distributed in definite zones, which has considerably facilitated investigations on the gland. It must be realised that in this group we are dealing with end-products of a line of evolution quite separate from the line that led to terrestrial vertebrates, so that it is not surprising that the pituitary gland should have evolved its radical specialisations.

Detailed reviews on the pituitary gland of teleosts have recently been published, and references for undocumented statements made in this chapter will be found in these reviews (Ball and Baker, 1969; Sage and Bern, 1971).

THE PITUITARY GLAND IN GENERAL

The pituitary gland at first sight appears to be almost as varied as the teleosts themselves, but closer examination shows that this variety can be reduced to a common anatomical and histological pattern. Two species in which the pituitary has been studied in detail are the European eel, *Anguilla anguilla*, and the molly, *Poecilia latipinna*, a small euryhaline and viviparous cyprinodont which lives in Atlantic coastal regions of the southern USA and Central America. The pituitaries of these two teleosts will serve as basic types, and notable departures from them will then be considered.

The adenohypophysis develops as a solid anlage, but a hypophysial cleft may arise later as a schizocoel, a development found in some primitive teleosts such as the herring. Remnants of the cleft are found in the adult of some primitive forms. The fact that the anlage is solid obscures embryological comparisons with other vertebrates, but nevertheless the relationships between the various regions of the gland in teleosts and tetrapods are now well established and generally accepted (Wingstrand, 1966a).

THE PITUITARY OF THE EEL, *Anguilla anguilla*

The two primary divisions of the gland are obvious in sagittal section (fig. 10.1), with the central neurohypophysis interdigitating with the adenohypophysis. The latter is divisible into a posterior *pars intermedia* and an anterior *pars distalis*, but the two are more closely fused than in tetrapods to form a compact adenohypophysis. The pars distalis is divisible on the basis of its histology into rostral and proximal regions. The interdigitations of the neurohypophysis with the pars intermedia are very deep and elaborate, a common feature in teleosts, while the interdigitations with the pars distalis are less pronounced. The extensive penetration of the pars distalis by neurohypophysial processes is a teleostean specialisation, foreshadowed in holostean fishes (chapter 9), but found nowhere else. The adenohypophysis and neurohypophysis are separated by an elaborately folded basement membrane which is probably always double and incorporates an intervascular space (Vollrath, 1966; Knowles and Vollrath, 1966a, b). It is likely that this structure occurs in all teleosts (see Leatherland, 1970a, b, c; Nagahama and Yamamoto, 1970).

The rostral pars distalis contains three cell-types. Most numerous are the η cells, shown experimentally to secrete LTH. In the eel these cells are arranged in follicles, as in other primitive teleosts. Between the follicles are masses and cords of δ cells, secreting TSH, and at the posterior border of the rostral pars distalis with the neurohypophysis is a layer of ϵ (ACTH) cells. The proximal pars distalis includes two cell-types arranged in vertical cords. The bulk of the cords is formed of α cells, which secrete STH, and they are mixed with gonadotropes. The pars intermedia includes two cell-types, the functions of which are not precisely known. The infundibular stem is extremely short in the eel, and grades into the neurohypophysis, which is enclosed by the adenohypophysis except dorsally (fig. 10.1). The neurohypophysis is not clearly divisible into median eminence and neural lobe, but it does show some differentiation in that the posterior region, in contact with the pars intermedia, contains much more AF + NSM than the anterior region, in contact with the pars distalis; there are reasons for thinking that the anterior region corresponds to the median eminence, the posterior region to the neural lobe.

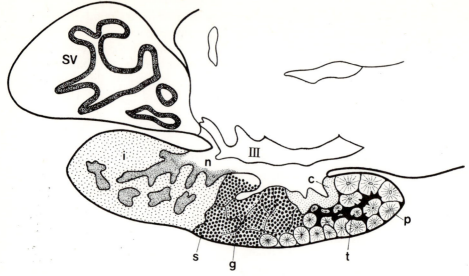

Fig. 10.1 *Anguilla anguilla*. Diagram of midsagittal section through the eel pituitary, anterior to the right. Follicles of lactotropes (p), mixed with TSH cells (t), and bordered posteriorly by ACTH cells (c), form the rostral pars distalis. The proximal pars distalis comprises cords of cells below the neurohypophysis (n), mainly composed of somatotropes (s) in the sexually immature fish, with scattered immature gonadotropes (g). Posteriorly is the pars intermedia (i), deeply invaded by processes of the neurohypophysis which in this region displays masses of AF+ neurosecretory material (fine stipple). The saccus vasculosus (SV) projects behind the pituitary. III, third ventricle. From Olivereau (1967a).

In the eel, as in most fishes, there lies posterior to the pituitary a thin-walled median downgrowth of the floor of the infundibular recess, the saccus vasculosus (fig. 10.1). In embryology this is derived from the aboral or dorsal surface of the saccus infundibuli, and so has been regarded by some authorities as homologous with the tetrapod neural lobe (Wingstrand, 1966a). Despite its close proximity to the pituitary, the saccus vasculosus seems to have no functional endocrine connections with the gland.

THE PITUITARY OF THE MOLLY, *Poecilia latipinna*

The pituitary of *Poecilia* is much deeper and shorter than the gland in the eel (colour plate), and it differs in some other respects. The rostral pars distalis contains only two endocrine cell-types, a mass of LTH cells, showing no trace of a follicular arrangement, and a posterior border of ACTH cells against the neurohypophysis. In contrast to the eel, the TSH cells in *Poecilia* lie in the proximal pars distalis, in a dorsal zone in which they are mixed with STH cells. The ventral pars of this region is occupied by a mass of gonadotropes. The neurohypophysis penetrates the glandular regions more extensively than in the eel, especially in the proximal pars distalis. The pars intermedia is much smaller than in the eel, and is not penetrated as deeply by neurohypophysial processes. It contains two cell-types, corresponding to those in the eel. *Poecilia* does not have a saccus vasculosus. The pituitary of another cyprinodont, *Oryzias latipes*, is virtually identical with that of *Poecilia* (Aoki and Uemura, 1970).

OTHER TELEOSTS

Departures from the general morphology and cell distribution seen in the eel and the molly are widespread and various, most obvious being the wide variations in the shape of the pituitary and in the proportions of its component parts. A common type has a much shorter longitudinal axis, and is much deeper dorso-ventrally (colour plate). In such cases (e.g. cyprinids, salmonids), the gland in the juvenile fish may have the flattened bun-shape seen in the eel and molly, but its shape changes as the fish grows (Olivereau, 1954, 1968). In these deeper glands, the neurohypophysis usually forms an elongated axis, more-or-less vertical, with the three regions of the adenohypophysis arranged in layers around it, the pars intermedia lying most ventral, with the proximal pars distalis immediately above, and the rostral pars distalis forming an incomplete ring embracing the neurohypophysis anteriorly (Olivereau, 1968). In this type of pituitary the ramifications of the neurohypophysis into the large pars intermedia are very elaborate (colour plate).

One of the most important variables in the teleostean gland is the location of the TSH cells, which may, as in *Poecilia*, lie in the proximal pars distalis (e.g. *Astyanax*, *Caecobarbus*, cyprinodonts, *Gasterosteus*, *Cichlasoma*, *Anoptichthys*), or they may be rostrally placed among the LTH cells, as in the eel (e.g. clupeoids, goldfish and other cyprinids). There are teleosts in which the TSH cells lie in an intermediate position, some in the rostral and some in the proximal regions (e.g. some cichlids, *Mugil*, salmonids). This variable position of the TSH cells is one of the reasons why the rostral/proximal division of the pars distalis is only a matter of descriptive convenience, and is not of fundamental morphological importance. Another variable is the position of the gonadotropes, which usually lie in the proximal pars distalis but in the trout occur in both rostral and proximal zones. Even in the eel, some gonadotropes invade the rostral pars distalis at full sexual maturity.

Another variation, and one that seems to be correlated with phylogeny, concerns the structure of the rostral pars distalis. In the more primitive teleosts (the isospondylous forms, including clupeoids, salmonids and apodes), the LTH cells are arranged in follicles (colour plate), as in the eel, and as in the living ganoid fishes which are related to the ancestors of teleosts (chapter 9). In certain juvenile clupeoids (including the herring) and in the young of some other primitive teleosts, an orohypophysial duct is present, like that in palaeoniscoids (chapter 9). The duct persists in the adult of a few primitive forms (e.g. *Elops*, *Hilsa ilisha*; Sathyanesan, 1963; Wingstrand, 1966*a*; Olsson, 1967), and the follicles of the rostral pars distalis in isospondylous fishes probably represent derivatives of the duct, and as such should be regarded as remnants of the hypophysial cleft, which arises as a schizocoel and persists as the orohypophysial duct in the herring (see Wingstrand, 1966*a*; Olsson, 1967). In most teleosts the orohypophysial duct is never developed, and the only widespread remnant of the system is seen in the follicles of primitive forms. In all the more advanced teleosts the lactotropes form a compact mass, with no trace of a follicular organisation (colour plate).

Despite these and other variations in the morphology of the gland, the teleost pituitary when studied in detail usually presents the principal regions described for the eel and *Poecilia*. In certain cases, however, the morphology of the gland is more unusual. For example, a Japanese goby, *Lepidogobius lepidus*, is reported as having four tinctorially distinct zones in the pars distalis, with no indications of how these relate to the usual bipartite pattern of this region; another curious feature of this fish is that there is little interdigitation of neurohypophysis and adenohypophysis, which recalls the juvenile condition in other teleosts (p. 203).

In many teleosts the infundibular stem is virtually absent, and the pituitary is pressed closed to the hypothalamic floor. An extreme example of this 'platybasic' type of gland is seen in the gobiidae (including *Lepidogobius*), in which the pituitary is pressed up into the hypothalamus, almost occluding the third ventricle and necessitating a devious course for the PON-neurohypophysial tract. At the opposite extreme are those teleosts with a distinct infundibular stem (the 'leptobasic' type), which may be extremely long and attenuated, as in *Lophius* bringing the pituitary forward to lie ahead of the brain (Wingstrand, 1966*a*). Another peculiar arrangement is seen in the sea-horse, *Hippocampus*, in which the neuro-hypophysis extends to enclose the pars intermedia, so that the posterior part of the gland consists of a central core of intermedia enclosed in a sleeve of neurohypophysial tissue.

No fish has a typical pars tuberalis, nor is there any evidence of its homologue in teleosts.

HISTOPHYSIOLOGY OF THE PARS DISTALIS

Experimental work in many laboratories and on many different species has shown that the teleost pituitary secretes the usual complement of hormones, though probably only a single gonadotropin (Pickford and Atz, 1957; Ball and Olivereau, 1966; Ball, 1969; Burzawa-Gérard and Fontaine, 1972; Chester Jones *et al.* 1973). Each of the hormones has been allocated by experimental work to one of the various cell-types. In contrast to the situation in amphibians (chapter 12), there is little disagreement about the functions of the morphological cell-types, so that it is possible to use a functional terminology for the cells of the teleost pars distalis.

LTH CELLS (LACTOTROPES, PROLACTIN CELLS, η CELLS)

Despite earlier controversies it is now certain that the pituitary secretes a prolactin-like hormone (sometimes called paralactin or fish prolactin), which plays a role in osmoregulation in many teleosts (Ball, 1969; Ensor and Ball, 1972). Evidence discussed below shows that this hormone originates from the η cells.

The lactotropes lie mainly in the rostral region, forming the compact mass that in most teleosts defines the rostral pars distalis. These cells also extend ventrally and laterally for a variable distance around the edge of the proximal pars distalis. The secretory granules stain red with erythrosin in Aliz BT and Cleveland–Wolfe trichrome, or with the azocarmine or acid fuchsin in other techniques such as Azan, Mallory and Masson. They are totally negative to PAS, AF and AB. In the living gland the granules are opaque, so that it is easy to locate the lactotropes as a dense white mass. In the primitive forms in which the lactotropes are arranged in follicles, the follicular lumen usually contains a colloidal material with variable staining properties, some taking OG, some PAS, AF, aniline blue and light green. EM studies have shown that some of this material is derived from degenerating cells (Knowles and Vollrath, 1966b, d). In such fishes (e.g. eel, salmonids, herring) the LTH cells are columnar, with apical cilia and microvilli projecting into the follicular lumen. Adjacent cells may be joined by desmosomes, and interspersed between them are occasional non-secretory 'neck cells', which are probably part of the stellate cell system (p. 191). The secretory granules are usually concentrated at the outer (basal) pole of the cell, a region rich in RNA and RER, while the Golgi complex lies on the follicular side of the nucleus (Knowles and Vollrath, 1966b; Ball and Baker, 1969; Hopkins and Baker, 1968; Nagahama and Yamamoto, 1969a). The membrane-bound spherical secretory granules are 280 nm in diameter in freshwater *Anguilla*, but smaller (200 nm) in elvers and adults caught at sea (Knowles and Vollrath, 1966b, d; Hopkins and Baker, 1968), and they increase from 140 to 260 nm in diameter as elvers ascend the rivers from the sea (Vollrath, 1966); they are 350 nm in diameter in the marine *Conger* (Knowles and Vollrath, 1966b) and 200 to 350 nm in the freshwater stage of the salmon *Oncorhynchus* (Nagahama and Yamamoto, 1969a). The Golgi complex in immature freshwater *Anguilla* consists of six to eight parallel cisternae, forming a bowl- or cup-shaped body, and EM studies suggest that the secretory granules are formed here, the outer convex surface of the Golgi complex perhaps receiving newly synthesized protein from the RER, the concentrated material then being released as membrane-bound granules at the inner concave surface (Hopkins and Baker, 1968).

The lactotropes of more advanced teleosts, not arranged around follicles, may be rather elongated in some species, but are more usually rounded cells as in *Poecilia* (colour plate). They are generally evenly granulated with no indications of the intracellular polarisation seen in *Anguilla*. In cyprinodonts such as *Poecilia* and *Fundulus* the nucleus is often indented or kidney-shaped, and with the light microscope the Golgi complex is easily visible in active cells as one or more clear tubules amongst the granules, curved in a U- or C-shape. The cytoplasmic RNA (=RER) forms a cap or halo on the nucleus. Fluorescent antibody to ovine LTH locates specifically on the granules of the lactotropes in various teleosts (*Fundulus, Oncorhynchus, Cichlasoma, Carassius, Leucisus, Anguilla, Salmo, Clupea*) (Ball and Baker, 1969; McKeown and van Overbeeke, 1971; Mattheij and Sprangers, 1969; Emmart, 1969; Aler, 1970, 1971a, b), confirming that the granules themselves do contain LTH.

The LTH granules are membrane-bound structures, which vary in size according to external salinity. In freshwater specimens of the cyprinodonts *Poecilia (Lebistes) reticulata, Xiphophorus helleri* and *Poecilia (Mollienesia) sphenops* the granules measured between 200 and 250 nm in diameter (Follénius and Porte, 1960), and in *Xiphophorus maculatus* from 200 to 300 nm (Weiss, 1965). Abraham (1971) found in *Mugil cephalus* that the diameter of the granules was inversely related to salinity, the median values being 260 nm in freshwater, 230 nm in seawater and 180 nm in a hypertonic seawater. In *Gasterosteus aculeatus* in freshwater, the LTH granules measure 200–260 nm in diameter (Follénius, 1968) and juveniles of the same species in seawater had granules 220–270 nm in diameter (Leatherland, 1970a). In *Tilapia mossambica*, the LTH granules in freshwater fish cover a wide size range (100–400 nm in diameter), with a median of *c*. 240 nm, but in seawater fish the larger granules were missing, and the range was 100–*c*. 340, median *c*. 200 nm (Dharmamba and Nishioka, 1968). In a study on *Poecilia latipinna*, Hopkins (1969) related granule size to the turnover-rate of LTH. Seawater *P. latipinna* had many mature granules, *c*. 300 nm in diameter, and smaller, probably immature, granules close to the Golgi, 150–250 nm in diameter. Seventy-two hours after transfer to freshwater, the granules were fewer in number and smaller (200–250 nm), and like the immature granules in seawater fish they had a translucent rim between the dense core and the membrane, an indication that the hormone in freshwater was being released more rapidly without attaining the mature storage phase represented by the larger granules in seawater. It should be noted that Hopkins (1969) was dealing with *P. latipinna* during adaptation to freshwater, in which the granule size was less than in seawater; in all the other cases, in which granule size was *greater* in freshwater than in seawater, the fish were adapted to each medium (see above).

One way in which the granules are secreted from the cell in *Xiphophorus maculatus* is by exocytosis, the granule membrane fusing with the cell membrane and the granule escaping through the resulting opening. This process usually occurs in bud-like projections of the cell into the cytoplasm of adjacent stellate cells or against a basement membrane. A similar secretory process occurs in other cyprinodonts, including *P. latipinna* (Weiss, 1965). In *Gasterosteus* the lactotropes display a synthetic area, with Golgi complex and a few granules, and a storage area containing many dense secretory granules. Granule extrusion occurs by exocytosis and bud formation, mainly close to stellate cells (Leatherland, 1970a).

Histochemical data show that the LTH cells contain SS/SH groups in *Anguilla*, *Mugil* and *Xiphophorus*, but their failure to react with AB indicates that they are not particularly rich in cysteine, although *Mugil* lactotropes do in fact incorporate radio-cysteine. Intense protein synthesis in these cells in goldfish in freshwater is indicated by their rapid accumulation of radio-acetate. EM studies showed that the eel lactotropes contain acid phosphatase at various sites, including the Golgi region and some developing secretory granules. The amount of acid phosphatase increased when LTH secretion was reduced by transfer of eels to seawater (Hopkins and Baker, 1968). Similar results have been obtained for acid phosphatase in the LTH cells of *P. latipinna*, and this enzyme is probably involved in the destruction of hormone synthesised in excess of secretory requirements (Hopkins, 1969).

EVIDENCE FOR THE SECRETION OF LTH BY THE η CELLS

The similar staining properties of the teleost η cells and the mammalian lactotropes were emphasised by Olivereau and Herlant in 1960, but at that time too little was known about the physiological role of LTH in teleosts to suggest an approach to identifying the function of the η cells. More recently evidence has accumulated that shows fish LTH to play a role in osmoregulation, reducing the exchange of sodium across the body surface, especially the gills, and also in some species increasing the water permeability of the gills and increasing renal water excretion. The importance of LTH in the electrolyte economy varies with species. In some teleosts (e.g. cyprinodonts such as *P. latipinna*, *Oryzias latipes*, *Xiphophorus*, *Fundulus heteroclitus*) the action of LTH in reducing sodium outflux is absolutely necessary for life in freshwater, but is not essential for life in seawater or dilute (isosmotic) seawater. In other teleosts (e.g. *Anguilla*, goldfish, minnow, catfish) LTH is not essential for life in freshwater, but nevertheless in species investigated (e.g. *Anguilla*, goldfish) the hormone does reduce sodium outflux in freshwater, but this action is not so important in overall sodium metabolism as in fish such as *P. latipinna* (Ball, 1969; Ensor and Ball, 1972).

In various species studies of the η cells in relation to environmental salinity have shown them to be more active in freshwater than in seawater, and usually no other cell-types show this correlation (Olivereau and Ball, 1970; Ensor and Ball, 1972). Activation of the η cells when *P. latipinna* is moved from seawater to freshwater has been followed in detail in relation to changes in plasma sodium levels, sodium movements in and out of the body, and the pituitary content of LTH. Not only do the cells display signs of greater synthetic and secretory activity in freshwater than in seawater, but the pituitary LTH content is much higher in freshwater, and changes in the η cells correlate closely with changes in the secretion of LTH and the concomitant adjustment of sodium metabolism during adaptation to new salinities (Ball and Ingleton, 1973). EM studies on *P. latipinna* have shown that the secretory mechanism of the η cell is stimulated on entry to freshwater and inhibited on entry to seawater; the latter event is accompanied by an increase in acid phosphatase in the Golgi complex and by the formation of a variety of lysosome-like bodies containing acid phosphatase (Hopkins, 1969). During the early stages of adaptation to freshwater, the number of stored secretory granules is reduced (Ball and Ingleton, 1973; Hopkins, 1969), and there is an increase in the number of small vesicles coated with spines, 40–80 nm in diameter, corresponding to junctional vesicles and probably concerned in the transport of newly-synthesised protein from the RER to the Golgi complex. The increase in the number of junctional vesicles and the reduction in the number of mature secretory granules led Hopkins (1969) to suggest that the turnover-rate of LTH is increased when *P. latipinna* moves from seawater to freshwater, a suggestion in line with other results for this species (Ball and Baker, 1969; Ball and Ingleton, 1973).

Mugil cephalus is another euryhaline teleost that has been studied. The η cells show classical morphological signs of greater secretory activity in freshwater, and low activity in seawater; the LTH content of the gland is high in freshwater specimens, and very low in seawater fish (Blanc-Livni and Abraham, 1970; Abraham, 1971). The different size of the granules in the different habitats has been mentioned (p. 176). Surprisingly, the RER was well developed not only in freshwater but also in specimens taken from a hypersaline lagoon, but poorly developed in seawater fish (Abraham, 1971). In many euryhaline teleosts, these cells have been shown to be active in freshwater and relatively inactive in seawater (see Ball and Baker, 1969; Olivereau and Ball, 1970; Ensor and Ball, 1972).

Other kinds of experiments which show that LTH is secreted by the η cells include the selective surgical removal of these cells and ectopic autotransplantation of pituitary fragments consisting mainly of η cells in *Poecilia* (see Ball, 1969); and the specific localisation of antibody to ovine prolactin on the η cell granules in various teleosts (see Chester Jones *et al.* 1973, and p. 176). The identification of the teleostean η cell as the lactotrope is probably as secure as the functional identification of any pituitary cell.

A few observations have been made on the lactotropes in relation to the life history. They are strongly granulated and erythrosinophilic in newly-born *P. latipinna*, and are already differentiated in the gland of the embryo within the maternal ovarian follicle. They differentiate early in gestation in the guppy, *Poecilia reticulata*, at first with secretory granules smaller than in the adult and with an active type of RER. Viviparous cyprinodonts, such as *Poecilia* and *Xiphophorus*, gestate the young within the ovarian follicles, and this type of pregnancy does not appear to require LTH, judging from the absence of structural changes in the lactotropes during gestation. In contrast, the marine fish *Zoarces viviparus* gestates its young within the ovarian cavity, and in this case the lactotropes become extremely active during pregnancy. A more curious parental role for fish LTH is indicated in the sea-horse, *Hippocampus*. The male sea-horse incubates the eggs in a ventral brood-pouch, which is maintained in part by LTH. The lactotropes in the male fish display an annual cycle which is correlated with the development and function of the brood-pouch, the cells being particularly active during the first half of the incubation period (Boisseau, 1967).

In migratory salmonids moving between the sea and freshwaters the lactotropes become rapidly activated during the upstream migration from sea to spawning ground (Olivereau, 1954; van Overbeeke and McBride, 1967). In the Atlantic salmon, *Salmo salar*, the cells are already active and proliferating in the brackish waters of the estuary (Olivereau, 1954), and in the Pacific salmon, *Oncorhynchus keta*, the lactotropes are already activated in sexually-maturing fish caught at sea, the activity increasing in the estuary and during migration up the river (Nagahama and Yamamoto, 1970). In the juvenile eel or elver (*Anguilla*), migrating from the sea, the lactotropes become increasingly active on entering the estuary and moving up the river (Vollrath, 1966).

Since LTH plays a role in retaining sodium within the body, it is curious that the lactotropes of *Anguilla* become inactive in de-ionised water (Olivereau and Ball, 1970). In contrast, de-ionised water activates the lactotropes of *Anoptichthys* and *Cichlasoma* (Mattheij and Sprangers, 1969; Mattheij, Stroband and Kingma, 1971).

There is evidence of some interaction between the lactotropes and other endocrine functions. The cells are activated after radio-thyroidectomy in the eel and goldfish, though not distinctly activated in the trout; however, antithyroid drugs had no marked effects on the lactotropes of *P. latipinna*,

Mugil (Ball and Baker, 1969) and *Cichlasoma* (Mattheij, Stroband and Kingma, 1971), though in each case the treatment induced pronounced alterations in the TSH–thyroid axis. In the male sea-horse, *Hippocampus*, ACTH treatment inactivates the lactotropes (Boisseau, 1967).

ACTH CELLS (ADRENOCORTICOTROPIC CELLS, CORTICOTROPES, ε CELLS)

Although these cells have been described for many years by workers on the teleost pituitary, only quite recently has any evidence of their function been available. Characteristically they lie as a sheet or layer at the posterior interface between the LTH cells and the neurohypophysis, although they may form islets dispersed among the lactotropes, as in catfish and tench (Olivereau, 1970a). In all cases, even when they form islets among the lactotropes, the ACTH cells lie close to processes of the neurohypophysis. There is now considerable evidence (p. 215) that neurosecretory type B fibres end close to the corticotropes, on the adjacent basement membrane; this recalls the way in which the cortico-tropes of amphibians and reptiles are always closely related to some of the first branches of the portal vessels (chapters 12, 13).

The ACTH cells commonly stain only faintly, so that some workers have habitually referred to them as chromophobes (see Follénius, 1968a). They may stain rather non-specifically and faintly with OG (Mattheij, 1968a, b), but most important is the fact that their granules characteristic-ally stain grey, black or dark blue with PbH and purple with Aliz BT (Olivereau, 1970a). In *P. latipinna* these cells are nearly chromophobic, with a fine powdery granulation, Aliz B+ or erythrosin+, and a fusiform nucleus containing a fine scattering of chromatin. The nucleolus is usually insignificant (colour plate). In the carp (*Cyprinus carpio*), the ACTH cells and interrenal are normally active, the ACTH granules strongly PbH+ and Aliz B+; however, after fasting for eight months the interrenal became relatively inactive and the corticotropes were atrophied and almost chromophobic (Olivereau, 1970a). *Anguilla* has large cortico-tropes, with a coarse and dense granulation that stains heavily with PbH and Aliz B and more faintly with erythrosin; the cells and their nuclei are usually oval, not fusiform as in cyprinodonts, and the nucleoli are usually indistinct.

In most cases the corticotrope granules do not stain with PAS, unlike the ACTH granules in many tetrapods, and they are also AF− and AB− (Ball and Baker, 1969; Olivereau, 1970a). However, in *Anoptichthys* they are faintly PAS+ and AB+ (Mattheij, 1968a, b). In *Anguilla* they are rich in SS/SH groups. The tendency towards chromophobia shown by the corticotropes of most teleosts is probably in part a result of stress when the animals are killed, which would tend to deplete the cells of ACTH and visible granules (see Ball and Baker, 1969).

EM studies on the corticotropes of *Anguilla* showed a moderately electron-dense cytoplasm containing numerous fine vesicles or micro-tubules, a diffuse RER and a poorly-defined Golgi complex. The cytoplasm is evenly packed with electron-dense granules, spherical in *Anguilla* and 200–250 nm in diameter, elongated in the related marine *Conger* (Knowles and Vollrath, 1966*b*). In *Perca fluviatilis* the granules are 120–160 nm in diameter (Follénius and Porte, 1961), and in *Gasterosteus aculeatus* 150–220 nm, located mainly in the part of the cell adjacent to the basement membrane against the neurohypophysis (Follénius, 1968; Leatherland, 1970*a*), the RER and Golgi complex being at the other pole in marine animals (Leatherland, 1970*a*) or scattered, with no polarisation, in freshwater animals (Follénius, 1968). In *Oncorhynchus nerka* and *O. keta*, the secretory granules are 150–250 nm in diameter, of varying electron density, and the limiting membrane is often widely separated from the dense core (Nagahama and Yamamoto, 1969*a*, 1970). ACTH granules in mammals often have this vesicular form (Farquhar, 1971). *Mugil* corticotropes also have vesicular granules, 120–250 nm in diameter in freshwater specimens, 110–220 nm in seawater. The plasma membranes of the cells are folded to form a series of channels, continuous with the space between the double basement membrane that forms an interface with the neurohypophysis. These channels, probably playing some role in transport, appear to be connected to the series of stellate cells between the nearby lactotropes (Abraham, 1971). *Tilapia mossambica* has rather large vesicular secretory granules, of 240 nm mean diameter in freshwater and 200 nm in seawater (Dharmamba and Nishioka, 1968; Sage and Bern, 1971).

EVIDENCE FOR THE SECRETION OF ACTH BY THE ε CELLS

Allocation of corticotropic function to the ε cells was accomplished simultaneously for *Anguilla* and *P. latipinna* by use of the adrenocortical inhibitor Metopirone (SU 4885, Ciba); in both fishes, this inhibitor of steroidogenesis induced increased ACTH secretion (shown by morphological stimulation of the interrenal cells) and a specific initial activation of the ε cells (Olivereau and Ball, 1963; Ball and Olivereau, 1966). With longer treatment, the TSH cells and thyroid were activated, and other side-effects of the drug have been observed (see Ball and Baker, 1969). The ACTH cells have been identified in the same way in *Anoptichthys* (Mattheij, 1968*b*). The effects of surgical removal of the interrenal in *Anguilla*, and of various treatments designed to alter ACTH secretion, have all confirmed the corticotropic function of the ε cells (see Ball and Baker, 1969). McKeown and van Overbeeke (1971) have shown that fluorescent-labelled antibodies to porcine ACTH and synthetic β 1–24 ACTH locate specifically in the ε cells of *Oncorhynchus nerka*.

The corticotropes of *Anguilla* and trout are slightly inactivated after radio-thyroidectomy, and thyroxine treatment leads to their slight stimulation in the eel. In *Mugil* also, the ACTH cells are stimulated by thyroxine and inhibited by chemical thyroidectomy. In the male sea-horse *Hippocampus*, in which the brood-pouch is dependent upon LTH and ACTH, the corticotropes show an annual cycle of activity, becoming most active when eggs are being brooded in the pouch (Boisseau, 1967). In the freshwater *Cichlasoma*, the corticotropes are stimulated by exposure of the fish to de-ionised water or to salt water (Mattheij, Stroband and Kingma, 1971), and in *Anguilla* they are temporarily activated on entry to seawater from freshwater (Olivereau and Ball, 1970), in parallel with a transitory increase in plasma cortisol levels (Ball *et al.* 1971). They are also more active in *Mugil* in freshwater than in seawater (Olivereau and Ball, 1970; Abraham, 1971).

STH CELLS (SOMATOTROPIC CELLS, SOMATOTROPES, GROWTH HORMONE CELLS, α CELLS)

The somatotropes are the most prominent acidophil in the pars distalis, especially in marine teleosts in which the lactotropes are inactive. They occupy much of the proximal pars distalis. These are the classical acidophils, staining selectively and intensely with OG in various trichrome and tetrachrome techniques. With Aliz BT, the lactotropes stain red and the somatotropes yellow (colour plate); as in other vertebrates this distinction is not always easily achieved, but it is usually possible with careful technique. With Azan, the somatotropes of *P. latipinna* are orange but with Aliz BT they usually stain a clear yellow. This tinctorial distinction between red LTH cells and yellow or orange STH cells has been made in many teleosts (Ball and Baker, 1969; Mattheij, 1968a; Mattheij, Stroband and Kingma, 1971).

In *P. latipinna* the somatotropes occupy the centro-dorsal region of the proximal pars distalis, intermingled with the much scarcer TSH cells. The somatotropes are usually large and rounded, sometimes elongated, and typically filled with fine secretory granules, often so densely packed as to appear homogeneous. The ovoid nucleus is frequently placed eccentrically at one pole of the cells, and nuclear size seems to vary within the same gland. The nucleolus is usually prominent, as is the Golgi image in the form of a ring or crescent. In *P. latipinna* the cells show a tendency towards sexual dimorphism. In the adult female, they are numerous and very active, while the adult male usually has relatively few somatotropes, poorly granulated or entirely agranular, with nucleus, nucleolus and Golgi image indicating low activity. In the female, the continuous cup-shaped mass of somatotropes is easily visible in the living gland, the α granules being a dense white in contrast to the more trans-lucent ventral gonadotropes. In the male fish, however, the STH cell mass is thinner and discontinuous, and generally not visible in the living gland. *Anguilla*, when sexually mature, displays a similar dimorphism, the female having larger and more active somatotropes than the male.

The somatotropes are typical acidophils, with granules negative to AB and AF. They are virtually PAS— also, but they can be faintly stained with PAS in various species, recalling the faint PAS reaction shown by the mammalian acidophil granules (chapter 3); this slight PAS reaction may reflect the presence of lipid in the granules (Purves, 1966). In *Anguilla* the cells contain SS/SH groups and in *Mugil* they incorporate radio-cysteine avidly. Goldfish somatotropes display their intense protein synthetic activity by rapid accumulation of radio-acetate and amino acids.

At the ultrastructural level, adult *Anguilla* STH cells are seen to be filled with membrane-bound secretory granules about 400 nm in diameter, with no clear indication of RER or Golgi complex, and with few mito-chondria (Knowles and Vollrath, 1966*b*). The granules are rather smaller (270–400 nm) and the RER well-developed in the elver (Vollrath, 1966). *Cymatogaster* somatotropes show granules 400 nm in diameter (Leather-land, 1969), and in *Gasterosteus* the RER is well-developed and the granules 180–300 nm in diameter in freshwater (Follénius, 1968) and 250–350 nm in the marine form (Leatherland, 1970*b*). STH granules are the same size (250–330 nm) in *Perca* (Follénius and Porte, 1961), and *Oncorhynchus* (200–350 nm), and in this salmon the Golgi complex showed stages in the elaboration of secretory granules (Nagahama and Yamamoto, 1969*a*, 1970). There are some indications in *Perca* that the somatotropes may have a cycle of activity, in that cells rich in RER are poor in secretory granules and *vice versa*. As in salmon, perch STH granules have been observed in the process of formation in the Golgi complex, and they are secreted by exocytosis from the cell surface (see Ball and Baker, 1969).

EVIDENCE FOR THE SECRETION OF STH BY THE α CELLS

The functional identification of these cells is not as well-founded as that of the other cell types. It depends largely on the fact that all other pars distalis functions have been allocated to other sites by experimental work, and only STH remains to be secreted by the α cells. In confirmation, fluorescent antibody to mammalian STH was found to locate specifically in the α cells of *Oncorhynchus nerka* (McKeown and van Overbeeke, 1971). Various circumstantial observations add support to this identifi-cation. The α cells are very numerous in the Atlantic salmon (*Salmo salar*) during the rapid growth of the smolt, and they are also very active during the rapid growth of adult Pacific salmon (*Oncorhynchus*) in the sea (Ball and Baker, 1969). A similar correlation between bodily growth and α cell activity has been established for the marine stickleback, *Gasterosteus* (Leatherland, 1970b). The greater numbers and activity of these cells in female *P. latipinna* and *Anguilla* may be related to the greater size usually attained by the female in these species. Again, the α cells become extremely active during periods of prolonged starvation in *Anguilla* and *Cyprinus carpio*, a reaction which can be explained by analogy with mammalian physiology as indicating increased STH secretion to adjust metabolism during fasting (Olivereau, 1970b). In *Poecilia formosa*, the scarcity and degranulation of α cells in ectopic pituitary autotransplants that secrete little STH, but normal amounts of LTH, also argue for the somatotropic nature of these cells.

Unfortunately, there have been few observations on the somatotropes in relation to life history. In *P. reticulata* they differentiate later in gestation than the lactotropes, but they are present and very active in the newly-born and rapidly growing *P. latipinna*. The EM observations described on p. 183 suggest that these cells are more active in the rapidly growing elver than in the adult eel (*Anguilla*). Concerning collateral endocrine interactions, it has been claimed that chemical thyroidectomy increased the storage of STH granules in *P. reticulata*, an effect opposed by simultaneous treatment with thyroxine. As in the rat, normal thyroid function may be necessary for normal secretion of STH, and in addition there is evidence of a peripheral synergism between thyroxine and STH in promoting body growth in teleosts (Pickford and Atz, 1957; Ball, 1969).

In *Anguilla*, treatment with cortisol causes regression of the somatotropes, and they are activated by surgical stress, though not by the stress of anaesthesia and bleeding. At sexual maturity in the female eel STH cells are reduced in number, which may relate to the reduction in growth that commonly accompanies sexual maturation in many teleosts (Olivereau, 1967a).

Observations that are difficult to explain at present are that eels with small skin lesions exhibit hyponatraemia accompanied by strong activation of the somatotropes, and that these cells are extremely activated in eels maintained in de-ionised water (Olivereau and Ball, 1970). What role fish STH may play in osmoregulation is as yet unknown.

GONADOTROPIC CELLS (GTH CELLS, GONADOTROPES)

When adequately identified, the gonadotropes are usually found to lie in the proximal pars distalis, generally in the ventral and lateral regions. However, GtH cells also spread into the rostral pars distalis at sexual maturity in various teleosts, including the eel, salmon and trout (Olivereau,

1972). They are typical basophils, containing glycoprotein secretory granules that are strongly PAS+, AF+, AB+ and aniline blue+. The appearance of the gonadotropes varies a great deal during the cyclical development and regression of the gonads. An important question is whether teleosts possess one or two types of gonadotropes. Mammals, in which the pituitary undoubtedly secretes two gonadotropins, FSH and LH, have generally been found to have two types of gonadotropes, the β cell secreting FSH and the γ cell secreting LH (chapter 3). There is in fact no very definite evidence that lower vertebrates secrete two gonadotropins, and indeed recent work on teleosts points to there being only a single gonadotropin with both FSH- and LH-like physiological properties (Burzawa-Gérard and Fontaine, 1972; Sundararaj, Anand and Sinha, 1972; Chester Jones *et al.* 1973). Two kinds of gonadotropic cells have been described in some teleosts, but they cannot be designated β and γ cells.

The eel, *Anguilla*, the Pacific salmon, *Oncorhynchus*, and the goldfish *Carassius* are some of the teleosts in which the GtH cells can be divided into two categories according to tinctorial properties, location, granule size and morphological features such as vacuolisation. It has been shown that the two types are probably equivalent in male and female eels. At the EM level, two types of gonadotropes have been described in the immature eel, one with dense granules, *c.* 190 nm in diameter, the other with lucent granules, *c.* 130 nm in diameter (Knowles and Vollrath, 1966*b*). These authors suggested these were LH and FSH cells respectively, but this dualism ran far ahead of the then-current physiological information, and is counter to the present biochemical and physiological information (Chester Jones *et al.* 1973). Two types of gonadotropes have been distinguished by light microscopy in *Mugil* spp., separated not only by staining properties, size and location, but also by differential precipitation of their granules by different concentrations of trichloracetic acid. Two ultrastructurally different GtH cells have also been described in the viviparous *Zoarces*, one kind being active during ovarian development, the other during pregnancy. The staining combination PbH–PAS separates the two gonadotropes of birds and mammals, and it also separates the two types of gonadotropes in *Anguilla* and *Mugil*, one being PAS+, the other PbH+ (see Ball and Baker, 1969).

It is difficult to be certain that these two kinds of gonadotropes might not be two stages in the activity cycle of a single cell-type. It is easier to reconcile this interpretation with all the evidence that the teleosts and other lower vertebrates secrete only a single gonadotropin, than it would be to suppose that a second hormone has gone undetected by the sophisticated biochemical techniques employed in recent years by various laboratories to extract gonadotropic hormones from teleost pituitaries (see Chester Jones *et al.* 1973).

In addition to glycoprotein secretory granules, the mature eel GtH cells also contain very large granules, probably lysosomes, with variable staining affinities, OG+, AB+, AF+, aniline blue+, and erythrosin+ (Olivereau, 1967*a*). The gonadotropes in several teleosts have been shown to be rich in SS/SH groups, and in *Poecilia sphenops* and goldfish they incorporate radio-sulphur more rapidly than any other cell-type, probably forming sulphate esters of acid mucopolysaccharides. Carp gonadotropes are rich in sialic acid, known to be a constituent of carp gonadotropin as of mammalian FSH and LH (Burzawa-Gérard and Fontaine, 1972).

GtH cells have been identified in many teleosts, usually in relation to the sexual cycle. It is generally accepted that pars distalis basophils that are quiescent or undifferentiated before sexual maturity, and that show pronounced secretory changes correlated with the gonadal cycle, are gonadotropes. The literature on this subject is voluminous (see Ball and Baker, 1969), and a detailed recent account was given by Mattheij (1970) for *Anoptichthys*. Apart from this mass of 'correlative' studies, there have been reports of characteristic activity changes in teleost gonadotropes following surgical gonadectomy or administration of gonadal steroids. A detailed account is available of the cyclic changes in the GtH cells of the adult viviparous *Poecilia latipinna* which demonstrates the extreme range of morphological changes shown by these cells during the monthly cycle of oocyte development and pregnancy (Ball and Baker, 1969). The activity of the gonadotropes in this fish relates to vitellogenic oocyte growth, but not to pregnancy; the cells are quiescent during most of gestation, which proceeds to completion independently of the pituitary (Ball, 1962). As in many teleosts, maximal activity in the gonadotropes of *P. latipinna* is characterised by complete or partial loss of glycoprotein secretory granules, and the development of large vacuoles in conjunction with cytological evidence of strong synthetic and secretory activity. In addition to secretory granules the active GtH cell contains a few very large amphiphilic globules, PAS+, OG+ and erythrosin+. These are AB−, so that after AB–PAS–OG they stand out red against the smaller dark blue secretory granules. These large *R granules* or globules, like those in the eel, are probably lysosomes, resembling those in the gonadotropes in amphibians and reptiles (chapters 12, 13). They occur in many teleosts (Ball and Baker, 1969), often lining the vacuoles of the gonadotropes towards the end of vitellogenesis. Presumably the lysosomal enzymes serve at this stage to remove excess secretory products, which would explain their marked development during early gestation in *P. latipinna*, when vitellogenesis is suddenly inhibited; a condition analogous to the arrest of LTH secretion that occurs when *P. latipinna* moves from freshwater to seawater, which also involves an increase in 'scavenger' acid phosphatase in the Golgi complex and in the number of lytic organelles in the lactotrope (Hopkins, 1969).

Fluorescent-labelled antibody to purified carp gonadotropin located specifically on granules in large vacuolated basophils in the peripheral proximal pars distalis (Billard, Breton and Dubois, 1971), but did not locate on the PAS+ material inside the vacuoles that presumably corresponds to lytic R granules. The addition of excess carp gonadotropin to fluorescent antiserum against crude carp TSH allowed these cells to be identified as gonadotropes, in distinction from TSH cells, but only a single type of gonadotrope could be distinguished (Billard, Breton and Dubois, 1971).

The GtH cells of *Oncorhynchus nerka* contain a few large granules (3000 nm in diameter), of low electron-density, and many secretory granules, 300–500 nm in diameter. The large bodies are PAS+, AF+ and aniline blue+, and presumably are lytic R granules. The cells have a well-developed RER and Golgi complex (Nagahama and Yamamoto, 1969a), and resemble those described with the light microscope in this species (van Overbeeke and McBride, 1967). *O. keta* has similar gonadotropes (Nagahama and Yamamoto, 1970), but with rather smaller secretory granules (200–300 nm in diameter). Similarly in the goldfish, the GtH cells contain large amphiphilic R granules, 500–3000 nm in diameter, together with many smaller PAS+ secretory granules, 200–300 nm in diameter. When these cells are extremely active, the RER cisternae become remarkably dilated, resulting in the vacuolation seen with the light microscope and producing 'signet ring' cells (Nagahama and Yamamoto, 1969b). Secretory granules of about the same size occur in the gonadotropes of *Cymatogaster* (200–300 nm, Leatherland, 1969) and *Gasterosteus* (235–270 nm, Follénius, 1968; 260–290 nm, Leatherland, 1970b); in *Gasterosteus*, both investigators describe the development of dilated RER cisternae containing amorphous dense material.

Little is known about the responses of teleost gonadotropes to collateral changes in endocrine functions. Of great interest is evidence that suggests that GtH secretion in various teleosts is inhibited by stress and by injection of ACTH or corticosteroids such as would mimic stress (see Ball and Baker, 1969). These responses have important ecological implications, in that under unfavourable (stressful) conditions such as overcrowding, reproduction would be inhibited and the population ultimately reduced. Other work, both *in vivo* and *in vitro*, indicates that poeciliid gonadotropes are inhibited by thyroxine (Sage and Bromage, 1970).

TSH CELLS (THYROTROPIC CELLS, THYROTROPES, δ CELLS)

In mammals, it is usually possible by tinctorial means to separate two basophilic cell-types in the pars distalis, the gonadotropes and thyrotropes. Most workers on teleosts have found the gonadotropes and thyrotropes to have similar staining properties, and these cells must be differentiated by other means. However there are some exceptions: in *Phoxinus*, *Rutilus*, *Caecobarbus*, *Brachydanio*, *Barbus* and *Anoptichthys* the thyrotropes show a stronger affinity for AF and AB (pH 0.2) than the gonadotropes (Ball and Baker, 1969; Mattheij, 1968a; Mattheij, Stroband and Kingma, 1971) while in *Cichlasoma* (Mattheij, Kingma and Stroband, 1971; Mattheij, Stroband and Kingma, 1971) and *P. latipinna* (Ball and Baker, 1969), the thyrotropes have less affinity for AB (pH 0.2) than the gonadotropes, and a stronger affinity for PAS. In *Anguilla*, the thyrotropes have a stronger affinity for AF than the gonadotropes (Olivereau, 1967a).

Fortunately, visual distinction between the two kinds of teleost basophils depends not only on tinctorial differences, but also on a spatial separation that is usually marked. When the TSH cells lie among the lactotropes in the rostral pars distalis, they are far removed from the gonadotropes in the proximal region (p. 184). In the teleosts such as *Poecilia*, with TSH cells in the proximal pars distalis, there is usually a spatial separation of the two in that the TSH cells lie dorsally and centrally, the GtH cells ventrally and laterally. This spatial separation is not always as clear as in *Poecilia*, where the gonadotropes form a homogeneous peripheral zone (colour plate). In *Anoptichthys*, for example, gonadotropes and thyrotropes are mixed throughout the proximal pars distalis (Mattheij, 1968a), and in *Cichlasoma* strands of the mainly peripheral gonadotropes project inwards amongst the TSH cells (Mattheij, Stroband and Kingma, 1971). In conditions of strong stimulation, such as iodine deficiency or after radio-thyroidectomy, the rostrally-located thyrotropes in *Oncorhynchus tshawytscha* may spread to a limited extent into the ventral area of the proximal pars distalis, and in juvenile *O. kisutch* the thyrotropes are localised entirely in the proximal pars distalis, exceptional among salmonids, in which they usually are confined to the rostral region as in *Anguilla* (Ball and Baker, 1969; Olivereau, 1972).

The thyrotropes of the immature male eel, *Anguilla*, are small angular cells, lying in the rostral pars distalis between the follicles of lactotropes. Occasional TSH cells interpose between the lactotropes in the follicle walls. They have very fine secretory granules with typical staining reactions, AF +, PAS +, AB +, aldehyde thionin +, aniline blue +. In the female the thyrotropes are similar, but have a greater tendency to form large masses in the middle of the rostral pars distalis (Olivereau, 1967a). In *Poecilia* spp. they lie, usually in groups of a few cells, in the finger-like projections of the proximal pars distalis into the neurohypophysis, mixed with the more numerous somatotropes. They are often angular in shape, and have the same staining reactions as the thyrotropes of *Anguilla*. Teleost thyrotropes always display these staining properties, but there is little information about their histochemistry. They incorporate radio-cysteine in *Mugil*, and the presence of SS/SH groups has been demonstrated in *Poecilia reticulata*, though not in *Anguilla*, and goldfish thyrotropes incorporate radio-glucose very rapidly, presumably an indication of glycoprotein synthesis, since there is biochemical evidence that teleost TSH is a glycoprotein (Chester Jones *et al.* 1973).

EM studies on various teleosts have revealed differences in the size of the TSH granules. In immature *Anguilla* the granules are about 140 nm in diameter (Knowles and Vollrath, 1966*b*), and they are about the same size (140–190 nm) in *Cymatogaster* and *Gasterosteus* (Leatherland, 1969, 1970*b*; Follénius, 1968). The granules are larger (250–330 nm) in *Perca* (Follénius and Porte, 1961), and in *Zoarces* the presumptive thyrotropes contained large granules (*c.* 400 nm), sometimes together with smaller granules (120–160 nm) within the cisternae of the RER. Trout TSH granules vary greatly in size, from 100 to 800 nm (see Ball and Baker, 1969). The granules in *Oncorhynchus nerka* measure 100–200 nm, and in *O. keta* 200 nm, and are often found within the dilated RER cisternae, a characteristic feature of thyrotropes (Nagahama and Yamamoto, 1969*a*, 1970). Goldfish thyrotropes contain granules 60–220 nm in diameter, and after chemical thyroidectomy the RER cisternae distend to form vacuoles, the Golgi complex hypertrophies and the number of stored secretory granules is reduced (Nagahama and Yamamoto, 1969*b*). In *Cymatogaster*, TSH cells appear to release granules into the basement membrane adjoining the neurohypophysis (Leatherland, 1970*c*).

EVIDENCE FOR THE SECRETION OF TSH BY THE δ CELLS

A great deal of work has resulted in the allocation of thyrotropic function to the δ cells, the most detailed being that of Olivereau on the eel (see Olivereau, 1967). Surgical removal of the thyroid is impossible in most teleosts, because the gland takes the form of scattered follicles in the pharyngeal region, closely associated with the ventral aorta. However, partial destruction of the eel thyroid was achieved by massive doses of radio-iodine. Following this 'partial thyroidectomy', the δ cells displayed signs of progressively increasing activity during the seven-month period of the study. In addition to exhibiting signs of increased protein synthesis, the δ cells became degranulated, in agreement with an independent demonstration of the loss of nearly 80 per cent of pituitary TSH in such radio-thyroidectomised eels (see Ball and Baker, 1969). In a complementary experiment eels were treated with thyroxine, which induced involution of the thyroid gland accompanied by inactivation changes in the δ cells. Partial or total radio-thyroidectomy of the trout, goldfish and Pacific salmon has yielded results similar to those for the eel (Olivereau, 1972).

Another approach to the identification of the δ cells has been the induction of a state of thyroid deficiency with various drugs which inhibit the synthesis of thyroid hormone. These drugs (thiouracil, thiourea) have been administered to various teleosts, with consistent results including hyperactivity of the δ cells and morphological stimulation of the 'blocked' thyroid gland as a result of increased TSH secretion (Ball and Baker, 1969; Mattheij, 1969; Mattheij, Stroband and Kingma, 1971). Under appropriate conditions thyroxine can suppress the activity of the δ cells, accompanied by reduction in thyroid activity (Ball and Baker, 1969; Mattheij, 1969; Mattheij, Stroband and Kingma, 1971; Higgins, Ball and Wigham, 1973). By use of fluorescent antibodies to carp gonadotropin and to carp TSH, the small polygonal scattered δ cells of carp (*Cyprinus carpio*) have been identified as thyrotropes (Billard, Breton and Dubois, 1971).

Changes have been recorded in the activity of thyrotropes during the life history. In viviparous cyprinodonts these cells differentiate before birth, several months before the gonadotropes can be identified, and old age in cyprinodonts appears to be associated with reduced activity of the TSH cells and the thyroid (Ball and Baker, 1969). Thyrotropes are present in only small numbers during the freshwater (parr) stage of young Atlantic salmon, and the pituitary contains little TSH. In the next migratory (smolt) stage, which travels downriver to the sea, the TSH cells become very numerous and the thyroid is strongly stimulated; it has been known for many years that the change from parr to smolt in salmonids is at least partly dependent on thyroid hormone (see Chester Jones *et al.* 1973). EM studies indicate that the TSH cells are more active in the adult migratory silver eel than in the younger freshwater (yellow) stage (Knowles and Vollrath, 1966*b*, *c*, *d*).

For many years there has been great interest in interactions between gonads and thyroid. No generalisations have emerged from studies in this field, but some interesting facts have been reported. Thus, male eels can be made sexually mature by injections of human chorionic gonadotropin, and this treatment simultaneously activates the thyrotropes and the thyroid gland, possibly because of some interplay between gonadotropin, sex hormones and TSH at the hypothalamic level (see Ball and Baker, 1969). The TSH cells of *Xiphophorus* were inhibited by both androgens and oestrogens *in vitro*; however, oestrogen *stimulated* the thyrotropes of *Poecilia reticulata in vivo*, while androgen inhibited them both *in vivo* and *in vitro* (Sage and Bromage, 1970). These indications of complex interplay between steroids, the thyroid and the thyrotropes recall observations on the hypophysectomised catfish *Mystus vittatus*, in which oestrogen and progesterone restored thyroid activity and testosterone raised it to double the normal level; cortisone also restored thyroid activity (Singh, 1969). Since in the catfish all the steroids must have acted directly on the thyroid, without the intervention of TSH, it is not surprising that in-vitro and in-vivo effects of steroids on the thyrotropes should not always be the same.

The adrenocortical inhibitor su 4885, used to identify corticotropes, activates the TSH cells after long treatment in the eel and *P. latipinna* (Ball and Olivereau, 1966). However, this response was not produced in *Anoptichthys* during a treatment similar to that given to *P. latipinna* (Mattheij, 1968*b*), and in *Anguilla* it is not seen after surgical removal of the interrenal. Thus, the effect of su 4885 on the thyrotropes is probably a direct pharmacological one rather than the result of depressed blood cortisol levels (see Ball and Baker, 1969).

In *Anguilla*, but not in *P. latipinna* and *Cichlasoma*, chronic treatment with ovine LTH produces histological signs of activation in the TSH cells and the thyroid (Ball and Baker, 1969; Mattheij, Stroband and Kingma, 1971; Higgins and Ball, 1972), an action that recalls the goitrogenic effect of LTH in anuran amphibians (chapter 12). However, it appears that LTH does not act as a goitrogen in *Anguilla*, but that it releases TSH and causes a genuine functional activation of the thyroid (see Ball and Baker, 1969; Ball *et al.* 1972), in the same way that LTH apparently releases TSH in the newt *Triturus* (chapter 12). There are also indications that the thyrotropes may respond to stress and elevated levels of circulating corticosteroids, but the nature of the response is not clear (Ball and Baker, 1969). Although histological studies suggest that the thyrotropes are less active in seawater than in freshwater in *Anguilla*, salmon and *Cichlasoma* (Olivereau and Ball, 1970; Mattheij, Kingma and Stroband, 1971), physiological work on other teleosts, including *P. latipinna* and *F. heteroclitus*, indicates a generally higher rate of thyroid hormone secretion in seawater than in freshwater. However in *P. latipinna* the thyroid is hyperplastic in freshwater, though circulating thyroid hormone is at a lower level than in dilute seawater, and this may represent a 'compensatory work hypertrophy' in an iodine-poor environment, in its turn dependent on higher TSH secretion in freshwater (Higgins, Ball and Wigham, 1973). If this observation could be generalised, it would explain the otherwise paradoxical association of low thyroid activity in freshwater with hyperactivity of the thyrotropes.

STELLATE CELLS IN THE PARS DISTALIS

Interspersed among the LTH cells in the rostral follicles of *Anguilla* are a few small cells lying adjacent to fine channels which connect the follicular lumen with the intervascular space between the follicles. Because of their position, these have been called *neck cells*, and the suggestion was made that by altering their size and shape they could regulate the passage of substances along the channels (Knowles and Vollrath, 1966*b*). In all probability these neck cells belong to the system of stellate (follicular) cells, which are a general feature of the adenohypophysis (Vila-Porcile, 1972). Stellate cells have been illustrated in the elver pars distalis (Vollrath, 1966), and apparently occur in all regions of the adenohypophysis of teleosts, usually with their fine processes penetrating between the endocrine cells (Leatherland, 1969, 1970*a*; Abraham, 1971). They lie between the lactotropes of *P. latipinna* and *Xiphophorus*, and exhibit signs of being concerned in the transport of LTH to capillaries (Hopkins, 1969; Weiss, 1965), and similar appearances have been reported for *Gasterosteus* (Follénius, 1968), in which the cell bodies lie at the periphery of the rostral pars distalis and adjacent to blood capillaries, and send their processes amongst the lactotropes (Leatherland, 1970*a*). In *Mugil*, Abraham (1971) described channel cells, penetrating between the lactotropes with attenuated processes, and possibly involved in transport of LTH and of material from neurosecretory terminations to the lactotropes. These various cells (neck cells, chromophobes, interstitial cells) probably all belong to the stellate cell system, though they are not always stellate in shape. It is significant that in *Gasterosteus* the chromophobe (stellate) cells in the rostral pars distalis often surround extracellular colloidal masses (Leatherland, 1970*a*), called pseudofollicles by Follénius (1968). This morphological feature characterises the 'follicular' form of the cells in mammals (Vila-Porcile, 1972). In addition, histiocytes or macrophages have been described in cultures of the lactotrope cell mass of *Fundulus heteroclitus*, moving between the lactotropes, possibly in response to some chemical signal from the endocrine cells which they contact briefly (Emmart and Mossakowski, 1970).

HYPOTHALAMIC CONTROL OF THE PARS DISTALIS: PHYSIOLOGICAL ASPECTS

The anatomical apparatus by which the hypothalamus could exert control over adenohypophysial activities is considered later (pp. 214–20). At this point, we will deal with the physiological evidence that this control operates in teleosts. Experimental investigations in this field are not numerous, but have been accumulating over the past decade. The subject has been reviewed several times (Ball *et al.* 1965; Olivereau and Ball, 1966; Olivereau, 1967*b*; Ball and Baker, 1969; Peter, 1970; Ball *et al.* 1972; Hawkins and Ball, 1973).

CONTROL OF LTH

Like the mammalian lactotrope, the LTH cell of *Poecilia* spp. remains active if the pituitary is ectopically transplanted. This activity is manifested both functionally (tolerance of freshwater, maintenance of normal sodium metabolism) and cytologically. Furthermore, in ectopic transplants as in the normal pituitary, the lactotropes are rapidly activated when *P. latipinna* enters freshwater from dilute seawater. Thus, hypo-thalamic connections are not necessary for the activation of these cells in response to reduced salinity, nor for their continued activity in freshwater. By incubating the pituitary of *P. latipinna* on media of different osmotic pressure, it was shown that low osmotic pressure directly activates the synthesis and secretion of LTH (Ball *et al*. 1972). Thus, in cyprinodonts it is possible that activation of the lactotropes when the fish moves from seawater to freshwater is a direct response to the transitory fall in plasma sodium and osmotic pressure that occurs during adaptation (Ball and Ingleton, 1973). Many in-vitro observations have emphasised the auto-nomy of the lactotropes, and in *Fundulus heteroclitus* new cells have been shown to arise by mitosis in organ culture, these new cells elaborating and releasing LTH granules (Emmart and Mossakowski, 1967). In addition, there are some indications of hypothalamic influences on LTH secretion. A long photoperiod stimulates LTH secretion in *Gasterosteus*, an obser-vation suggestive of a central nervous mechanism channelled through the hypothalamus, and the lactotropes of several teleosts usually appear to be cytologically more active in ectopic transplants than in the normal gland (Ball *et al*. 1972). The study of LTH-dependent characters in *Anguilla* has suggested that the ectopic gland in fact releases less LTH than normal, and reserpine seemed to induce some inhibition of LTH release. There must certainly be differences among teleosts in the details of control of the pituitary, and at present it is only possible to say that LTH secretion seems to have a large degree of autonomy, but that there may be a hypothalamic LTH-inhibiting factor, with hints of an LTH-stimulating factor, the balance between the two being probably different in different species (Ball *et al*. 1972).

CONTROL OF ACTH

Results from transplanting the pituitary gland indicate that ACTH secretion depends almost completely on hypothalamic connections. In *Poecilia formosa* ectopic transplants maintained interrenal structure only to a limited extent, and the corticotropes in the grafts were hypoactive (Ball *et al*. 1965; Olivereau and Ball, 1966). Plasma cortisol levels in *P. latipinna* with pituitary autotransplants are at hypophysectomy levels after one or three weeks. Thus hypothalamic connections are essential to maintain 'resting' secretion of ACTH. Nevertheless, stress can elevate plasma cortisol to normal levels in *P. latipinna* bearing an ectopic pituitary, but not in hypophysectomised fish, indicating that ACTH secretion is elicited from the transplant by the stress stimulus. This most probably acts via the hypothalamus, since the response can be blocked by prior treatment with betamethasone, a synthetic corticosteroid known to inhibit secretion of hypothalamic ACTH-releasing factor (CRF) in mammals. This interpretation is supported by the findings that beta-methasone given to intact *P. latipinna* can reduce plasma cortisol to hypophysectomy levels, but median eminence extracts from hypo-physectomised rats (containing *inter alia* rat CRF) can overcome the betamethasone block, producing high plasma cortisol levels within forty-five minutes (Ball *et al.* 1972; Hawkins and Ball, 1973). The goldfish resembles *Poecilia*, in that ectopic pituitary grafts only partly maintain the interrenal, but transplants in *Anguilla* and *Gambusia* apparently secrete enough ACTH to maintain normal interrenal structure, even though the ACTH cells in the case of *Anguilla* look hypoactive (Ball *et al.* 1972).

In-vitro work suggests rather more autonomy of ACTH secretion than would appear from the work on transplants. On cytological grounds the ACTH cells in both *Anguilla* and *Salmo* remained continually active in culture, with enhanced radio-uridine uptake by *Salmo* corticotropes after three weeks (Ball *et al.* 1972). Goldfish pituitaries incubated for $1\frac{1}{2}$ hours secreted ACTH spontaneously, but this release was enhanced by adding crude extracts of goldfish hypothalamus (Sage and Purrott, 1969). There is also some evidence that part of the negative feedback action of cortico-steroids may be exerted at the level of the ACTH cells, as well as on the hypothalamus.

In summary, the ACTH cells appear to depend for full secretory activity on stimulation by the hypothalamus, although their degree of autonomy probably varies with species and may be quite high. Stress in *P. latipinna* can elicit ACTH secretion from the ectopic pituitary, possibly by activating a hypothalamic mechanism, CRF then reaching the ACTH cells by way of the general circulation. Part of the feedback action of cortisol is exerted at the pituitary level.

CONTROL OF STH

In pituitary homotransplants in *Poecilia formosa*, somatotropes were sometimes identifiable and moderately active in appearance though reduced in numbers (Olivereau and Ball, 1966). This modest activity relates to the slight linear growth displayed by fish bearing the transplants, in contrast to the shrinkage in length always seen after hypophysectomy (Ball *et al.* 1965). Similarly, in *P. latipinna* bearing pituitary autotrans-plants slight STH secretion is suggested by the slight growth or reduced shrinkage detected over periods of three to eight weeks. The somato-tropes in the *latipinna* autotransplants always seem to be better preserved and more active than in the *formosa* homotransplants. However, there is evidence that the activity of the cells in *latipinna* autotransplants diminishes with time. In *Anguilla*, autotransplants always contain some STH cells after two months, usually displaying signs of moderate secretory activity. *Anguilla* somatotropes cultured for two or more weeks *in vitro* look active, with abundant cytoplasmic RNA, and incorporation of radio-uridine into the nucleus and of radio-leucine into STH which is released into the medium. In contrast, *Salmo gairdneri* pituitaries, cultured in the same way for up to six weeks, displayed histological signs of regression of the somatotropes starting as early as one week (Ball *et al.* 1972).

In summary, any conclusions about hypothalamic control of teleost STH must be tentative. For *Poecilia* and *Salmo* the evidence is consistent with the hypothalamus producing an STH-releasing factor, but in *Anguilla* STH secretion appears strongly autonomous. In addition, we have no information about non-hypothalamic factors, such as metabolic products, which very possibly might influence STH secretion.

CONTROL OF GONADOTROPIN

Gonadotropes, though usually present, are consistently regressed in ecotopic pituitary homotransplants in hypophysectomised *Poecilia formosa*, in agreement with the failure of vitellogenesis in fish bearing the transplants (Ball *et al.* 1965). A similar regression of the gonadotropes occurs in pituitary autotransplants in *Anguilla* and *P. latipinna*. Pituitary autotransplants in goldfish fail to maintain gonad weight (Ball *et al.* 1972), and in this fish lesions in the NLT, but not in other parts of the hypothalamus, induce gonadal regression (Peter, 1970). The evidence, then, indicates a stimulatory hypothalamic influence on GtH secretion, centred on the NLT. Following the development of a radioimmunoassay for carp gonadotropin (Breton, Kann, Burzawa-Gérard and Billard, 1971), in-vitro experiments showed that acid extracts of carp hypothalamus stimulate the secretion of gonadotropin by carp pituitaries (Breton, Jalabert, Billard and Weill, 1971); sheep hypothalamic extracts had the same effect and, very interestingly, carp and trout hypothalamic extracts stimulate the secretion of sheep LH *in vitro* (Breton *et al.* 1972). This work provides the clearest demonstration we have of a substance in the teleost hypothalamus that resembles the mammalian releasing factors, in this case a gonadotropin-releasing factor probably synthesised in the NLT.

CONTROL OF TSH

Brain involvement in control of the TSH cells has been indicated by the finding that an increasing photoperiod at a constant low temperature leads to elevated thyroid activity in the salmon (see Higgins, Ball and Wigham, 1973). It is difficult to see how this effect of light could be mediated without participation of the hypothalamus. Histological study of the thyroid and thyrotropes in various teleosts bearing ectopic pituitary transplants has shown that TSH secretion may be normal or higher than normal. Even in those experiments in which TSH secretion from ectopic glands was on average normal, some individuals displayed frank thyroid hyperactivity associated with the presence of many active thyrotropes in the grafts. Extension of this type of investigation in *Poecilia latipinna*, using physiological as well as histological parameters for assessing thyroid activity, has confirmed that TSH secretion may be greater than normal when the pituitary is removed from direct connections with the hypothalamus: thus there may exist a TSH-inhibiting factor (TIF), a postulate supported by the fact that reserpine treatment of intact *P. latipinna* strongly enhances TSH secretion (Higgins, Ball and Wigham, 1973). Work on the goldfish, involving lesions of parts of the hypothalamus, also indicated a predominantly inhibitory hypothalamic control of the thyrotropes in this teleost, and located the source of TIF in the NLT (Peter, 1970).

In organ culture the thyrotropes of *Xiphophorus*, *Anguilla* and trout remain active, even becoming hyperactive in the trout. These results suggest the lack of some normal tonic inhibition (i.e. TIF) in the culture medium. Thyroxine appears to suppress TSH secretion at the pituitary level, since addition of thyroxine to the culture medium suppresses the activity of the TSH cells (Ball *et al.* 1972). Work on *P. latipinna* agrees with this last finding, in showing that thyroxine depressed thyroid activity in pituitary-autotransplanted fish to the same or greater extent as in intact fish (Higgins, Ball and Wigham, 1973). On the other hand, thyroxine implants in either the pituitary or the NLT suppress thyroid activity in the goldfish, which suggests that thyroxine exerts its negative feedback action at the pituitary level (in agreement with the in-vitro work) and has a positive feedback at the NLT, enhancing TIF secretion. Damage to the pituitary stem, which presumably prevented TIF from reaching the thyrotropes, masked the suppressive action of thyroxine implants in the pituitary (Peter, 1971).

In summary, despite species variation it is possible to generalise and state that the teleost hypothalamus, unlike that of mammals, does not seem to stimulate TSH secretion, which is either autonomous or is primarily influenced by a TIF. It is still possible that a TRF may also be elaborated, and that it may be found to predominate in some teleosts.

HISTOPHYSIOLOGY OF THE PARS INTERMEDIA

The pars intermedia partly or completely surrounds the distal (posterior) region of the neurohypophysis, and is usually extensively invaded by neural processes. Its relative size varies a good deal. It may be the smallest region of the adenohypophysis, as in cyprinodonts, or together with the enclosed posterior neurohypophysis it may form as much as two-thirds the volume of the entire pituitary, as in salmonids (frontispiece). Cells from the pars distalis may invade the pars intermedia (e.g. *Hippocampus*), and pars intermedia cells are sometimes found in the pars distalis (e.g. cyprinodonts).

Two cell-types can usually be distinguished by staining reactions and often also by differences in shape and position. Staining with PAS followed by PbH usually gives clear differentiation between the two, one cell-type being PAS +, the other PbH +. PAS and PbH appear to be mutually exclusive in staining the pars intermedia, but there is no correlation between the reactions of the cells to the classical trichrome stains or Aliz BT on the one hand, and to PAS on the other; the PAS + cells may be cyanophilic (*Hippocampus, Phoxinus, Anguilla*), OG + (cichlids, *Blennius, Zoarces, Anoptichthys*), or amphiphilic (cyprinodonts), and the response of these cells to any particular staining method seems more than usually sensitive to slight variations in technique. The PbH + cells have been variously described as chromophobic, acidophilic or weakly basophilic. Older accounts, in which the pars intermedia was said to contain only chromophobes, obviously need to be checked against investigations with the PAS–PbH technique. In some species (e.g. *Mugil, Anguilla*), the PbH cells are usually club-shaped, with the 'handle' stretching to the boundary membrane between the neurohypophysis and pars intermedia (colour plate). The PAS + cells of cyprinodonts occur in small numbers as intrusive islets in the pars distalis, especially in the rostral zone, and the number of islets seems to increase with age (colour plate). In contrast, the PbH + cells do not occur outside the pars intermedia.

Not all teleosts display these two typical cell-types. Salmonids appear to lack the PAS + cell, and have a PbH + cell together with a second type that is totally chromophobic.

Acidophilic droplets, colloidal in appearance, often occur amongst the pars intermedia cells, as in other vertebrates. They have amphiphilic staining properties, commonly being strongly OG +, and their function is uncertain.

Few ultrastructural studies have been made on this region. In *Anguilla* Knowles and Vollrath (1966a) described two main cell-types. Type I probably represents the PAS + cell, and is oval, with diffuse RER and a large nucleus and nucleolus. It contains membrane-bound electron-dense granules mainly 180 nm in diameter or less. Type II, probably the PbH + cell, is elongated, with an extensive RER at its inner end, away from the basement membrane. It often contains many membrane-bound electron-dense granules measuring 270–360 nm in diameter, and also a much larger membrane-bound inclusion measuring about 1000 nm, which may correspond to the colloid vesicles seen with the light microscope. A third cell-type is found rarely, with small nucleus and dense cytoplasm; its equivalent with the light microscope is not known. In *Gasterosteus*,

Follénius (1968) distinguished the two cell-types with the light microscope, and with the EM could recognise with certainty only the PAS+ type, with secretory granules 240–260 nm in diameter; the PbH+ cell in this teleost contains mainly electron-lucent vesicles together with a few electron-dense granules, according to Leatherland (1970*b*). In *Perca*, the PAS+ cell has granules 250–300 nm in diameter, and the PbH+ cell contains only rare granules (Follénius and Porte, 1961). In some teleosts the PAS+ cells have the larger granules (*Hippocampus*), in others the PbH+ cell granules are the larger (*Anguilla*, *Zoarces*). In *Anguilla*, the size of the granules in both cell-types increases with age (Vollrath, 1966).

THE FUNCTIONS OF THE PARS INTERMEDIA CELLS

The presence of two cell-types suggests that the pars intermedia may secrete two distinct hormones. While this may be so, it is by no means certain at present. There is no doubt that this region is the source of MSH (Ball and Baker, 1969), but it is not possible to state with certainty which of the two cells secretes this hormone, though most of the evidence favours the PbH+ cell (Baker and Ball, 1970; Olivereau, 1969*a*, 1971). Older work suggested that the teleost pituitary might secrete two antagonistic melanotropic hormones, MSH (intermedin) and melanophore-concentrating hormone (MCH) (Pickford and Atz, 1957). It has been suggested that the two cell-types correspond to these two hormones; however, this bi-hormonal theory of pituitary control of the melanophores is not now generally accepted (see Bradshaw and Waring, 1969), the observed effects being explicable in terms of only a single pituitary hormone (MSH) interacting with direct sympathetic innervation of the pigment cells. On the hypothesis that the cell that secretes MSH should be more active in fish on an illuminated black background than on white, several workers have examined the pars intermedia in relation to background adaptation. The results are confusing. In some species the PAS+ cell is activated on a black background, in other species it is the PbH+ cells that respond to background, and in a few species no cytological responses could be detected (Ball and Baker, 1969; Baker and Ball, 1970). *Anguilla* has been intensively studied in this type of experiment. Taking the results together with the effects of pituitary autotransplantation and treatment with reserpine and metopirone, it seems certain that the PbH+ cell is the source of MSH in this teleost (Olivereau, 1969*a*, 1971; Baker and Ball, 1970). The evidence concerning *P. latipinna* is confusing. The PAS+ cells are activated and more numerous on a black background in this fish, and simultaneously the secretion rate of MSH is increased, pointing to the PAS+ cells as the source of MSH. Nevertheless, during three weeks' culture *in vitro*, the pituitary of *P. latipinna* releases MSH continuously, and it is the PbH+ cells that are active in the cultures, and the PAS+ cells that are regressed (Baker and Ball, unpublished observations).

Non-pigmentary functions of the pars intermedia have been indicated. There is growing evidence that in some teleosts, in which the PbH+ cells appear to secrete MSH, the PAS+ cell may have an osmoregulatory function. These cells are more active in freshwater than in seawater, and are most active in de-ionised water, in *Anguilla* (Olivereau and Ball, 1970), and Olivereau (1969*b*) has suggested that they may secrete a hormone concerned in calcium regulation. The PAS+ cells are also activated by transfer from seawater to freshwater in *Mugil*, and in *Oryzias* are activated in de-ionised water (Olivereau and Ball, 1970).

Various observations relate the pars intermedia to reproductive changes. For example, in the marine *Zoarces viviparus* the PAS+ cells increase in number and activity during oogenesis and breeding, and in the freshwater goldfish the PbH+ cells multiply during gonad maturation and the PAS+ cells multiply after spawning (Ball and Baker, 1969).

HYPOTHALAMIC CONTROL OF THE PARS INTERMEDIA

In both pituitary transplants and in culture the PAS cells of *Anguilla* and *Poecilia* spp. display reduced activity or become completely atrophied, suggesting that some stimulatory hypothalamic factor is necessary to maintain these cells, no matter what their function may be. More details are available about the PbH+ cells. In homotransplants in *P. formosa* these cells become atrophied (Olivereau and Ball, 1966), and though they are better-maintained in three-week autotransplants in *P. latipinna*, the fish behave like hypophysectomised animals in that they lose melanin and appear to be deficient in MSH (Ball *et al.* 1972).

Pituitary autotransplants in *Anguilla* after two months display some maintenance and activity of the PbH+ cells varying from regression to normal activity, the varying state of the cells being correlated with the degree of maintenance of melanin content and its dispersion within the melanophores (Olivereau, 1969*a*). Metopirone treatment of intact *Anguilla* causes rapid skin darkening and activation of the PbH+ cells. These same responses can be elicited in eels with pituitary autotransplants, but to a lesser degree, suggesting the existence of a hypothalamic stimulatory factor (MSH-releasing factor, MRF) necessary for maximal activation of the PbH+ cells. However, treatment of intact eels with reserpine, which depletes hypothalamic amines, also causes rapid darkening of the skin, together with rapid nuclear hypertrophy and degranulation of the PbH+ cells, results which have been interpreted as indicative of a hypothalamic MSH-inhibiting factor (MIF), which may be a monoamine (cf. amphibians, chapter 12) or under monoaminergic control. It seems then, that there is a dual control of MSH in *Anguilla* (Olivereau, 1971).

Culture of the pituitary and bioassay of the culture medium has shown that MSH is released continuously during the culture period (*P. latipinna, Carassius, Anguilla, Salmo gairdneri*), and that in all species the PbH+ cells are very active, alongside regressed PAS+ cells (see Ball *et al.* 1972). These observations, like those of Olivereau, point to the existence of a hypothalamic MIF that inhibits the PbH+ cells *in vivo*, for example in a fish on a white background (Baker and Ball, 1970). In agreement with this hypothesis, lesioning of the hypothalamo-neurohypophysial tract in the catfish *Ictalurus* impairs white-background adaptation but does not affect adaptation to a black background (see Ball *et al.* 1972).

In summary, the evidence points to a hypothalamic inhibitory influence on the PAS+ cell, while the PbH+ cell is probably controlled by a dual hypothalamic mechanism.

THE HYPOTHALAMUS AND NEUROHYPOPHYSIS IN TELEOSTS

HYPOTHALAMIC NUCLEI

Many different hypothalamic nuclei occur in teleosts, but only two have been studied in any detail, the *preoptic nucleus* (PON) and the *nucleus lateralis tuberis* (NLT). The 'unknown' nuclei may in fact play some part in control of the adenohypophysis, but we have no positive evidence on this point (see Peter, 1970).

The *preoptic nuclei* have been described in detail in many teleosts, and exhaustive reviews have recently been published (Perks, 1969; Dodd, Follett and Sharp, 1971). They are sheets of neurons lying above the optic chiasma and just below the ependyma of the third ventricle, and lie in an L- or arc-shape (fig. 10.2). In general the PON can be divided into a dorsal *pars magnocellularis* and a ventral *pars parvocellularis*, and the cells are bipolar or multipolar, with short processes projecting between the ependymal cells into the third ventricle (Perks, 1969; Haider and Sathyanesan, 1972*a*); these processes may secrete into the ventricle, but more probably they receive material from the cerebrospinal fluid (Dodd, Follett and Sharp, 1971) (fig. 10.2). All the cells of the PON contain AF+ NSM. Tracts from the PON are often described as diffuse, but there seem usually to be several which converge in mid-ventral line to form the PON-neurohypophysial tract. The tract runs into the pituitary, and expands to form the greater part of the neurohypophysis (Perks, 1969; Dodd, Follett and Sharp, 1971).

Two kinds of cells, dark cells and light cells, have been found in both parts of the PON in *Anguilla*, and these probably give rise to the two kinds of type A fibres found in the tract and the neurohypophysis. The

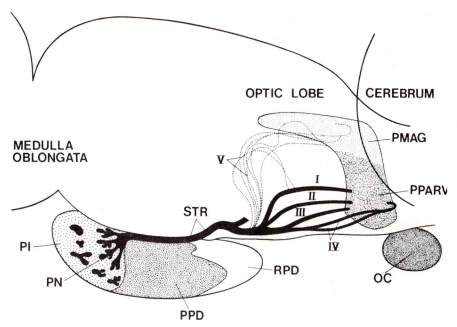

Fig. 10.2. *Anguilla anguilla*. Diagram of midsagittal section of brain and pituitary (anterior to the right), to show the PON-neurohypophysial system. PMAG, preoptic nucleus, pars magnocellularis; PPARV, preoptic nucleus, pars parvocellularis; I–V, component preoptico-neurohypophysial tracts; STR, sub-terminal region of the common preoptico-neurohypophysial tract; OC, optic chiasma; RPD, rostral pars distalis; PPD, proximal pars distalis; PI, pars intermedia; PN, posterior neuro-hypophysis. The nucleus lateralis tuberis, not shown in this diagram, lies in the floor of the hypothalamus, above the pituitary gland. From Leatherland, J. F., Budtz, P. E. and Dodd, J. M. (1966). *Gen. comp. Endocr.* **7**, 234–244.

dark cells, with the larger secretory granules, 215 nm in diameter, are the probable source of type A1 fibres, and the *light cells*, with granules 163 nm in diameter, probably give rise to type A2 fibres (Leatherland and Dodd, 1969). Type A secretory granules are greater than 100 nm in diameter, and their electron-dense contents completely fill the boundary membrane. These are the classical neurohypophysial elementary neurosecretory granules (ENG) and stain with AF, CAH, AB and aldehyde thionin (Knowles and Vollrath, 1966a, b; Ball and Baker, 1969; Bern, Zambrano and Nishioka, 1971).

The *nucleus lateralis tuberis* (NLT) is usually present as a pair of crescentic structures lying around the anterior and lateral regions of the infundibular stem base. It can be divided into various regions, differing in different teleosts. Its cells are generally AF−, although in some species some of the NLT cells are AF+ (Perks, 1969; Ball and Baker, 1969; Haider and Sathyanesan, 1972b). A detailed account of the

NLT of *Mugil* has recently been given. It is divisible into pars lateralis, containing dense groups of polygonal neurons, and a pars medialis, with smaller cells, adjacent to the infundibular cavity. The NSM material is AF−, CAH−, AB− and aldehyde thionin−, but it stains with 'acid' dyes, such as phloxine, acid fuchsin and azocarmine (Blanc-Livni and Abraham, 1970). Dendritic processes of the neurons may project into the infundibular recess (Haider and Sathyanesan, 1972b). Axons from the NLT seemingly pass into the neurohypophysis in the main tract alongside the type A PON axons (Knowles and Vollrath, 1966b).

The NLT gives rise to the 'non-stainable' type B neurosecretory fibres that are found in the teleost neurohypophysis (Ball and Baker, 1969). The course of these fibres has not often been traced, but the perikarya of the NLT neurons contain type B secretory granules (Knowles and Vollrath, 1966b; Zambrano, 1970a, b), although cases have been reported where the NLT secretory granules are larger than those in pituitary type B fibres (*Salmo, Gasterosteus, Leuciscus*; see Ball and Baker, 1969; Follénius, 1970; Ekengren, 1972). The staining reactions of type B fibres are generally found to be similar to those of the NLT neurons. However, it is probably premature to conclude that all type B fibres originate in the NLT. With the EM, type B secretory granules are 100 nm in diameter or less, with their electron-dense core usually separated from the bounding membrane by a clear space; they are termed large granulated vesicles (LGV) (Zambrano, 1970a; Bern, Zambrano and Nishioka, 1971).

Type B fibres without perikarya have been found in the PON region of *Anguilla*; the origin of these fibres is unknown, but it was suggested that they could act as a link between NLT and PON (Knowles and Vollrath, 1966b).

Other hypothalamic nuclei have not been studied in any detail. However, the goldfish hypothalamus has been found to contain two aminergic nuclei in the posterior hypothalamus, which appear to secrete nor-adrenaline into the third ventricle and to give rise to four tracts which end in the hypothalamus (see Dodd, Follett and Sharp, 1971).

The nature of the various hypothalamic fibres has been intensively studied recently, and most evidence shows that the PON and type A fibres are peptidergic, while the type B fibres are usually shown to be aminergic (see Zambrano, 1970a, b; Bern, Zambrano and Nishioka, 1971; Zambrano, Nishioka and Bern, 1972). The cells of the NLT have been shown to be aminergic in *Gillichthys* (Zambrano, 1970a; Bern, Zambrano and Nishioka, 1971), but are not aminergic in the roach, *Leuciscus rutilus*, nor do any of the five kinds of cells contain type B secretory granules in this fish (Ekengren, 1972).

THE NEUROHYPOPHYSIS

The neurohypophysis consists largely of axonal nerve fibres, mostly non-myelinated, which originate in hypothalamic nuclei. Many axons terminate on capillaries in the neurohypophysis, and these mainly belong to the PON system and are type A fibres. Many other fibres terminate on the basement membrane separating neurohypophysis and adenohypophysis; this membrane is probably always double, containing an intervascular space which extends to surround capillaries (Nagahama and Yamamoto, 1970; Leatherland, 1970*a*, *b*, *c*). The basement membrane around capillaries in the posterior neurohypophysis of *Cymatogaster* is elaborated to form a complex three-dimensional network around the capillary remarkably similar to the arrangement around the short loops of the toad median eminence (see chapter 12). These elaborate extensions of the basement membrane seem to serve as an increased area for contact with neurosecretory fibres and pars intermedia endocrine cells (Leatherland, 1970*c*), and may occur in other teleosts and in other parts of the neuro-adenohypophysial interface. Yet other fibres, especially type B, penetrate beyond the basement membrane and directly innervate the pars distalis as well as the pars intermedia.

In the more primitive teleosts such as *Anguilla*, tube-like extensions of the third ventricle bordered by ependymal cells penetrate into the posterior neurohypophysis, forming a hollow centre to each finger-like projection of the neural tissue into the pars intermedia; pituicytes, similar to ependymal cells, are widespread both in these primitive fishes and in more advanced forms in which no hollow processes penetrate the neurohypophysis. EM studies of the eel neurohypophysis have indicated that the pituicytes are secretory, releasing a PAS+ substance into the extensions of the infundibular recess (Knowles and Vollrath, 1966*a*). It is not known how general this secretory activity of pituicytes may be, and it is possible that there may be two kinds of pituicytes at least, glial and ependymal elements (see Ball and Baker, 1969). In trout and salmon, and probably in other teleosts, the neurohypophysis scarcely penetrates the adenohypophysis at hatching, the penetrations developing as the fish grows (see Ball and Baker, 1969).

The neurohypophysis can usually be easily divided into two parts, the anterior region containing mainly AF− type B fibres and rather few pituicytes, in contact with the pars distalis; and the posterior region containing mainly AF+ type A fibres and many pituicytes, in contact with the pars intermedia. On functional, anatomical and embryological grounds, evidence has recently become available that confirms the long-held concept that these two regions correspond to the median eminence and neural lobe respectively (Ball and Baker, 1969; Perks, 1969; Vollrath, 1972). In most teleosts there is no definite boundary between the two parts, and a few type A fibres occur in the anterior region and a few type B fibres posteriorly. *Cymatogaster, Gasterosteus* and *Anguilla* seem to have clearer division of the neurohypophysis than most teleosts (Leatherland, 1970c; Follénius, 1968; Olivereau, 1967a). The NSM in the posterior neurohypophysis often forms large bodies (Herring bodies), which represent accumulations of granules within swollen nerve endings (see Ball and Baker, 1969; Perks, 1969).

The hypothalamus and neurohypophysis include at least two functionally and morphologically distinct systems which are less clearly separated anatomically in teleosts than in other groups. These are the hypothalamo-neural lobe system, corresponding at least approximately to the PON–type A fibre–posterior neurohypophysis; and the hypothalamo–type B fibre system, corresponding approximately to the NLT–type B fibre–anterior neurohypophysis, though we should emphasise that nuclei other than the NLT may contribute to this system. Both systems are concerned with the elaboration, transport, storage and release of NSM, but the first is probably chiefly concerned with the secretion of neuro-hypophysial octapeptides into the blood, while the second is concerned with the control of the adenohypophysial cells.

THE PON–TYPE A FIBRE SYSTEM

Two octapeptides with characteristic biological properties occur in teleosts, arginine vasotocin (AVT) and isotocin or ichthyotocin (IT), and these are thought to be the neurohypophysial hormones of these animals although their physiological roles are ill-defined (Perks, 1969). In *Anguilla* both AVT and IT are present in the PON, as well as in the neurohypophysis. Eels in freshwater showed a preponderance of AVT over IT in both regions, but in eels caught in brackish water the PON was richer in IT than AVT, and the neurohypophysis contained more AVT than IT (Holder, 1969a, b). After hypophysectomy, AVT and IT migrate along the PON-neurohypophysial tract in the same way as the elementary neurosecretory granules, AVT moving more slowly than IT (Holder, 1970). This adds to older evidence that the octapeptides are associated with type A granules, and are formed in the PON (see Perks, 1969; Ball and Baker, 1969). The two different kinds of neurons in the PON (p. 200) presumably correspond to the two different octapeptides, and recent evidence suggests that AVT occurs in the larger (type A1) granules, and IT in the smaller (type A2) granules (Rodríguez, 1971). Two kinds of type A fibres, defined on the basis of granule size, have been reported from several teleosts in addition to the eel.

The posterior neurohypophysis contains mainly type A fibres, together with a few type B (Ball and Baker, 1969; Leatherland, 1970c). The great majority of the AF+ type A fibres enter the finger-like projections of the neurohypophysis in the pars intermedia, and often have swollen terminations which appear as Herring bodies under the light microscope. With the EM, the terminations are seen to contain accumulations of secretory granules, and also many clear 'synaptic' vesicles. At these endings in *Anguilla* the secretory granules appear to break down, lose their electrondensity, and perhaps release small particles into their surroundings (Knowles and Vollrath, 1966a). The majority of type A fibres probably terminate within the neurohypophysis itself, in its posterior region at one of three sites: on pituicytes, around capillaries, or against the basement membrane separating the neuro- from the adenohypophysis. This last category might include fibres concerned in adenohypophysial control. Synapses with pituicytes have been described in *Anguilla*, *Gasterosteus* and *Cymatogaster* (Knowles and Vollrath, 1966a; Leatherland, 1970b, c). In *Anguilla*, the number of synaptoid contacts between type A1 endings and pituicytes appeared to increase when the animals were transferred to seawater.

Type A endings on capillaries have been described mainly at the border of the neurohypophysis, against vessels included within expansions of the basement membrane (Henderson, 1969). With the light microscope, it is commonly observed that regions of the neurohypophysis around capillaries are poor in stainable NSM, and it seems likely that this appearance represents degranulated type A fibres (e.g. *Gasterosteus*, *Cymatogaster*; Leatherland, 1970b, c). Type A endings near capillaries occur in *Tilapia*, but flattened processes of stellate perivascular cells intervene between axon and capillary so that the contact is indirect (Bern, Zambrano and Nishioka, 1971). Synaptoid endings of type A fibres on capillaries, or on the elaborated basement membrane close to capillaries, are found in the neurohypophysis in *Cymatogaster* (Leatherland, 1970c). In *Anguilla*, by far the majority of type A1 and type A2 fibres end on the basement membrane between neuro- and pars intermedia. This double membrane encloses an intervascular channel, which widens at points to accommodate the capillaries of the plexus intermedius; in common with most vertebrates, there is little direct vascularisation of the intermedia, but this elaborate 'boundary' plexus lies at the border with the neurohypophysis. The terminations on the boundary membrane could be points where octapeptides are released, and transferred via the intervascular channel to capillaries (Knowles and Vollrath, 1966a). Most such type A endings in the eel and in *Cymatogaster* occur in the region adjacent to the pars intermedia, but in the eel a few type A fibres end on the basement membrane close to the pars distalis, and in *Tilapia* and *Gillichthys* type A endings occur in relation to capillaries in the anterior neurohypophysis (Bern, Zambrano and Nishioka, 1971). In the case of endings on the basement membrane, it is not possible to know for certain whether the neurosecretory material is destined for the neighbouring endocrine cells, or for transport to the general circulation; however, if the details of the blood supply to the pituitary in the trout (p. 211) can be generalised to other teleosts, it seems possible that type A endings on the basement membrane in the posterior neurohypophysis release material which passes into the general circulation for systemic actions, but the few type A fibres ending on the intervascular space or capillaries in the anterior region will release material which passes into capillaries of the pars distalis, and hence probably acts on the endocrine cells. Type A fibres in the anterior neurohypophysis of *Mugil* accompany capillaries in the neural pene- trations into the rostral pars distalis. These neural processes contain stainable NSM, and with the EM it appears that the type A fibres dis- charge their secretory granules into the capillaries before entry into the rostral pars distalis itself; whether this type A NSM passes into the general bloodstream via the rostral pars distalis to act systemically, or whether it is destined to influence the activity of the LTH cells, is uncertain (Abraham, 1971).

Many type A fibres in some of the species studied pass beyond the boundary membrane and terminate in the pars intermedia, and a few terminate in the pars distalis. These are considered in the next section (p. 214).

Light-microscope accounts of changes in NSM in the neurohypophysis nearly all refer to AF+ type A material, and so, probably, to the octa- peptides AVT and IT. The physiological role of these factors is uncertain. Various observations relate them to the control of osmoregulation (especially AVT) on the one hand, and to reproductive activities (possibly IT?) on the other (Perks, 1969; Heller, 1969, 1972).

The amount of NSM in the neurohypophysis commonly alters in relation to osmotic stimuli. Some teleosts show loss of this material (and of measurable AVT) when transferred to a hypertonic medium, and at the same time lose NSM from the PON (see Ball and Baker, 1969), though other species show no such changes. *Mugil* contains more type A granules, and more stainable NSM in the rostral processes of the neuro- hypophysis in freshwater than in seawater, findings which Abraham (1971) related to control of the nearby LTH cells rather than to systemic actions of the octapeptides. When *Misgurnus* was exposed to a hypotonic medium or to dehydration, stainable NSM increased in the pars magno- cellularis of the PON but decreased in the pars parvocellularis, indicating different functions for the two regions (see Ball and Baker, 1969). Changes such as these have usually been interpreted as indicating release or retention of octapeptides in response to osmotic demands. However, some recent work casts doubts on this interpretation. In goldfish, the electrical activity of the PON was increased by salt solution perfused through the nasal cavity, and this also induced depletion of AF+ NSM from the PON, the PON-neurohypophysial tract, and the neurohypophysis. Similar depletion of the system followed immersion for several days in 1 per cent saline and short periods of electrical stimulation of the olfactory tract (Jasinski, Gorbman and Hara, 1967). Electrical stimulation of the olfactory tract or systemic perfusion with Ringer's solution also altered the NSM content of the trout PON (Kreitner and Laget, 1971). Thus the responses of the PON-neurohypophysial system to changes in external salinity might represent responses to chemo-olfactory stimulation, and may or may not be related to adaptive osmoregulatory adjustments. In addition, experiments in which fish are transferred between different salinities might provoke non-specific stress responses. Bearing in mind these reservations, there is, however, enough evidence that octapeptides are involved in teleost osmoregulation to allow us to accept that at least some of the observed changes in the PON-neurohypophysial complex relate adaptively to control of water and electrolytes (see Ball and Baker, 1969; Heller, 1969; Perks, 1969).

Many workers have observed fluctuations in the amount of AF+ NSM in the neurohypophysis which can be related to the reproductive cycle. Most cases involve a depletion of material during gonad maturation and spawning. This depletion in female *Fundulus heteroclitus* is associated with a reduction in pituitary content of IT, but not of AVT (see Ball and Baker, 1969), and during sexual maturation of *Oncorhynchus tschawytscha* the ratio of IT to AVT in the neurohypophysis declines, possibly indicating preferential release of IT (Wilson and Smith, 1971). Changes in the PON, type A fibres and AF+ NSM are also related to the gonadal cycle in *Oryzias latipes*, the system being depleted during the spawning period (Kasuga and Takahashi, 1971). There is now strong evidence that neurohypophysial hormones – though whether AVT or IT is not known – stimulate contractions of the ovary and oviduct in teleosts, and this might explain the apparent involvement of the PON-neurohypophysial system in reproduction (Heller, 1972).

Changes in background colour or illumination have been found to alter the PON-neurohypophysial system in some cases, and these effects are probably related to the control of the pars intermedia, considered on p. 218.

THE HYPOTHALAMO–TYPE B FIBRE SYSTEM

The 'non-stainable' fibres in the pituitary are usually considered to arise in the NLT, though other sources in the hypothalamus remain possible (Ball and Baker, 1969; Perks, 1969; Follénius, 1970*b*). They have occasionally been described as AF+, but generally they are AF– and CAH–, though they can be stained with dyes such as azocarmine, eosin, light green, phloxin, PAS, aniline blue or by silver impregnation. Similar staining reactions are seen in the cells of the NLT. The pathways of these fibres are difficult to follow with the light microscope, but they have been traced between the cells of the proximal pars distalis in eel, and of the pars intermedia in trout.

These axons seem to correspond to the type B fibres seen with the EM. The secretory granules in these fibres are large granulated vesicles (LGV), with a clear space between the granule and the bounding membrane (figs. 10.3, 10.4), and are less than 100 nm in diameter. Similar LGV occur in the NLT in *Gillichthys* (Zambrano, 1970*a*) and *Anguilla* (Knowles and Vollrath, 1966*b*), but the granules in the NLT are bigger than type B LGV in *Gasterosteus* (Follénius, 1970*a*) and *Leuciscus* (Ekengren, 1972). Type B fibres have been shown to be aminergic in *Gasterosteus* (Follénius, 1970*a*), *Gillichthys* and *Tilapia* (Zambrano, 1970*a*; Bern, Zambrano and Nishioka, 1971; Zambrano, Nishioka and Bern, 1972), and their LGV resemble vesicles which are considered to be storage sites of biogenic amines in other systems. These LGV in type B fibres of *Tilapia* and *Gillichthys* probably contain at least two substances in the dense core, a protein and an active catecholamine; it is not certain whether or not they contain acetylcholine (Zambrano, 1970*a*; Bern, Zambrano and Nishioka, 1971; Zambrano, Nishioka and Bern, 1972). The 'synaptic' vesicles of type B (and type A) fibres in *Gasterosteus*, but not the LGV, probably do contain acetylcholine (Follénius, 1970*b*). Incubation with 5-hydroxydopamine resulted in the LGV of *Gillichthys* type B fibres showing a higher density than controls, while injections of 6-hydroxydopamine caused these fibres to degenerate, confirmatory evidence that they are monoaminergic, in *Gillichthys* (Zambrano, Nishioka and Bern, 1972), and *Gasterosteus* (Follénius, 1972*a*).

Primary catecholamines (detected by the Falck–Hillarp fluorescence technique) occur in the neuron cell-bodies of the lateral and rostral NLT of *Gillichthys*, and in the NLT of other teleosts (*Cyprinus*, *Anguilla*), though whether noradrenaline or adrenaline predominates is not known (Zambrano, 1970*a*); the NLT of *Anguilla japonica* and *Oryzias latipes* contains monoamine oxidase activity (Urano, 1971*b*), further evidence of its aminergic nature. However, the NLT of the goldfish (see Zambrano, 1970*a*) and of *Leuciscus* (Ekengren, 1972) does not contain catecholamines, which introduces a note of caution in attempting to generalise about this system. Ultrastructural, cytochemical and specific impregnation methods used on the hypothalamic region of *Gillichthys* demonstrated similarities between the LGV in the type B fibres and those in the perikarya of the median and lateral neurons of the NLT, and after hypophysectomy only these neurons underwent retrograde degeneration (Zambrano, 1970*b*). Thus in *Gillichthys*, and probably other teleosts, the aminergic type B fibres seem definitely to originate in the NLT. There is, however, some doubt that the type B fibres associated with the rostral pars distalis of *Gasterosteus* do originate in the NLT, and it seems improbable that they

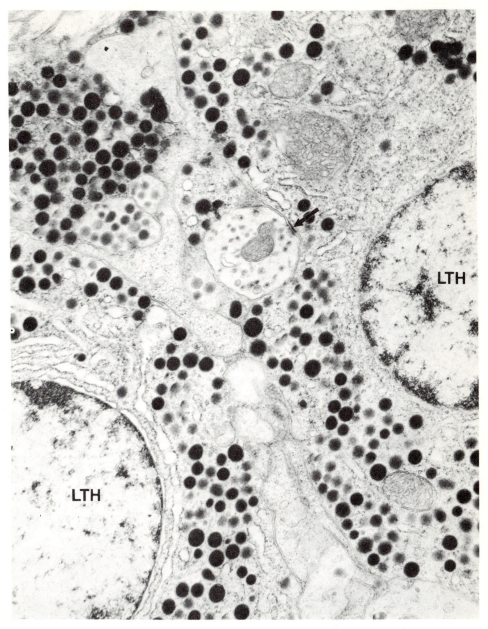

Fig. 10.3. Electron micrograph of the rostral pars distalis of the mullet, *Mugil platanus*. A type B fibre makes synaptoid contact (arrow) with a lactotrope (LTH). Photograph and information kindly supplied by Dr D. Zambrano.

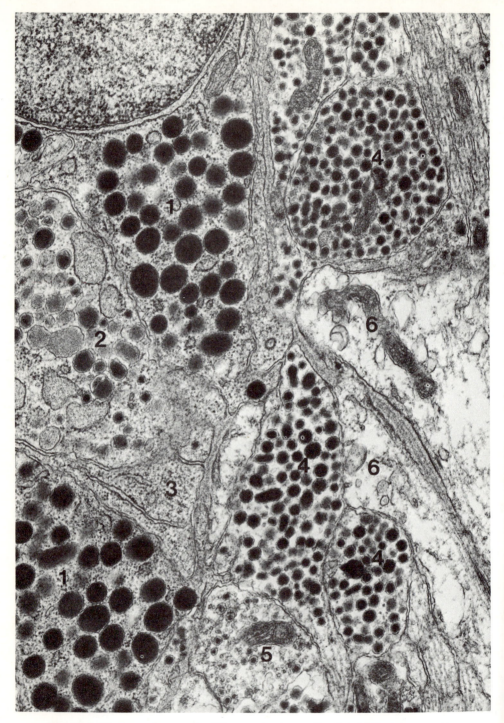

Fig. 10.4. Electron micrograph of the proximal pars distalis of *Tilapia mossambica*, a female fish adapted to freshwater. 1, STH cell; 2, gonadotrope; 3, process of stellate cell; 4, type A fibre; 5, type B fibre; 6, glial element. Photograph and information kindly supplied by Drs R. S. Nishioka and H. A. Bern.

are adrenergic, since they do not accumulate injected radio-noradrenaline, in contrast to the type B fibres associated with the proximal pars distalis and the pars intermedia (Follénius, 1970*a*). However, they accumulate selectively another neurotransmitter, γ-aminobutyric acid (Follénius, 1972*b*).

BLOOD SUPPLY TO THE PITUITARY

Many workers have studied the blood supply of the pituitary complex in teleosts (Ball and Baker, 1969). The arterial supply from the internal carotids enters the gland by a single median hypophysial artery or a pair, penetrating the anterior neurohypophysis after running for a variable distance along the ventral surface of the hypothalamus. In the neuro-hypophysis the arteries give rise to a capillary plexus lying close to the neuro-adenohypophysis interface; this plexus seems to lie within the neural tissue and its processes in the region of the pars distalis, but often seems to be mainly enclosed by the double basement membrane in the region of the pars intermedia, forming a typical plexus intermedius (Ball and Baker, 1969; Henderson, 1969; Knowles and Vollrath, 1966*a*, *b*; Leatherland, 1970*c*). The details probably vary in different teleosts. From this plexus (the *primary longitudinal plexus*), capillaries pass into the pars distalis and form an elaborate network of vessels, sinusoidal in appearance, between the endocrine cells, the *secondary centrifugal plexus*. It seems that in the pars intermedia region there is little or no penetration of the glandular tissue, the vascular basement membrane together with its associated plexus intermedius penetrating between the intermedia cords in association with neural processes. Blood is collected into a superficial venous plexus on the surface of the gland, and from there into posterior vessels that drain ultimately into the anterior cardinal veins (fig. 10.5).

A recent account of the vascular system in the pituitary of the brook-trout, *Salvelinus fontinalis*, has been given by Henderson (1969). She emphasised that there are in effect two independent vascular beds within the gland (fig. 10.6). The anterior hypophysis is supplied by a pair of ventral hypothalamic arteries, which divide into a superior ramus to the hypothalamus, particularly the NLT region, and an inferior ramus to the pituitary. The inferior ramus divides into arterioles which loop to and fro in the meninx overlying the hypothalamus; these loops, like the pre-portal loops in the median eminence of other vertebrates, may act to retard the flow of blood and facilitate neurovascular exchanges in the neurohypophysis. The arterioles enter the anterior neurohypophysis, and together with a few vessels from the superior ramus they give rise to the primary longitudinal plexus, overlying the pars distalis interface (fig. 10.6). Numerous branches from this plexus extend into the pars distalis, supplying the sinusoid-like capillaries of the glandular parenchyma, and blood drains into the superficial venous plexus.

0.1 mm

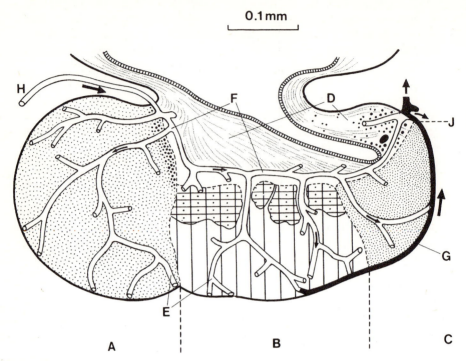

Fig. 10.5. Diagram to illustrate the main features of the blood supply to the cyprinodont pituitary. Anterior to the left. A, rostral pars distalis; B, proximal pars distalis; C, pars intermedia; D, neurohypophysis. Blood enters the gland from the hypophysial artery (H), and passes to the primary longitudinal plexus (F) in the neurohypophysis. From here it is distributed to the adenohypophysis in the second-ary centrifugal plexus (E), and is then collected into a superficial venous network (black) (G) and passes to the hypophysial vein (J). Modified from Follénius (1965).

The posterior part of the pituitary receives most of its vascular supply from the caudal hypothalamic artery, which also supplies the saccus vasculosus (fig. 10.6). A number of small branches of this artery extend into the posterior neurohypophysis, to supply the vascular plexus in the neuro-intermedia interface, the plexus intermedius; only a few vessels penetrate the pars intermedia glandular tissue directly. Venous drainage is by large channels originating at the ends of the neural interdigitations, and passing into the superficial venous network (fig. 10.6).

A minor arterial supply to the adenohypophysis is by peripheral arteries from the internal carotids, and the dorso-caudal region of the neurohypophysis sometimes receives a small supply from the anterior primary longitudinal plexus and from the caudal hypophysial artery.

As Henderson (1969) emphasises, the two vascular systems appear to

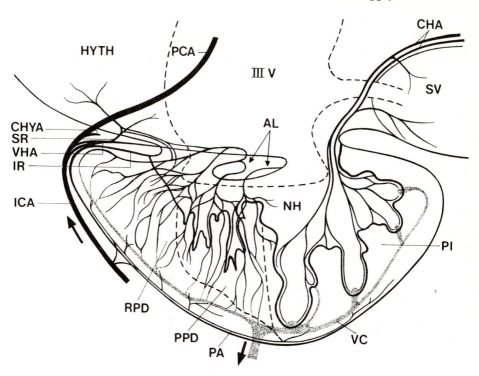

Fig. 10.6. *Salvelinus fontinalis*. Diagram of the vascularisation of the pituitary region of the brook trout in parasagittal view, anterior to left. The course of the caudal hypophysial artery is not shown. This vessel (which is often absent) passes directly to the caudal region of the neurohypophysis and there gives rise to a few capillaries. Abbreviations: AL, arterial loops; CHA, caudal hypothalamic artery; CHYA, origin of caudal hypophysial artery; HYTH, hypothalamus; ICA, internal carotid artery; IR, inferior ramus; NH, neurohypophysis; PA, peripheral artery; PCA, posterior cerebral artery; PI, pars intermedia; PPD, proximal pars distalis; RPD, rostral pars distalis; SR, superior ramus; SV, saccus vasculosus; VC, venous channels; VHA, ventral hypothalamic artery; IIIV, third ventricle. The extent of the third ventricle and the boundaries between parts of the adenohypophysis are indicated by broken lines. Solid vessels, arteries and capillaries; stippled vessels, principal venous channels. From Henderson (1969).

be essentially independent, and this situation may be more common in teleosts than has previously been recognised (Jasinski, 1969). The anterior primary longitudinal plexus with its ramifications probably has the functions of a hypophysial portal system, and as in the median eminence of other vertebrates most of the neurosecretory axons associated with this plexus are type B. Some fibres end on these capillaries (Bern, Zambrano and Nishioka, 1971), but most probably penetrate into the pars distalis. The 'portal vessels' connecting this plexus to the secondary plexus in the pars distalis are short capillaries rather than large vessels, but the pattern

8

is similar to that in urodeles with short infundibular stems (chapter 12). The plexus intermedius is comparable to that in tetrapods, and in *Salvelinus*, as in other teleosts, it appears to be a major site for AF+ fibre terminations (Henderson, 1969). It seems that the vascular pattern of trout, and perhaps of other teleosts, conforms to the usual vertebrate arrangement (separation of median eminence and neuro-intermedia vascular beds) more closely than has been thought.

From time to time there have appeared descriptions of what are claimed to be more typical median eminence–portal vessel components in teleosts (see Ball and Baker, 1969). The earlier accounts are generally not convincing. Recently, a portal system has been described in the Indian catfish *Heteropneustes fossilis*, in which a capillary plexus on the infundibular floor is said to be closely associated with a network of neurosecretory axons from the PON, vessels from this plexus passing into the adenohypophysis (Sathyanesan and Haider, 1971). A similar system has been described in *Clarias batrachus* (Sathyanesan, 1972). In neither case was the capillary plexus shown to receive terminations of neurosecretory fibres, and comparing the accounts with that of Henderson (1969) quoted above it seems possible that this plexus is, in fact, the system of arteriole loops which supply the primary longitudinal plexus in the anterior neurohypophysis, its association with neurosecretory fibres being a case of mere proximity. For *Heteropneustes fossilis*, another account published at about the same time (Sundararaj and Viswanathan, 1971) concluded that there is no trace of a portal system and median eminence. Neither group of investigators used the EM, which is critical in trying to evaluate their findings.

It will be seen that all blood from the neurohypophysis drains through the adenohypophysis before reaching venous channels; this has clear functional implications in the case of the capillary plexus of the pars distalis, but it seems likely that in the pars intermedia the vessels passing through the glandular tissue are venules, and that no exchange with the pars intermedia cells takes place across their walls. However, EM work is needed to clarify this point.

ANATOMICAL ASPECTS OF
HYPOTHALAMIC CONTROL

The physiological evidence that adenohypophysial functions in teleosts are controlled by the hypothalamus was summarised on pp. 192–200. It will have become apparent from the accounts of the neurohypophysis and the blood supply to the gland that there are two main anatomical pathways by which the hypothalamus can exert its control: neuroglandular, by direct innervation of the endocrine cells; and neurovascular, by way of the intrinsic vessels of the primary longitudinal plexus and the plexus intermedius. The former is probably the more important route, and represents essentially an extension – almost literally – of the more usual median eminence neurovascular route.

1. NEUROGLANDULAR CONTROL, BY NEURO-SECRETORY TERMINATIONS IN THE ADENOHYPOPHYSIS

Both type A and type B fibres terminate in various ways in relation to the endocrine cells (fig. 10.7). Type A endings predominate in the pars intermedia, and type B in the pars distalis, but there are overlaps in each case (see, for example, fig. 10.4).

The evidence summarised by Ball and Baker (1969), Bern, Zambrano and Nishioka (1971) and Leatherland (1970b, c) demonstrates the range of neuroglandular junctions between neurosecretory fibres and endocrine cells. The fibre may contact the cell directly, sometimes in a synaptoid manner (fig. 10.3); or it may terminate on a single or double basement membrane separating it from the endocrine cells, which sometimes includes cytoplasmic processes of interstitial (stellate?) cells (fig. 10.7). Among the more recent findings it is interesting to note that in *Tilapia* no direct neuro-endocrine contacts are found against LTH and ACTH cells, the type B fibres instead terminating on the basement membrane between neurohypophysis and the endocrine cells (fig. 10.7), but type B fibres do contact the STH, TSH and GtH cells of the proximal pars distalis (Bern, Zambrano and Nishioka, 1971). In *Cymatogaster*, type B fibres end on the boundary membrane adjacent to both ACTH and TSH cells, with synaptoid structure, and they also end less commonly in synaptoid fashion on the STH cells and on the boundary membrane with the pars intermedia, and more frequently on pituicytes in the posterior NHP (Leatherland, 1969, 1970c). In *Gasterosteus*, type B fibres contact GtH cells, and make synaptoid contact with TSH and STH cells, and with the basement membrane adjacent to the ACTH cells (Leatherland, 1970a, b; Follénius, 1968). *Gillichthys* (fig. 10.7) has direct synaptoid contacts between type B fibres and all the adenohypophysial cells (Zambrano, 1970b; Bern, Zambrano and Nishioka, 1971). Thus the type B fibre system has all the anatomical attributes required for control of the pars distalis cells by the hypothalamus.

We have seen that the type B fibres contain large granulated vesicles which include catecholamines and proteins. Originating, as they appear to do, in the NLT, which has been shown to be the source of inhibition of TSH and stimulation of gonadotropin in the goldfish (Peter, 1970), these fibres are obvious candidates as mediators of hypothalamic control of the adenohypophysis. The NLT has often been described as showing structural changes in correlation with gonadal cycles in teleosts (Ball and

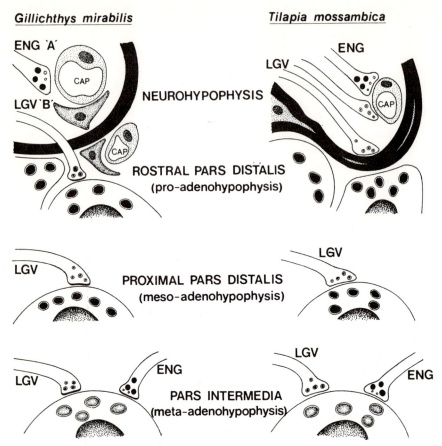

Fig. 10.7. Diagrammatic summary of the relationship between neurosecretory fibres and endocrine cells in the various regions of the pituitary of two teleosts, *Gillichthys mirabilis* and *Tilapia mossambica*. ENG, type A fibres, containing typical elementary neurosecretory granules; LGV, type B fibres containing large granulated vesicles (dense-cored vesicles). Note the presence of presynaptic membrane modifications in *Gillichthys* and their absence in *Tilapia*. From Bern, Zambrano and Nishioka (1971) and Sage and Bern (1971).

Baker, 1969), and recently more direct evidence has implicated this nucleus in pituitary control. After hypophysectomy, only the neurons of the medial and lateral NLT degenerated in *Gillichthys* (Zambrano, 1970*b*), and there is a direct relationship between the gonadal state and the neurosecretory activity of the type B fibres innervating the gonadotropes. After castration, the lateral NLT neurons and the type B fibres to the GtH cells became very active and these changes were abolished by androgen treatment (Zambrano, 1971). This evidence that the NLT lateral neurons and type B fibres stimulate the gonadotropes agrees with the results from the lesioning work of Peter (1970). After destruction of type B fibres with 6-hydroxydopamine, the lactotropes of *Gillichthys* became hypertrophied and showed signs of increased synthetic activity. A study of the parr and smolt stages of the Pacific salmon (*Oncorhynchus*) indicated an inverse relationship between the neurosecretory activity of type B fibres and the secretory activity of the LTH cells that they innervate (Zambrano, Nishioka and Bern, 1972), indicating an inhibitory influence on LTH secretion mediated by the type B fibres. Treatment of *Gillichthys* with the catecholamine-depleting agent 6-hydroxydopamine caused the ACTH cells to become hyperactive, and produced elevated plasma cortisol levels; the same treatment also caused the MSH cells to become highly active, and in the vicinity of both cell-types type B fibres were observed in stages of degeneration (Zambrano, Nishioka and Bern, 1972). Although the exact relationship of these findings to the physiological work on hypothalamic control is not entirely clear (for example, most evidence suggests hypothalamic *stimulation* of ACTH), nevertheless these results certainly implicate type B fibres and the NLT in control of adenohypophysial functions. As Zambrano (1970b) points out, the demonstration of a protein component in the LGV of type B fibres raises the possibility that hypophysiotropic factors, synthesised in the NLT, may be present in the LGV together with a catecholamine that somehow controls the release and storage of the hypophysiotropic factor at the fibre terminal; this would be in line with physiological work on mammals (McCann *et al.* 1972), including evidence that LGV from equine hypophysial stalks are rich in protein and are the probable site of storage of LH releasing factor (Ishii, 1970, 1972). The presence in carp hypothalamus of a gonadotropin releasing factor able to release sheep LH is highly relevant in this context (p. 195). The neurosecretory endings in the mammalian median eminence are type B, and again their LGV contain both a protein and a catecholamine (Ishii, 1972; Scott *et al.* 1972). Thus, the teleost anterior neurohypophysis in many respects is very like the mammalian median eminence, and in all probability, as suggested by embryology, the median eminence is its true homologue.

The rather few type A fibres that penetrate the pars distalis (fig. 10.4) have been described as ending on intervascular spaces adjacent to the endocrine cells, and in some cases as making direct contacts, sometimes synaptoid, with the glandular cells (Ball and Baker, 1969; Leatherland, 1969, 1970c; Bern, Zambrano and Nishioka, 1971). According to Knowles and Vollrath (1966b, c) type A3 fibres in the rostral pars distalis of *Anguilla* are more numerous and contain more NSM in the silver (migratory) eel than in the yellow eel, which might be related to the greater activity of the rostral TSH cells in the silver eel. Once the silver eel reaches the sea, AF + NSM becomes scarce in fibres penetrating the proximal pars distalis (perhaps related to the maturing gonadotropes in that region), and the type A3 fibres, with 150 nm diameter granules, are replaced by fibres with smaller granules (100 nm in diameter). Type A fibres contact the gonadotropes in *Gasterosteus* (Leatherland, 1970*b*), and in *Mugil* these fibres appear to secrete their granular contents into capillaries supplying the LTH cell region, and behave in such a way as to suggest that they may be stimulatory to the LTH cells (Abraham, 1971).

The common termination of type A fibres on pars intermedia cells in various species has frequently been emphasised (Zambrano, 1970*b*; Bern, Zambrano and Nishioka, 1971; Sage and Bern, 1971; Zambrano, Nishioka and Bern, 1972), particularly in relation to the concept of a dual (type A and type B) innervation of the pars intermedia (Knowles and Vollrath, 1966*a*). In both *Tilapia* and *Gillichthys*, type A (and type B) fibres end in direct contact with the pars intermedia cells, the contacts being synaptoid in *Gillichthys* (Bern, Zambrano and Nishioka, 1971, fig. 10.7). In *Gasterosteus*, type A fibres have synaptoid endings on the PAS+ cells of the pars intermedia, and both type A and type B fibres have non-synaptoid endings on the PbH+ cells (Leatherland, 1970*b*). *Cymatogaster* has type A2 fibres, and a few type B, ending on the boundary membrane (Leatherland, 1970*c*), and *Salmo* and *Perca* display a similar arrangement (Ball and Baker, 1969). In *Anguilla* Knowles and Vollrath (1966*a*) found that the terminations of type A1 and A2 fibres are associated with the boundary membrane, apparently discharging their contents into the intervascular channel. The pars intermedia cells also appear to release their products into this channel, and the authors suggested that the type A fibres might influence the activity of the endocrine cells by way of the channel. The same kinds of type A1 and A2 fibres also make synaptoid contacts with neighbouring pituicytes (ependymal cells), and the contacts increased in number in eels that were briefly exposed to a white background. Knowles and Vollrath interpreted these observations as evidence that the pituicytes play some role in regulating the activity of the pars intermedia cells. The pituicytes seem to secrete a PAS+ material into the tube-like extensions of the infundibular recess with which they are associated, and the amount of this material increased in the eels on a white background; it was suggested that this material might form a feedback link between the pituitary and the PON, via the third ventricle. There is evidence from higher vertebrates (chapter 15) for an association between secretory neurons and ependymal cells, and of secretion by ependymal cells into the third ventricle. It may be that, in general, pituicytes (ependymal and glial elements) play some role in neurosecretory control.

Although no neurosecretory fibres penetrate the pars intermedia parenchyma in *Anguilla*, the related *Conger* shows some synaptoid junctions between type A fibres and pars intermedia cells (Knowles and Vollrath, 1966*a*).

In summary, all parts of the adenohypophysis are directly innervated by neurosecretory fibres, with type B fibres predominating in the pars distalis and type A fibres in the pars intermedia. The anterior neurohypophysial core, conveying type B fibres mainly to the pars distalis, has clear resemblances to the neural component of the median eminence.

2. NEUROVASCULAR CONTROL, BY FIBRE ENDINGS ON NEUROHYPOPHYSIAL CAPILLARIES

Apart from the various neuroglandular contacts, which have attracted great attention in recent years, many workers have described synaptoid or other contacts between neurosecretory fibres and the capillaries of the primary longitudinal plexus and the plexus intermedius. According to Follénius (1965), it is type B fibres that terminate on the anterior primary capillary plexus, while type A fibres mostly end in the posterior region, close to the boundary membrane and hence related to the plexus intermedius. However, in *Tilapia* both type A and type B fibres end on the primary plexus (Bern, Zambrano and Nishioka, 1971), and in *Mugil* type A fibres end on branches of the plexus passing into the LTH cell region. Such neurovascular links may play a part in transmitting hypothalamic control to the adenohypophysis, and clearly resemble the relay pattern in the median eminence of other vertebrates; but, despite only limited information, the indications are that in teleosts neurovascular links are less important than the neuroglandular contacts described in the previous section.

3. POSSIBLE ROLE OF THE THIRD VENTRICLE IN HYPOTHALAMIC CONTROL

Several workers have described processes of the cells in both the NLT and PON which penetrate the ependyma and project into the third ventricle, and some authors consider that these processes may be secretory. It has been postulated that material released at these points might be transported to the pituitary from the cerebrospinal fluid, either by capillaries (though there is little anatomical basis for this) or by way of certain specialised cells lining the infundibular recess, which appear to send AF+ or PAS+ fibres towards the gland (Ball and Baker, 1969). The ependyma of the mammalian median eminence contains cells (tanycytes) which appear capable of transferring substances from the cerebrospinal fluid into the primary portal capillaries (Scott *et al.* 1972; Porter, Kamberi and Ondo, 1972; Kobayashi, 1972), as well as some cells that may secrete into the third ventricle (Scott *et al.* 1972), and the specialised cells of the teleost infundibular recess may have analogous functions. However, some workers believe the dendritic processes of the

NLT and PON cells to be absorptive rather than secretory (Leatherland and Dodd, 1969; Dodd, Follett and Sharp, 1971), and the whole subject is largely speculative at the present time.

SUMMARY

The neurohypophysis of teleosts contains at least two neurosecretory systems, distinct morphologically and, as it now seems, in function. The *NLT–type B fibre system* (which might include nuclei other than the NLT) appears to be largely aminergic, and to innervate the pars distalis cell directly, or via intervascular channels in the boundary membrane between pars distalis and neurohypophysis, or by way of short capillaries between the neuro- and adenohypophysis. Type B fibres also innervate pars intermedia cells in some species, if not all. The *PON–type A fibre system* is peptidergic and terminates mainly on capillaries in the posterior neurohypophysis, including the vessels of the plexus intermedius. Since these capillaries in trout, and probably other teleosts, form part of a vascular bed independent of the supply to the pars distalis, and having direct venous drainage, it may be that the type A fibres at these sites release octapeptides directly into the systemic circulation. A complication, however, is that many type A fibres innervate pars intermedia cells, often, it seems, jointly with type B fibres, and some type A fibres innervate pars distalis cells. Clearly, it is possible that there are several kinds of type A fibres, some releasing octapeptides into the systemic blood, others (possibly with smaller secretory granules) releasing materials (octapeptides or other molecules?) which act on adenohypophysial cells. Type A fibres have also been reported as ending on capillaries of the primary plexus of the median eminence in other vertebrates (chapters 8, 11, 12), so that the teleosts are not alone in presenting this seemingly anomalous feature.

Finally, it may be said that the teleosts present, as it were, an alternative pituitary gland to the usual pattern, involving the direct neurosecretory innervation of the pars distalis. Comparable direct innervation of pars distalis cells has recently been discovered in a lungfish (chapter 11). It seems possible that the orderly regional arrangement of the pars distalis cells in teleosts is dictated by this specialised hypothalamo-adenohypophysial relationship.

11

THE PITUITARY GLAND
IN CROSSOPTERYGIAN FISHES

The class Crossopterygii forms a separate stock from the elasmobranchs and actinopterygians (fig. 7.1), and crossopterygian fishes first appear in the fossil record in the mid-Devonian, by which time three separate groups were already established, the Osteolepidoti, Coelacanthini and Dipnoi. The palaeontological evidence indicates that the land vertebrates – the tetrapods – evolved from the generalised osteolepid stock in the latter half of the Devonian; thus the surviving relatives of the extinct osteolepids – the single coelacanth genus *Latimeria* and the six species of lungfishes (Dipnoi) – have a special interest, in being closer than any other living fishes to the ancestors of the tetrapods. All coelacanths were thought to have perished some 50000000 years ago, until in 1939 *Latimeria* was dramatically found alive in the Indian Ocean. Coelacanths are probably more closely related to the tetrapod ancestors than the lungfishes, which were a Devonian offshoot from the main stock and early on became specialised in many ways. Unfortunately rather little is known about the pituitary of lungfishes, and even less about the gland in *Latimeria*.

ORDER DIPNOI

Despite the great interest of these creatures, there have been few studies on the pituitary using modern techniques. The work of Wingstrand (1956) and Kerr and van Oordt (1966) deals with the gland in the African lungfish, *Protopterus* spp. Less is known about the Australian *Neoceratodus* and the South American *Lepidosiren*.

The organisation of the pituitary is amphibian rather than fish-like, in having a well-marked neural lobe, a distinct median eminence, a mosaic arrangement of cell-types in the pars distalis and no saccus vasculosus (fig. 11.1). Fish-like features are the elaborate intermingling of neural and intermediate elements, the direct innervation of the pars distalis cells, the absence of a pars tuberalis and the large hypophysial cleft between pars intermedia and pars distalis. In *Neoceratodus* diverticuli from the cleft penetrate the pars distalis, as in *Acipenser* (Wingstrand, 1966a). The adenohypophysial anlage is solid, the hypophysial cleft appearing later as a schizocoel. In *Protopterus* there is practically no sella turcica and the

[221]

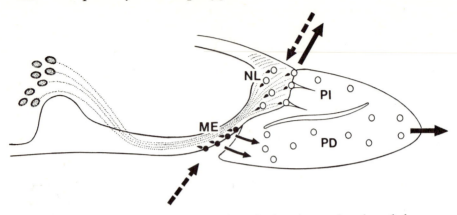

Fig. 11.1. Lungfish pituitary, diagrammatic sagittal section to show hypothalamo-hypophysial vascular and neurosecretory links. ME, median eminence; NL, neural lobe; PD, pars distalis; PI, pars intermedia. Dotted circles, neurosecretory cells of the preoptic nucleus; dotted lines, neurosecretory axons, with axon terminals marked in the ME and NL; filled circles, primary portal capillaries; empty circles, secondary portal capillaries and other intrahypophysial capillaries; interrupted arrows, arteries; solid arrows, veins; thin arrows, portal veins. From Jasinski (1969).

gland is flat, with the pars distalis behind the neural lobe as in many amphibians (chapter 12). *Neoceratodus* has a deep sella turcica, with the pituitary extended ventrally from the brain and the pars distalis anterior to the neural lobe. *Lepidosiren* exhibits an intermediate condition (Wingstrand, 1966*a*).

The *pars distalis* has nothing of the clear regional differentiation found in teleosts, but like the mosaic gland of many tetrapods it displays a vague zonation resulting from the greater or lesser abundance of different cell-types in different regions. The distalis cells are arranged in cords separated by sinusoidal capillaries; the cords are generally compact, but sometimes have a central lumen containing colloid. This feature is particularly marked in *Neoceratodus*, and recalls the colloid-filled follicles found in the pars distalis of turtles, birds and mammals (Wingstrand, 1956, 1966*a*). Five cell-types have been distinguished in the pars distalis. Lack of experimental investigations makes it impossible to allocate specific endocrine functions to any of these cells with certainty, but in their staining reactions and distribution the cells strongly resemble those of the amphibian gland, for which there is adequate histophysiological information (chapter 12). On the basis of these similarities, and considering the time at which the dipnoan cells differentiate during ontogeny, the most recent investigators (Kerr and van Oordt, 1966) have tentatively allocated functions to the dipnoan cells.

Two distinct acidophils are present. Type 1 acidophil is erythrosinophilic after Aliz BT and is distributed throughout the gland. Type 2 is more OG +, faintly PAS + and is confined to the caudal pars distalis, a region which becomes hyperplastic in very large adult fish (van Oordt, 1968). Presumably the acidophils secrete LTH and STH respectively. There are three basophil types. Type 1 and type 2 both have typical basophil staining reactions (PAS +, AF +, AB +, aniline blue +), but can be distinguished by details of size, distribution and granulation. Type 3 basophils are restricted to the anterior tip of the pars distalis, close to the entry of the portal vessels, and are violet (amphiphilic) after Aliz BT, PAS +, but AF − and AB −. The type 1 basophil appears very early in development, and may secrete TSH. Type 2 basophils are found only in adult fish, in which they may be very abundant, and are possibly gonadotropes, while type 3 basophil strongly resembles the amphibian ACTH cell in location and staining properties (chapter 12) and is probably the corticotrope. As far as we are able to compare the descriptions, it seems that Godet (1964) suggested similar functional identifications on the basis of the tinctorial properties of the cells. He observed that all three basophils regress during aestivation, correlated with regression of the thyroid, cessation of spermatogenesis and atrophy of the sexual accessories.

A surprising recent finding is that the pars distalis of *Lepidosiren* is directly innervated, a feature hitherto believed to be restricted to teleost fishes (Zambrano and Iturriza, 1973). Fibres from aminergic neurons in the median eminence region (p. 225) and possibly from other hypothalamic regions as well, run into the pars distalis and end among the endocrine cells. The EM shows that these fibres contain the typical type B large granulated vesicles (LGV); they associate with pericapillary spaces, but apparently end among the endocrine cells, though no synaptoid endings have been found (fig. 11.2).

The *pars intermedia* and neural lobe are closely associated to form a dorsal neuro-intermediate lobe, separated from the pars distalis by the hypophysial cleft. *Protopterus* has a massive intermedia, consisting of hollow cellular tubules interdigitating with neural lobe processes. The cavities of the intermedia often communicate with the hypophysial cleft, from which they probably derive, but in the adult fish many are closed. In *Neoceratodus* the hypophysial cleft also sends diverticuli into the pars distalis (cf. sturgeons, chapter 9), while in *Lepidosiren* the pars intermedia is quite different, often just a thin layer a few cells thick between neural lobe and hypophysial cleft, but in some specimens consisting of closed lobules or open follicles communicating with the cleft (Zambrano and Iturriza, 1972). Two cell-types occur in the pars intermedia of *Protopterus*; one is weakly PAS +, AB + and aniline blue +, while the other is strongly PAS +, AB − and OG + (Kerr and van Oordt, 1966). The second cell-type is more abundant in younger fish. There is some experimental evidence that MSH is secreted by the pars intermedia, and that its

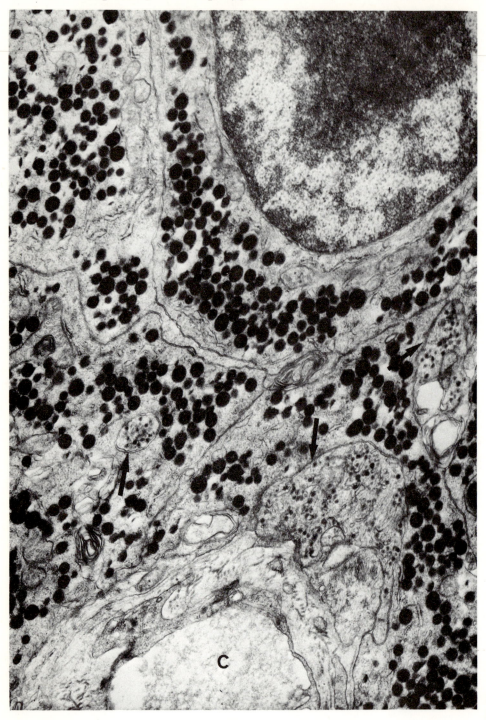

Fig. 11.2. *Lepidosiren paradoxa*. Electron micrograph of pars distalis, showing type B neurosecretory fibres (arrows) amongst the endocrine cells, and associated with a capillary (C). × 18 000. From Zambrano and Iturriza (1973).

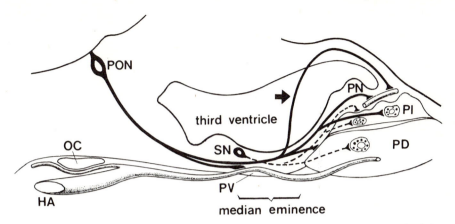

Fig. 11.3. *Lepidosiren paradoxa*. Diagram to represent the hypothalamo-hypophysial relationships. Anterior to left. Thick black lines represent the peptidergic type A fibres, originating from the preoptic nucleus (PON), which end around the primary portal capillaries (PV), on the plexus intermedius, and within both the neural lobe and the pars intermedia. Dotted lines represent the aminergic type B fibres, originating from small neurons (SN) of the median eminence, and mainly ending in the pars distalis (PD), pars intermedia (PI) and neural lobe (PN) close to the pars intermedia. OC, optic chiasma; HA, hypothalamic artery. The thick arrow indicates the upper part of the hypothalamo-hypophysial tract, which passes through the lateral wall of the infundibular cavity and constitutes the main bundle of type A fibres projecting into the neural lobe. From Zambrano and Iturriza (1973).

secretion may be under inhibitory hypothalamic control (see Ball and Baker, 1969). Two intermedia cell-types also occur in *Lepidosiren*, and these are directly innervated by type A1 fibres and a few type B fibres (Zambrano and Iturriza, 1973).

The *neurohypophysis* is clearly divisible into median eminence, short infundibular stalk (long in *Neoceratodus*) and neural lobe (Perks, 1969). There seems to be no account of any hypothalamic nuclei other than the PON, which lies relatively far anterior, dorsal to the optic chiasma, and is very short. However, in *Lepidosiren*, Zambrano and Iturriza (1973) have recently described numerous small aminergic neurons lying just below the ependyma of the median eminence (fig. 11.3). The perikarya contain LGV 90–100 nm in diameter, and these neurons resemble those of the NLT of teleosts and the infundibular and arcuate nuclei of tetrapods (Zambrano and Iturriza, 1973). The cells of the PON stain with the usual 'neurosecretory' techniques, and they send short dendrites between the nearby ependymal cells, terminating in small globules immersed in the ventricular cerebrospinal fluid (Wingstrand, 1956; Zambrano and Iturriza, 1973). In *Lepidosiren*, the perikarya of the PON have been observed to contain lysosomes and secretory granules 140–190 nm in diameter; only one kind of neuron could be distinguished (Zambrano and Iturriza, 1973). These neurons give rise to the axons of the PON-neurohypophysial tract. The pair of tracts run backwards and ventrally in the floor of the infundibular recess, and in the region of the median eminence each tract divides into dorsal and ventral components (figs. 11.1, 11.3). Many of the ventral PON axons terminate on the dense primary capillary bed of the *median eminence*. This neurovascular contact zone contains less stainable NSM than the neural lobe. The primary portal capillaries in *Lepidosiren* are supplied by branches of the hypothalamic arteries; the primary capillaries penetrate into the ventral (palisade) layer of the median eminence, and connect extensively with the capillaries of the pars distalis. In a few cases, minor connections can be found between the primary capillary bed and the vessels of the neuro-intermediate lobe, but the latter is essentially vascularised independently of the pars distalis, a tetrapod-like feature (Zambrano and Iturriza, 1972, 1973). The walls of the primary capillaries in *Lepidosiren* are characteristically fenestrated, and several kinds of neurosecretory nerve endings can be distinguished on the pericapillary spaces. The most common endings (type A1) have electron-dense, irregular secretory granules, 140–180 nm in diameter. A scarcer type (A2) has granules 120–130 nm in diameter, while type A3 contains paler granules, 140 nm in diameter. All endings contain clear 'synaptic' vesicles, and no type B or type C endings are visible (fig. 11.4). In the more posterior part of the median eminence, lying just above the pars distalis, type A1 fibres end on a thick avascular layer of connective tissue which separates them from the pars distalis cells. This condition resembles that in the 'median eminence' of the hagfish *Eptatretus* (chapter 7), and may be a case of the survival of a primitive arrangement alongside a more typical median eminence structure (Zambrano and Iturriza, 1973). From the primary capillary bed, short portal vessels run to the rostral tip of the pars distalis. The distribution of blood within the pituitary and its drainage are not known in any detail (Kerr and van Oordt, 1966; Wingstrand, 1966a; Perks, 1969), though the virtual separation of the vascular beds of the pars distalis and the neuro-intermedia has recently been demonstrated for *Lepidosiren* (Zambrano and Iturriza, 1973). As in sturgeons (chapter 9), it is obvious in these fish that the portal system is essentially a specialised area of the 'mantle plexus' between the infundibular floor and the pars distalis (Green, 1966; Kerr and van Oordt, 1966; Ball and Baker, 1969).

The fibres of the dorsal PON-neurohypophysial tract, together with a few from the ventral tract, run past the median eminence and into the *neural lobe*. This consists basically of a system of hollow neural tubules, shown by development to be diverticuli of the infundibular cavity, placed medially between the two large lateral primary branches of the infundibulum (Wingstrand, 1966a). In the adult the neural lobe is a mass of ramifying rods, the hollow ones lined by ependymal cells, the solid ones

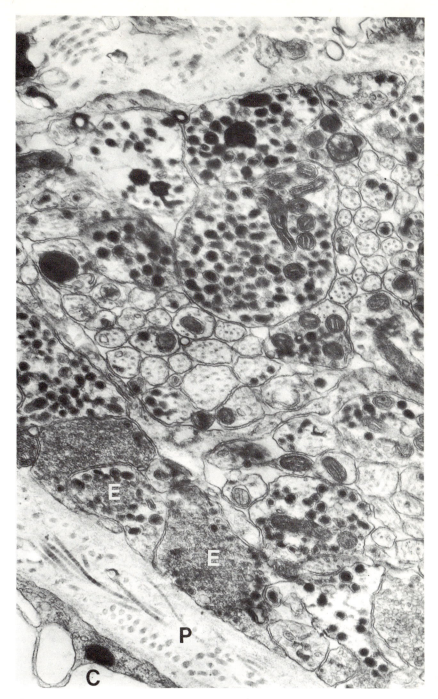

Fig. 11.4. *Lepidosiren paradoxa*. Electron micrograph of the neurohaemal region of the anterior median eminence, to show type A fibres, and their endings (E) on the capillary (C) perivascular space (P). Clusters of clear 'synaptic' vesicles appear in the type A endings, together with a few elementary secretory granules. × 21 000. From Zambrano and Iturriza (1973).

with a core of these cells (Wingstrand, 1956). These neural processes intertwine elaborately with the (primarily hollow) tubes of the pars intermedia, except in *Lepidosiren* with its simpler intermedia (Wingstrand, 1966*a*, *b*; Zambrano and Iturriza, 1972). Each neural process consists of an ependymal core, a fibrous layer with rare scattered pituicytes, a palisade layer, and an outer connective tissue membrane against the adjacent intermedia cells (Wingstrand, 1956; Kerr and van Oordt, 1966). PON axons, with plentiful AF+ NSM (i.e. presumptive type A fibres) are plentiful in these neural processes, and in addition some axons spread into the ependyma of the floor of the infundibular cavity, where Herring bodies can be seen close to the cerebrospinal fluid (Perks, 1969).

The connective tissue sheath between neural and intermedia tissues, enclosing a typical intervascular space, contains a rich capillary network, the elaborately folded plexus intermedius. This has its independent blood supply from the basilar arteries (Zambrano and Iturriza, 1972, 1973). The pars intermedia itself is virtually avascular. In *Lepidosiren*, a few capillaries from the plexus intermedius penetrate the neural lobe (Zambrano and Iturriza, 1973). Most of the PON fibres probably end on the plexus intermedius, judging from the accumulation of NSM in this region, though no EM work has been done in *Protopterus*. In addition there is evidence of direct innervation of the pars intermedia cells in *Protopterus*, as well as in *Lepidosiren* (p. 225), some nerve fibres passing from the neural lobe into the intermedia (Wingstrand, 1956). *Protopterus*, like amphibians, secretes arginine vasotocin and mesotocin (Perks, 1969; Sawyer, 1969) and probably the plexus intermedius capillaries drain in such a way that these octapeptides can reach the general circulation. Neurohypophysial hormones have been shown to cause renal diuresis with enhanced urinary sodium loss in *Protopterus*, together with an increase in total body sodium loss (Perks, 1969). It is not clear how these effects are related to the peculiar physiology of this lungfish, a freshwater animal which enters into a state of suspended animation when it aestivates during the dry season. That neurohypophysial hormones may be concerned physiologically with aestivation is suggested, however, by the report that the neural lobe contains more stainable NSM in aquatic *Protopterus* than in aestivating (aerial) fish in their cocoons and that the amount of this NSM decreases in fish transferred from water to aerial cocoons; furthermore, blowing air into the mouths of aquatic *Protopterus* caused a marked increase in neural lobe NSM after three hours (see Ball and Baker, 1969). These findings implicate neurohypophysial hormones in the aquatic/aerial metabolic changes, but without specifying exactly what they do.

The above account of the neural lobe deals mainly with *Protopterus*. A recent paper gives details of the ultrastructure of this region in *Lepidosiren* (Zambrano and Iturriza, 1972). In this genus the neural lobe is composed of several hollow lobules or follicles. Each lobule contains a central closed or hollow core of ependymal cells (the hollows continuous with the infundibular recess), a fibrous layer (hilar region), and an outer palisade layer, rich in AF + NSM. The palisade layer is in contact with the plexus intermedius, enclosed as usual in a double basement membrane which includes a perivascular space. Thus the lobules have the same structure as the tubules of *Protopterus*. The *ependymal cells* contain spherical granules 140–200 nm in diameter, which may be ingested NSM. The cells produce long processes which traverse the hilar region and terminate in ependymal end-feet against the perivascular membrane. Occasional neurosecretory axons make non-synaptoid contacts with the ependymal cell membrane. The ependymal end-feet do not form a complete collar round the capillary, but leave gaps for the endings of neurosecretory fibres. Pinocytotic vesicles occur in the end-feet membrane in contact with the pericapillary membrane, and Zambrano and Iturriza (1972) suggest that NSM may be released into the perivascular space and some of it may then be transported through the ependymal cells (appearing as the intracellular granules) to be released into the infundibular recess. The extensions of the ependymal cells to form end-feet on pericapillary spaces exactly resembles the organisation of ependymal cells and pituicytes in the neural lobe and median eminence of many tetrapods. The *hilar region* contains little NSM and is composed of small axons and ependymal cell processes, and a few pituicytes lie beneath the ependymal cells, which they resemble. In the *palisade layer* are found numerous large neurosecretory fibres, some containing an exceptionally large number of secretory granules. Four kinds of nerve fibres can be recognised, all containing 'synaptic' vesicles. Three are scattered throughout the neural lobe: type A1 fibres have spherical electron-dense granules 150–180 nm in diameter, and probably contain and release mesotocin; type A2 fibres have irregular dense granules, 130–150 nm in diameter, and probably release arginine vasotocin; and type C (cholinergic?) fibres contain only clear 'synaptic' vesicles. Aminergic type B fibres, with LGV 90–100 nm in diameter, occur only in the region close to the pars intermedia and are probably concerned in the hypothalamic control of the intermedia cells, supplementing perhaps the rather few aminergic fibres that actually end in the pars intermedia (Zambrano and Iturriza, 1972, 1973).

The unusual median eminence in *Lepidosiren*, with type A fibres ending on capillaries anteriorly, but on avascular connective tissue posteriorly, has great evolutionary implications, not the least being the support that it offers for the concept that the latter arrangement, similar to that found in a hagfish (chapter 7), might be the primitive condition of the median eminence. The presence of direct aminergic innervation of the pars distalis cells, though less extensive than in teleosts, raises difficulties in interpreting the course of evolution of hypothalamic pituitary control.

If both portal link and direct innervation were present in the earliest gnathostomes, a proposition suggested by the occurrence of the portal system in all fish groups and in tetrapods, then why should the direct innervation have been lost, as far as we know, in elasmobranchs, most ganoids and tetrapods? If on the other hand the original gnathostomes had only a portal link, then why should direct innervation have developed, apparently independently, in both actinopterygians and crossopterygians, and why should this novel link have largely supplanted the portal link in teleosts? These are important questions, but unfortunately we do not have enough information to suggest any general answers.

ORDER RHIPIDISTIA, SUB-ORDER COELACANTHINI

The fossil coelacanths (upper Devonian – Jurassic) are considered to be more closely related to the central crossopterygian stock (osteolepids) than the Dipnoi, and for this reason the Osteolepidoti and Coelacanthini are usually classified as sub-orders of a single order, the Rhipidistia. However, studies on the living coelacanth *Latimeria* have shown that the creature has developed many specialisations during the 50 000 000 years or so since the extinction of its more conservative ancestors. Although little information is yet available about the coelacanth pituitary, any expectations that it may represent, as it were, a half-way stage between the gland of primitive fishes and that of amphibians seem likely to be disappointed. The dipnoan pituitary is in fact a more satisfactory intermediate type, despite the isolated phylogenetic position of the lungfishes. As far as we can tell, the gland in *Latimeria* is as peculiar as many of the other anatomical systems of this 'living fossil'. One point of interest is that in several features (heart, persistent notochord, retention of skeletal cartilage, etc.) *Latimeria* seems to betray neoteny, the retention of juvenile structures in the adult. This neotenous tendency seems to have affected the pituitary gland. Unfortunately, the only material so far available has been too badly preserved to allow detailed investigations of micro-anatomy and histology.

The pituitary is unique in its massive anterior extension (fig. 11.5). The main part of the gland, consisting of neuro-intermediate lobe and the principal part of the pars distalis, lies in the orthodox position behind the optic chiasma, the neural lobe being an anterior process of the infundibulum (fig. 11.6). The neural lobe interdigitates with the pars intermedia in the typical fish-like manner (Lagios, 1972). The principal part of the pars distalis lies in a dorsal depression of the neuro-intermediate lobe (fig. 11.6), and from it projects forwards a long cylinder of fibrous connective tissue, up to 10 cm in length and terminating far forwards in the roof of the buccal cavity (fig. 11.5). Inside this fibrous cylinder are found occasional well-vascularised islets of pars distalis tissue, while at

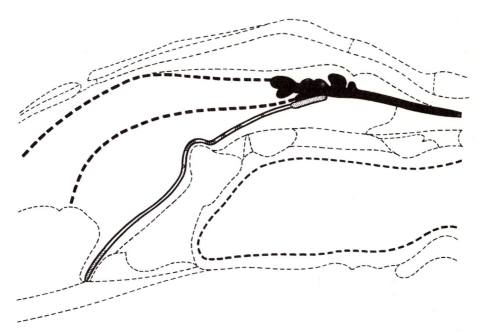

Fig. 11.5. *Latimeria chalumnae*. Diagrammatic median sagittal section of the head, buccal cavity at the bottom, anterior to left, to show the brain (black), and the cerebral and buccal parts of the adenohypophysis (stippled), joined by the connective tissue cylinder containing islets of pars distalis tissue. From Millot and Anthony (1965).

the anterior (buccal) end is a large mass of pars distalis parenchyma (Lagios, 1972). To avoid potentially misleading comparisons with other fishes, this anterior mass is best called the *buccal pars distalis*, and the posterior mass, in contact with the neuro-intermedia, the *cerebral pars distalis*.

The long fibrous cylinder probably represents part of the persistent and elongated stalk of Rathke's pouch (Millot and Anthony, 1965). The buccal pars distalis contains well-vascularised cords and follicles of acidophilic cells, with colloid in the follicular lumen. In addition there are central cystic spaces which may represent the residual hypophysial cavity (Lagios, 1972). In its position relative to the buccal cavity and in its follicular organisation, the buccal pars distalis resembles the Rachendachhypophyse of holocephalians (chapter 8).

The cerebral pars distalis is separated from the neuro-intermedia by thick fibrous tissue, and is divisible into an anterior part containing acidophils, and a posterior part in which the cell-types could not be characterised because of poor fixation (Lagios, 1972). No details are available about the neuro-intermedia, but a small saccus vasculosus is

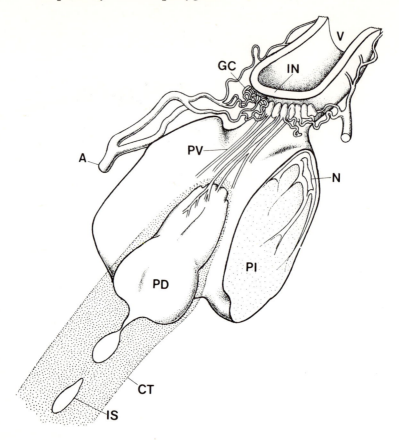

Fig. 11.6. *Latimeria chalumnae*. Diagrammatic reconstruction of the cerebral portion of the pars distalis (PD), neuro-intermediate lobe (N, neural lobe; PI, pars intermedia), and the median eminence region. V, third ventricle; IN, infundibulum; A, hypophysial artery. GC, glomeruloid capillary complexes of the primary portal capillaries (the three to the left drawn in detail, the rest indicated as swellings); PV, portal vessels; CT, connective tissue tube, enclosing islets of pars distalis tissue (IS), and also extending to cover the median eminence. Note the interdigitations of the neural lobe and pars intermedia on the cut surface to the right. From Lagios (1972).

evaginated from the posterior wall of the infundibulum (Millot and Anthony, 1965; Lagios, 1972).

The blood supply to this pituitary is very interesting. Internal carotid arteries enter the cranium close to the buccal pars distalis, and converge on the fibrous cylinder. It is possible that some fine branches may directly supply the buccal pars distalis, but these can be of only minor importance (Lagios, 1972). The internal carotids then ascend towards the optic chiasma, embedded in the tubular fibrous sheath, apparently without producing any branches *en route*. Ventral to the chiasma the arteries

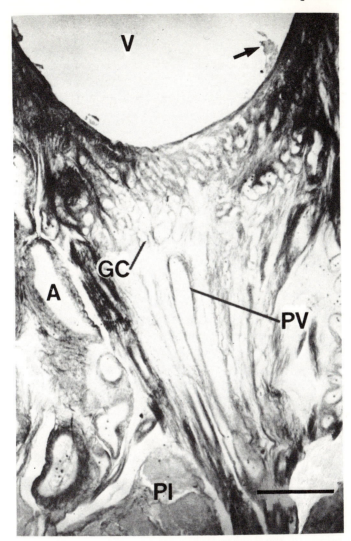

Fig. 11.7. *Latimeria chalumnae.* Thick (10 μm) transverse section of the median eminence. A, artery; GC, glomeruloid capillary complex of primary portal capillaries. Each of these complexes is separately ensheathed in fibrous connective tissue. V, third ventricle; arrow, remnant of infundibulum; PV, portal veins; PI, pars intermedia. Scale, 500 μm. From Lagios (1972).

bifurcate and give rise to a group of small convoluted arterioles, reminiscent of the pre-portal arterioles in other vertebrates (chapters 9, 12). These supply the primary capillaries of the median eminence, which take the form of perpendicular glomeruloid complexes embedded in dense connective tissue on the rostral face of the infundibulum (figs. 11.6, 11.7).

Capillary branches of this system closely approach the junction between the dense connective tissue and the infundibular wall; unfortunately the latter was extensively autolysed in the specimen available to Lagios (1972), but it must represent the median eminence itself, and may be presumed to contain neurosecretory fibres terminating on the primary capillaries. The latter merge with dilated vertical venous channels (fig. 11.7) which extend into the cerebral pars distalis and pass beyond in the fibrous cylinder towards the buccal pars distalis. Though not traced, these longer portal vessels must supply the buccal pars distalis, which is well-vascularised yet receives little or no blood from the neighbouring internal carotids (Lagios, 1972).

Though necessarily incomplete, this account suggests that the coelacanths preserve a well-developed median eminence and portal system, quite separate from the neural lobe which is intermingled with the pars intermedia (fig. 11.6). The glomeruloid complexes of the primary capillary bed lie embedded in connective tissue, a feature which resembles the neurohaemal contact area in acipenseroids (chapter 9), but differs from the glomeruloid primary capillaries of *Amia* (chapter 9) and elasmobranchs (chapter 8) which penetrate the median eminence neural tissue. Like the teleosts, the modern coelacanths are the end-product of a long period of evolution, in both cases from primitive ancestors which must have inherited the median eminence and portal system from the common gnathostome stock. Unlike the teleosts, the coelacanths have retained this primitive system, a fact which emphasises the extremely specialised nature of the hypothalamo–pars distalis connections of teleosts.

If we compare the gross anatomy of the coelacanth pituitary with that of ganoid fishes on the one hand, and of amphibians on the other, the coelacanth gland can at once be seen to be specialised, particularly in the great elongation of the pars distalis and its separation into two main parts. This specialisation may be less radical than it looks at first, in that it may simply be that Rathke's pouch becomes unusually elongated during development, giving rise to isolated islets of glandular tissue. On this interpretation, the large buccal pars distalis might be considered homologous with the Rachendachhypophyse of holocephalians, although unlike the latter it is supplied with blood from the portal system. What is certainly clear is that *Latimeria* has a pituitary as specialised as many other parts of its anatomy, for example the urinogenital system, swim bladder and heart, and that this living fossil is not likely to throw any light on the evolution of the tetrapod pituitary from the primitive piscine gland.

12

THE PITUITARY GLAND
IN AMPHIBIANS

The first vertebrates to attempt to leave the waters and colonise the land belong to the class Amphibia. The modern amphibians are in general only partly successful in this attempt, and are tied to water and damp places for purposes of respiration, water conservation and reproduction. It is, however, possible that the early amphibians, only imperfectly preserved as fossils, may have been more fully terrestrial than modern forms, although it is unlikely that they ever evolved a terrestrial mode of reproduction. Their early relatives that did solve the problems of terrestrial reproduction gave rise to the reptiles, and belong to the next chapter. Modern amphibians cannot be regarded in any way as ancestral to reptiles, birds and mammals, even in the vague sense in which this concept is employed by comparative physiologists. As A. S. Romer has written, 'a frog is in many ways as far removed structurally from the oldest land vertebrates as is man, and even a salamander must be regarded with suspicion'. Nevertheless, the amphibian pituitary is remarkably like the gland in the other tetrapods, strong evidence that the essential organisation of the tetrapod gland was evolved very early in evolution from the crossopterygian ancestors (fig. 12.1).

GENERAL ANATOMY OF THE AMPHIBIAN PITUITARY

There are three orders of living amphibians, the Anura (frogs and toads), Urodela (newts and salamanders) and Apoda or Gymnophiona, virtually blind worm-like burrowers which live in tropical regions. The evolutionary history of these animals from rhipidistian ancestors is exceptionally obscure, some authorities claiming that all modern amphibians evolved as a unit (monophyletic origin), others believing that the urodeles and apodans evolved together independently of the anurans (diphyletic origin), many of the close resemblances between modern urodeles and anurans being due to convergence. Whichever view is taken, many authorities consider that the urodeles, though highly specialised for a largely aquatic life, do preserve some primitive features, while the anurans, again specialised particularly in relation to their leaping locomotion, are usually regarded as more 'advanced'. The burrowing apodans are clearly

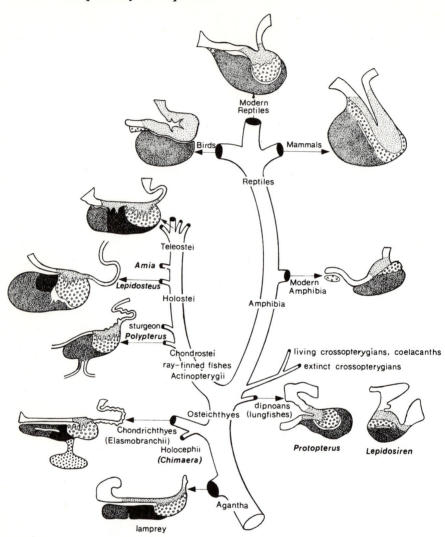

Fig. 12.1. Schematic representation of evolutionary relationships of the vertebrate groups and the structure of the pituitary gland in each group, as seen in sagittal section, anterior to the left. Sparse stippling, neural lobe; small circles, pars intermedia; small crosses, pars tuberalis; medium stippling, pars distalis (dipnoans, *Polypterus*, tetrapods) or rostral pars distalis (fishes); dense stippling, proximal pars distalis, where differentiated in fishes; coarse dots, ventral lobe of elasmobranchs. From Gorbman and Bern (1962).

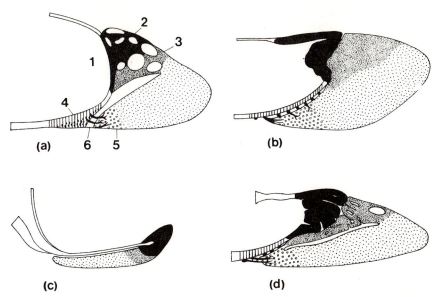

Fig. 12.2. General structure of the amphibian pituitary. Diagrammatic median sections of the pituitaries of (*a*) an anuran (*Bufo bufo*); (*b*) a urodele (*Ambystoma*); (*c*) an apodan (*Hypogeophis*); (*d*) a lungfish (*Protopterus*), for comparison. 1, saccus infundibuli; 2, neural lobe; 3, pars intermedia; 4, median eminence; 5, 'zona tuberalis'; 6, portal vessels. From Wingstrand (1966*a*).

the most specialised amphibians of them all. Examination of the pituitary gland does, indeed, show that the gland of urodeles (especially the neotenous forms) is more fish-like than that of anurans, while the apodan pituitary is the least fish-like.

Rathke's pouch develops as an epithelial bud, which remains compact in aurans and urodeles, but develops a transitory schizocoelic lumen in apodans. The development of the adenohypophysis from the anlage is more direct than in amniotes and does not allow for detailed comparisons. However, there are no real difficulties in recognising the homologies of the three major divisions of the adenohypophysis in the adult. The aboral face of the anlage contacts the infundibulum, and the zone of contact gives rise to the pars intermedia. This is an example of embryonic induction: the infundibulum normally induces the adenohypophysial anlage to differentiate into a pars intermedia (see Gorbman and Bern, 1962; Smoller, 1966; Jørgensen, 1968). The induction is prevented if infundibulum and adenohypophysis are experimentally kept apart. On the other hand, infundibular contact is not required for differentiation of the neurohypophysis in the infundibular element, nor for the differentiation of the pars distalis in the adenohypophysis, although there are indications that the median eminence may be induced by the adenohypophysial anlage (Smoller, 1966). However, the pars distalis must remain in contact with the infundibulum if its chromophilic cells are to develop normally during larval life, but this is because by this stage the hypothalamus exerts an endocrine influence on the differentiating adeno-hypophysis (Pasteels, 1957). The pars intermedia lies dorsal to the pars distalis in anurans and urodeles, but posterior in apodans (fig. 12.2). The pars tuberalis develops as a pair of anteriorly-directed outgrowths from the adenohypophysial anlage. These may remain in contact with the pars distalis (urodeles, apodans) or may become isolated as two patches of epithelial tissue on the ventral surface of the tuber cinereum (anurans).

The apodans have a long narrow infundibular stem, but the other amphibians display a wide posteriorly-directed saccus infundibuli which ends with a pair of diverticuli corresponding to the primary branches of the neural lobe of amniotes (Wingstrand, 1966*a*). The amphibian neural lobe develops from the postero-dorsal wall of the saccus infundibuli between these two primary branches, and from the medial wall of the branches themselves. It will be recalled that in fishes the postero-dorsal wall of the saccus infundibuli gives rise to the saccus vasculosus, the fish neural lobe developing from the ventral wall, a region that gives rise to the median eminence in amphibians (Wingstrand, 1966*a*).

THE PITUITARY OF ANURANS (ORDER ANURA, SALIENTIA OR BATRACHIA)

The pituitary gland is essentially similar in all frogs and toads. The adenohypophysis usually lies ventral and posterior to the neural lobe (fig. 12.2*a*). The *pars distalis* is flattened and often wider than long. Dorsally it is continuous with the *pars intermedia*, which together with the neural lobe forms a dumb-bell-shaped organ (fig. 12.3). There is no hypophysial cleft to separate intermedia and distalis. Anteriorly the pars distalis is connected to the median eminence by strands of connective tissue through which run the portal vessels (figs. 12.2, 12.3). The region of the pars distalis which receives the portal vessels appears to be homologous with the mammalian zona tuberalis. The *pars tuberalis* is represented by a pair of epithelial plaques attached on either side of the tuber cinereum, ahead of the median eminence.

The neurohypophysis is well-differentiated. The *neural lobe* is vascular-ised by numerous capillaries which run within the tissue and also lie in furrows on its surface, and contains abundant AF + NSM. The blood supply to the neural lobe is shared only by the adjacent pars intermedia, in the form of the usual plexus intermedius between the two regions (Wingstrand, 1966*b*). Anteriorly, the *median eminence* is an obviously thickened region in the infundibular floor (fig. 12.2*a*). Its ventricular wall is composed of ependymal cells, and below these are fibre bundles of the

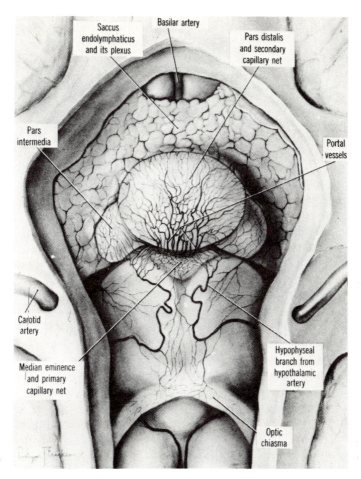

Fig. 12.3. Ventral view of the brain, pituitary and hypophysial portal circulation of the adult frog, *Rana catesbiana*. From Gorbman and Bern (1962).

hypothalamo-neurohypophysial tract, passing towards the neural lobe. Below is a fibrous layer, containing some AF+ NSM, though less than in the neural lobe. Processes of the pituicytes (glial cells) of this layer are arranged to form a palisade zone around the numerous capillaries that are partly embedded in the median eminence, and these primary portal capillaries are drained by portal vessels passing to the pars distalis.

Between the median eminence and the neural lobe the infundibular floor consists of a thin undifferentiated wall, which could be regarded as the ventral wall of an extremely short infundibular stem (fig. 12.2*a*). This area has some anatomical significance, in that it clearly separates the neural lobe from the well-developed median eminence, and it forms part of the roof of a large recess between pars distalis and pars intermedia (fig. 12.2*a*).

THE PITUITARY OF URODELES (ORDER URODELA OR CAUDATA)

The *pars distalis* lies in essentially the same position as in anurans, but it is more elongated and contains remarkably large secretory cells. The *pars intermedia* shows no special features, except that its lateral parts tend to be better developed than its median region, while the *pars tuberalis* is represented by two tongue-like outgrowths from the rostral parts of the pars distalis, which grow forwards and attach to the tuber cinereum (fig. 12.2*b*).

The neurohypophysis differentiates as in anurans. The *neural lobe* is vascular and contains AF+ NSM; in most urodeles it is compact, and often lobulated, but in *Necturus* and *Amphiuma*, which are to some extent aquatic neotenous larvae, the neural lobe is hollow and sends projections into the pars intermedia, as in Dipnoi (chapter 11). The urodele *median eminence* is always less well-developed than that of anurans. In the neotenous forms *Necturus*, *Cryptobranchus* and *Megalobatrachus* the floor of the infundibulum just above the pars distalis is covered by a capillary plexus which is continuous with, and drains into, the vascular bed of the pars distalis, with no large connecting portal vessels. The infundibular floor is not thickened to form a discrete median eminence, although the glial fibres may show a distinct palisade-like arrangement around the capillaries. In other urodeles, in which metamorphosis to a semi-terrestrial adult stage is complete (most newts, salamanders), the infundibular floor beneath the primary capillary plexus is thicker, definite portal vessels occur, and the primary capillaries are partly buried in the proliferated palisade zone. However, in contrast to the anurans, there is no undifferentiated area ('infundibular stem') separating median eminence from neural lobe, and the two structures grade into each other. Correspondingly, there is no recess separating the pars distalis from the pars intermedia, the two regions being broadly in contact (fig. 12.2*b*).

THE PITUITARY OF APODANS (ORDER APODA, GYMNOPHIONA OR CAECILIA)

The apodan pituitary is poorly-known. It is strikingly different from the gland of other amphibians in being very flattened, a modification found in other worm-like vertebrates, eels, snakes and some lizards (fig. 12.2*c*). The *pars distalis* lies in the orthodox position, anterior to the neural lobe. The latter is lodged in a dorsal depression of the pars distalis, and is encircled by the *pars intermedia*, which in sagittal section appears both in front of and behind the neural lobe (Gabe, 1972; fig. 12.2*c* does not show this feature); because of this it has been said 'la pars nervosa . . . est entourée de tissu adénohypophysaire, qui lui forme une sorte de "capuchon ventral"' (Gabe, 1972). The pair of *pars tuberalis* processes retain partial connections with the rostral pars distalis, a condition intermediate between that in urodeles and anurans. The very long *infundibular stem* fits into a dorsal groove on the pars distalis, and terminates in the compact *neural lobe* lodged in a widening of the groove. Though exceedingly narrow, the stem carries a fine recess from the third ventricle, which widens into a cavity in the base of the neural lobe. Above the anterior end of the pars distalis is the *median eminence*, a thickened region bearing the primary capillary plexus of the portal system. In its thickening and in its wide separation from the neural lobe the median eminence is at least as well differentiated as in the most advanced urodeles, but no details are available about its structure (Wingstrand, 1966*a*).

TAXONOMIC NAMES

There are certain difficulties concerning the correct taxonomic names of some amphibians, probably originating from the frequent use of these animals by experimental biologists who have perpetuated older names declared invalid by taxonomists. We have in some cases changed the taxonomic names used in papers dealing with amphibians which have since been renamed by taxonomists, but we have indicated the name used by the original author in the first reference to his work in the text.

HISTOPHYSIOLOGY OF THE
AMPHIBIAN PARS DISTALIS

Perhaps more than in other vertebrate groups, the situation now found in the literature on the pars distalis in amphibians illustrates very clearly the central dilemma that attends the study of pars distalis cells. The distinction between morphological and functional cell-types was discussed in chapter 3. Ideally, morphological identifications should correspond to functional identifications, but this is not always the case, and the amphibians illustrate very well the divergencies that can arise between the two ways of identifying pituitary cells. To illustrate what has happened in amphibian studies, we shall deal with both approaches in turn.

MORPHOLOGICAL CELL-TYPES

In 1963 van Oordt collated earlier work and concluded that in anurans and urodeles five morphological cell-types could be distinguished in the pars distalis by light microscopy. Subsequent studies, some with the EM, have confirmed this conclusion. For apodans, the only recent investigator (Gabe, 1972) has distinguished four cell-types. In addition to these chromophilic cells, most workers have noticed chromophobic cells in the pars distalis. Some of these are undifferentiated cells, some are stellate or follicular cells (see below, p. 249, and Cardell, 1969), while some are actually chromophils, but with too few granules to be recognised with the light microscope (Doerr-Schott, 1968a).

Kerr (1965) gave a detailed account of the gland in the primitive toad *Xenopus laevis*, which, following van Oordt (1968), may be taken as a basic type and source of terminology.

Acidophils type 1

Distinction between the two types of acidophils is difficult on a purely tinctorial basis, since as in all vertebrates, the red/yellow (erythrosin or azocarmine/orange G) staining distinction is not always easy to achieve. Largely because of this difficulty authorities on the amphibian pituitary have relied to a great extent on the location of the two acidophils for their definition, the A1 cells being scattered in the ventral or rostral pars distalis, the A2 cells being concentrated in the posterior or dorso-caudal region. The staining properties ascribed to these cells do not always agree with their distribution, and while the size of the secretory granules usually correlates with the location of the cells, the A2 cells having the smaller granules, it is impossible always to be certain that the elements described by different authors in different amphibians as A1 or A2 cells are truly homologous. Furthermore, some workers have confused the literature by using these names casually for the first and second acidophil in their accounts, without reference to the careful definitions of these cell-types proposed by Kerr (1965), van Oordt (1968) and Doerr-Schott (1968a).

In the strict sense, the A1 cells of *Xenopus* are large and densely filled with typical acidophilic granules, staining with OG, erythrosin and Luxol fast blue, but entirely PAS−, AF− and AB−. They occur in most parts of the gland but are most abundant in the rostro-central region (fig. 12.4; Kerr, 1965). In the frog *Rana* and the toad *Bufo* the A1 cells tend to be more generally scattered (van Oordt, 1968). Their staining properties vary. They are strongly erythrosinophilic in *Rana temporaria* and *R. esculenta* (van Oordt, van Dongen and Lofts, 1968; Rastogi and Chieffi, 1970a). They are also erythrosinophilic and carminophilic in *Bufo bufo* (= *B. vulgaris*) (Zuber-Vogeli, 1953; van Oordt, 1966; Mira-Moser, 1969a) and the midwife toad *Alytes obstetricans* (Rémy, 1969), but in another bufonid *Nectophrynoides occidentalis* they are OG+ (Zuber-Vogeli, 1968) and they are also OG+ in *Rana pipiens* (Ortman, 1961). They are PAS− in all the anurans investigated, and in

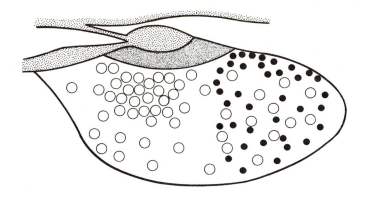

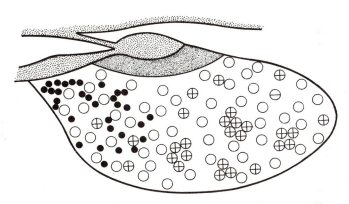

Fig. 12.4. *Xenopus laevis*. Diagrammatic sagittal sections of the pituitary to show the distribution of the pars distalis cell-types. Anterior to left. Top, acidophils (type 1, clear circles; type 2, solid circles); bottom, basophils (type 1, crossed circles; type 2, clear circles; type 3, solid circles). Pars intermedia, fine stippling; median eminence, neural lobe and hypothalamus, coarse stippling. From Kerr (1965).

R. temporaria they have been shown to be weakly PbH+ (van Kemenade, 1969*b*).

The urodele A1 cells tend to be more widely scattered in the pars distalis, though they are rostro-ventrally located in *Necturus* (Aplington, 1942) and are usually scarce in the dorsal region (Doerr-Schott, 1966*a*). They are carminophilic in *Necturus* (Aplington, 1942), but OG+ in *Triturus marmoratus, T. cristatus, T.* (*Diemictylus*) *viridescens, Taricha torosa* and *Pleurodeles waltlii* (Pasteels, 1960; Dent, 1961; Doerr-Schott, 1966*a*; Mazzi *et al.* 1966; Doerr-Schott, 1968*a*). Thus the A1 cells may be the erythrosinophil or the orangeophil in both anurans and urodeles.

Only a single acidophil could be distinguished in the apodan *Ichthyophis glutinosus* (Gabe, 1972).

In the few species studied with the EM, A1 cells have been found to have larger granules than A2 cells, the size range being about 200–500 nm in diameter in anurans, and 250–550 nm in urodeles (Doerr-Schott, 1968a, 1971; Clauss and Doerr-Schott, 1970). Apart from the size of the granules the two acidophils have identical ultrastructures (Doerr-Schott, 1968a).

Acidophils type 2

The A2 cells of *Xenopus* are smaller than the A1 cells, and are located in the dorso-caudal region (fig. 12.4). Unlike the A1 cells they have a slight affinity for PAS, so that after AB–PAS–OG the A1 cells are yellow and the A2 cells light brown (Kerr, 1965). Doerr-Schott (1968a) concluded that A2 cells occur in *Xenopus* only at certain times of the year, at other times appearing as chromophobes, and Kerr (1965) indicated that these cells readily transform into chromophobes.

A2 cells are not easily identified in *Rana*, but they can be distinguished from A1 cells with careful technique, and in *R. temporaria* they are small, elongated cells, OG+ and concentrated in the dorso-caudal region (van Oordt, van Dongen and Lofts, 1968); in this frog they are known to be PbH+ (van Kemenade, 1969b). The A2 cell is also OG+ in *R. esculenta*, in which at sexual maturity it develops unusually large OG+ granules which are gradually discharged during the breeding season (Rastogi and Chieffi, 1970a, b), but it is described as scattered, fuchsinophilic and strongly PAS+ in *R. pipiens* (Ortman, 1961).

In bufonids, A2 cells can be distinguished more readily than in frogs. In *Bufo bufo* they are arranged in groups of three or four, bordering blood capillaries in the dorso-caudal region, and they are OG+ and faintly PAS+ (Zuber-Vogeli, 1953; van Oordt, 1966; Doerr-Schott, 1968a; Mira-Moser, 1969a). In the viviparous toad *Nectophrynoides* they also form islets, often palisadic, along capillaries in the dorso-caudal region, but they are erythrosinophilic and occur only during the first part of gestation (Zuber-Vogeli, 1968). In another bufonid, *Alytes*, the A2 cells seem to occur in the tadpole as elongated cells, arranged as in *Nectophrynoides* but OG+, PAS− and PbH+ (Rémy, 1969). It seems that the A2 cells of bufonids always display an affinity for the large 'sinusoidal' capillaries in the dorso-caudal zone of the pars distalis.

This last characteristic is even more marked in urodeles, where dorso-caudally located A2 cells have nearly always been distinguished from A1 cells, and were described in *Triturus marmoratus* as 'erythrosinophilic, and often arranged like a palisade around capillaries' (Doerr-Schott, 1968a), a disposition even more marked in *Necturus*, in which they stain with the ponceau de xylidine rather than azocarmine in Masson's trichrome (Aplington, 1942). In other urodeles, the A2 cells are carmino-philic and erythrosinophilic (Copeland, 1943; Pasteels, 1960; Doerr-Schott, 1966a, 1968a). In *Pleurodeles* they contain lysosome-like globules, particularly large in old animals (Pasteels, 1960), a feature recalling the large OG + granules in the A2 cells of *Rana esculenta*.

The A2 granules have been shown in EM studies to be small, 100–300 nm in diameter in anurans, 100–250 nm in urodeles (Doerr-Schott, 1966a, 1968a, 1971; Clauss and Doerr-Schott, 1970).

Basophils type 1

The B1 cells in X*enopus* are large and often vacuolated, with very strongly staining granules, PAS+, AB+ but totally OG −. Thus, they stain a strong clear blue after trichrome or Aliz BT. They are AF + after oxid-ation with either acid permanganate or Lugol's solution. In *Xenopus* they form small groups in the centro-ventral region of the pars distalis (fig. 12.4; Kerr, 1965), and they are similarly distributed in species of *Rana*, though often small and difficult to find and generally rather widely scattered (Ortman, 1961; van Oordt, 1968; Rastogi and Chieffi, 1970). In *Bufo*, the B1 cells are present usually in small groups of a few cells each (Zuber-Vogeli, 1953; van Oordt, 1966, 1968; Mira-Moser, 1969a). *Nectophrynoides* has B1 cells scattered throughout the pars distalis (Zuber-Vogeli, 1968). Workers on anurans studied have all emphasised the relative scarcity of these cells.

B1 cells have not always been found in urodeles, probably because as in *Triturus cristatus carnifex* they become numerous and easily recog-nisable only after thyroidectomy (Mazzi *et al.* 1966). In the normal urodele, these are virtually chromophobic cells, with little cytoplasm and few weakly-staining granules, and are scattered throughout the ventral pars distalis. As such they occur in *Triturus cristatus carnifex*, *Salamandra atra* (Mazzi *et al.* 1966) and in *T. (Diemictylus) viridescens*, in which they become easily recognisable only at metamorphosis and after thyroid-ectomy (Copeland, 1943; Dent, 1961). In *Necturus* they are similarly modified by thyroidectomy, but normally they are scattered and virtually chromophobic, with only a thin rim of basophilic cytoplasma (Aplington, 1942, 1962; Aplington and Tedrow, 1968). Doerr-Schott (1968a) did not identify B1 cells in *Triturus marmoratus*, although she did describe scattered chromophobes with a developed RER and secretory granules, which might perhaps be inactive B1 cells. They are, in contrast, readily identifiable in the newt *Pleurodeles* (Pasteels, 1960).

The apodan *Ichthyophis* exhibits typical B1 cells (Gabe, 1972).

At the ultrastructural level, these cells have heterogeneous granules, spherical or elongated, varying in size within the range 120–500 nm in anurans (Doerr-Schott, 1968a; Clauss and Doerr-Schott, 1970; Mira-Moser, 1970), and 180–250 nm in the urodele *Triturus (Notophthalmus)*

9

viridescens (Cardell, 1964*a*; Dent and Gupta, 1967). Studies on *Xenopus* larvae indicated that the morphology and size of the granules may change with the activity of the cells (Pehlemann and Hemme, 1972).

In most amphibians, the B1 cells are the ordinary basophils, staining clear blue with trichrome and tetrachrome techniques, and showing no traces of the acidophilia which characterises the other two basophilic cell-types.

Basophils type 2

The B2 cells in *Xenopus* are large and numerous throughout the pars distalis, rostral cells being larger than caudal ones (Kerr, 1965; fig. 12.4). They differ in staining properties from the B1 cells in two important respects. Firstly, they stain brown, not magenta, with PAS–OG, because they have an affinity for OG as well as PAS; correspondingly, with Azan they take both azocarmine and aniline blue, and they can also be stained with Luxol fast blue and azofuchsin. Secondly, the B2 granules are AF + only in sections strongly oxidised with acid permanganate (Gabe's variant), not after mild oxidation with Lugol's solution (Gomori's or Halmi's variant).

B2 cells have been identified in all the amphibians investigated. They are the large 'globular' basophils described by many workers. This term is not appropriate for *Xenopus*, but in other amphibians the B2 cells clearly contain two kinds of inclusions; fine secretory granules, cyanophilic, PAS +, AF +, staining preferentially with AB in AB–PAS–OG; and large inclusions, the 'globules', PAS + and also staining with 'acid' dyes, OG, azocarmine, azofuchsin, etc. After AB–PAS–OG, the globules preferentially stain with PAS, so that the cells are readily seen to contain blue-violet fine granules with magenta globules (van Oordt, 1968; Mira-Moser, 1969*a*). If the globules are small, as in *Xenopus*, then the cells take on an overall intermediate colour, usually purple (Kerr, 1965; van Oordt, 1968; Doerr-Schott, 1968*a*; Zuber-Vogeli, 1968; Rastogi and Chieffi, 1970*a*). The globules resemble the R granules of teleostean gonadotropes (chapter 10), and have been shown in various anurans and urodeles to be rich in acid phosphatase and four other lysosomal enzymes (van Oordt, 1968; Doerr-Schott, 1968*a*; Masur and Holtzman, 1969). Thus they are apparently lytic bodies, like the R granules.

The EM shows that the B2 cells of both urodeles and anurans contain spherical or irregular secretory granules, 120–550 nm in diameter, together with large irregular bodies, the globular lysosomes, reaching as much as 3000 nm in diameter (Cardell, 1964*a*; Doerr-Schott, 1968*a*; van Oordt, 1968; Masur, 1969; Clauss and Doerr-Schott, 1970; Mira-Moser, 1970).

The apodan *Ichthyophis* has typical B2 cells, which occupy most of the cell cords in the lateral pars distalis (Gabe, 1972).

Basophils type 3

In *Xenopus*, the B3 cells are small and cuboidal or elongated, with a fine granulation that is both PAS+ and OG+. Thus, they are really amphiphils, but most workers have classified them as basophils. Unlike the B1 and B2 cells, they are AB−. An outstanding feature, found in other amphibians also, is that they have a strong affinity for AF, but only if preliminary oxidation is omitted or is mild; after strong acid permanganate oxidation, they are AF−, or only very faintly AF+ (Kerr, 1965; van Oordt, 1968; Doerr-Schott, 1968*a*). In other amphibians, permanganic oxidation similarly reduces whatever weak affinity they may show for AB (Doerr-Schott, 1968*a*). With trichrome, these cells in *Xenopus* stain a light blue or lavender. They have a characteristic distribution in a crescentic area around the rostral border of the pars distalis, always associated with primary branches of the portal vessels which enter the gland in this area (Kerr, 1965; fig. 12.4).

B3 cells have nearly always been observed in studies on the amphibian pituitary, always rostral and close to the portal vessels. Most workers have emphasised their fine granulation. A problem encountered in collating the literature is that they are essentially amphiphilic, so that their tinctorial responses are particularly sensitive to technical variations and probably also vary with species. Typical B3 cells stain with PAS, AF (without strong oxidation) and aniline blue on the one hand, and to a greater or lesser degree with OG, azocarmine, acid fuchsin, etc. on the other hand. Not surprisingly, many workers using trichrome or Aliz BT have termed them purple or violet cells (see van Oordt, 1968; Doerr-Schott, 1968*a*; Mira-Moser, 1969*a*). Typical B3 cells occur in *Rana temporaria*, *R. pipiens*, and *R. cyanophylyctis* (Ortman, 1961; van Oordt, 1968). They are more troublesome in *R. esculenta*: according to van Oordt (1968), Rastogi and Chieffi (1970*a*) and Doerr-Schott and Dubois (1972), the B3 cells in this frog are typical, with the emphasis in their staining towards the 'basophilic' side. But workers in another laboratory, using AB–PAS–OG and Aliz BT, find that the B3 cells in *R. esculenta* behave like acidophils, only faintly PAS+ and quite strongly OG+ and erythrosinophilic, so that they are orange after PAS–OG and red after Aliz BT (Dupont, 1967, 1968; Dupont and Peltier, 1970). They have been termed acidophils (Dupont, 1967), but they do have some affinity for Aliz B, so that after Aliz BT they may appear purple-violet, and in ectopic pituitary transplants their affinity for OG diminishes and they become more strongly PAS+ (Dupont, 1971). In *R. temporaria* and *Bufo bufo*, the B3 cells are strongly PbH+ (van Oordt, 1968; van Kemenade, 1969*a*, *b*).

Amongst the bufonids, typical B3 cells bordering portal capillaries occur in *Bufo bufo* and *Nectophrynoides* (van Oordt, 1966, 1968; Zuber-Vogeli, 1968; Mira-Moser, 1969*a*), and also in other *Bufo* spp. although in *B. arenarum* they are unusual in being strongly AB+, staining blue with

9-2

AB–PAS–OG (see van Oordt, 1968). The tadpole of *Alytes obstetricans* is unusual in having B3 cells which are purely acidophilic, though not investigated in detail (Rémy, 1969). These cells appear early in this toad, in which the pars distalis differentiates precociously, but in *Bufo bufo* they appear rather later, just before (Mira-Moser, 1969a) or during (van Oordt, 1966) metamorphosis, when the median eminence and portal system is differentiated; according to van Oordt (1966) some individuals do not develop recognisable B3 cells until well after metamorphosis.

Most studies on the urodele pituitary have identified the B3 cells, in the typical rostral location in association with secondary portal capillaries. They tend to form well-marked homogeneous cell-cords (Doerr-Schott, 1966a, 1968a). The neotenous mud-puppy, *Necturus*, has B3 cells which extend further laterally and caudally than in other amphibians, but they are typical in other respects, PAS +, AF + (after mild oxidation with Lugol's solution), purple after Masson's trichrome and usually bordering sinusoidal blood spaces (Aplington, 1942, 1962). The unusually wide distribution of these cells in *Necturus* is probably related to the diffuse median eminence and numerous portal connections in this species (p. 240). That the B3 cells are in fact functionally determined in relation to the portal vessels was elegantly shown in work on the newt *Pleurodeles waltlii* by Pasteels (1960). By rotating the pars distalis through 180°, the portal vessels were made to regenerate and connect with what was originally the posterior end of the gland. The original B3 cells degenerated, and new B3 cells differentiated in contact with the newly-formed portal connections in what was the original caudal region.

Because of this experimental work, the variable staining properties of the B3 cells create little difficulty, since we can identify these cells by their location. *Triturus viridescens*, for example, displays a condition opposite to that described above for *R. esculenta* and *Alytes*, in having B3 cells that are purely basophilic, PAS +, AF + (after Lugol), and purely blue after Azan, but with the typical location (Copeland, 1943; Dent, 1961).

The newt *T. cristatus carnifex* provides a further example of the capricious staining properties of these cells. They are usually finely granulated and only weakly PAS +, but occasionally they contain strongly PAS + granules together with an erythrosinophilic perinuclear zone (Mazzi *et al.* 1966).

Rostrally located B3 cells are found in the apodan *Ichthyophis*. They are violet after Aliz BT, strongly PAS +, and AF − after permanganic oxidation (Gabe, 1972).

EM studies show the B3 cells to contain small secretory granules, of variable electron density, 100–200 nm in diameter in *R. temporaria* and *Bufo bufo*, 100–220 nm in *Xenopus*, 130–240 nm in *Bombina variegata*, and 150–300 nm in *Triturus marmoratus* (Doerr-Schott, 1968a; Clauss and Doerr-Schott, 1970).

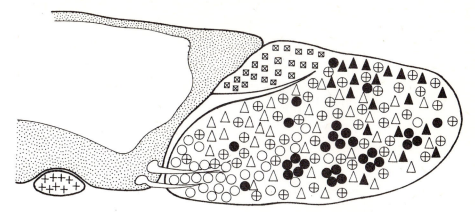

Fig. 12.5. Diagrammatic median sagittal section of a typical anuran pituitary showing the distribution of the cell-types in the adenohypophysis: ●, basophils type 1; ⊕, basophils type 2; ○, basophils type 3; △, acidophils type 1; ▲, acidophils type 2; ⊠, basophils of the pars intermedia; +, chromophobes of the pars tuberalis. Anterior to left, with portal vessels indicated from median eminence to pars distalis. From van Oordt (1968).

The distribution of the various cell-types in a typical anuran pituitary is shown in fig. 12.5. Three further features of the amphibian pars distalis should be mentioned at this point. (1) Histochemical studies have shown that protein-bound SS/SH groups are found only in the acidophils, apart from the lysosomal bodies of the B2 cells (van Oordt, 1968). (2) Stellate cells, virtually agranular, occur in the pars distalis, with long fine processes passing between and contacting the endocrine cells, and linked to each other and to the endocrine cells by desmosomes. Stellate cell processes also form end-feet against the outer basal membrane of pericapillary spaces in the gland, and are associated with the connective tissue capsule of the pars distalis (fig. 12.6) (Cardell, 1964a, 1969; Masur, 1969; Bunt, 1969; Compher and Dent, 1970). The function of these elements in amphibians is not certain. They appear first in the young larva of *Triturus viridescens*, and become more numerous and their processes longer during metamorphosis and terrestrial life (Dent and Gupta, 1967). Cardell (1969) pointed to the evidence that these cells are sustentacular, viz. their association with the external connective tissue capsule, and their desmosome linkages with each other and with endocrine cells, forming a reticular framework for the cellular parenchyma (fig. 12.6). It is not likely that they are secretory, since they have little RER, a small Golgi complex, and few granules. However, current opinion about these cells in vertebrates in general is that they may have some role in transport of material between blood vessels and endocrine cells (see Vila-Porcile, 1972).

(3) Doerr-Schott (1968a) has pointed out that secretion in amphibian

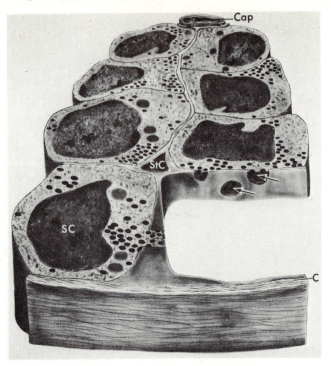

Fig. 12.6. Salamander (*Triturus viridescens*). A diagrammatic summary of the fine structure of the stellate cell and its relationships with other elements of the pars distalis. Processes from the stellate cell underlie the capsule (C) of the gland in such a way as to provide a continuous sheath beneath the capsule. Expanded regions of the stellate cell processes (end-foot processes) contact the pericapillary space of the capillary (Cap) and follow the contour of the pericapillary space for a considerable distance. Several chromophilic cells (SC) are shown in contact with the processes from a single stellate cell (StC). This drawing illustrates the interpretation that the processes are sheet-like extensions of the cell and are characterised by large fenestrations at frequent intervals (arrows). Adjacent chromophilic cells contact each other through these fenestrations. From Cardell (1969).

basophils appears to involve a lysis of the granules within the cytoplasm, whereas the acidophils exhibit the classical signs of secretion by exocytosis, in which the granules are extruded intact and then dissolve outside the cells (cf. Bunt, 1969).

FUNCTIONAL CELL-TYPES

The amphibian pars distalis secretes the usual complement of hormones, though as in other lower vertebrates there is no evidence for two distinct gonadotropins (Gorbman, 1964; van Oordt and De Kort, 1969).

Most work attempting to allocate functions to cell-types in the amphibian pituitary has been based on observations of parallel changes in target organs and pituitary cells under three conditions: experimental alterations in target organ activity; changes during the life history, especially the dramatic changes that occur during the thyroid-dependent metamorphosis of tadpole to adult; and changes during the annual physiological cycle of the adult. The last approach was particularly used by earlier workers, who often followed seasonal changes in a single target organ – usually the gonad – and related any correlated alterations in the pars distalis to the control of that single target. However, in *Rana temporaria*, and probably in other amphibians, seasonal changes in gonads, thyroid, adrenal cortex and growth-rate all run in parallel, and correspondingly all the pituitary cell-types show parallel changes during the year (van Oordt, van Dongen and Lofts, 1968). Obviously, observations of this kind have only limited usefulness unless supplemented by other approaches.

Some of the more recent work has been based on regional assays of the pituitary for biological activity, an approach that has been especially useful in identifying the thyrotropes and corticotropes.

In collating the literature, we have had to re-interpret some of the earlier findings in the light of more recent information. This has meant that in some cases we have arrived at conclusions about the allocation of endocrine functions that differ from those reached by the original authors. It seems preferable to take this approach rather than to perpetuate identifications of functional cell-types that now can be seen to be erroneous. With this in mind, each pituitary function will now be considered in turn.

Lactotropic hormone (LTH, prolactin)

LTH has been detected by bioassay in the pituitary glands of various anurans and urodeles (Bern and Nicoll, 1968; Nicoll and Nichols, 1971; Sage and Bern, 1972), and is secreted *in vitro* by the glands of *Necturus* and *Bufo* (Bern and Nicoll, 1968; Nicoll, 1971). This hormone seems to be involved in the control of larval growth.

The pituitary is necessary for growth in larval anurans (see Brown and Frye, 1969*a*). LTH has been found to promote growth in intact anuran tadpoles, and STH is relatively or totally ineffective; LTH also promotes growth in hypophysectomised *Alytes* tadpoles (see Bern and Nicoll, 1968). In *Rana pipiens*, LTH is effective in the hypophysectomised tadpole (Etkin and Gona, 1967), and only high doses of STH are active, probably because the preparations contain contaminating LTH (Brown and Frye, 1969*a*). Thus in *R. pipiens*, and probably in other anurans, LTH is the larval growth-promoting pituitary factor, secreted even before the development of functional hypothalamo-adenohypophysial connections

(Bern and Nicoll, 1968; Etkin, 1970). This is to be correlated with the fact that A1 cells are the only acidophils in larval *R. pipiens* (Ortman and Etkin, 1963). Ectopic pituitary transplants in larval *R. pipiens* prevent metamorphosis – an effect of LTH (Etkin, 1970) – and result in gigantic tadpoles (Etkin and Lehrer, 1960), and these transplants contain few cells other than active-looking A1 cells (Etkin and Ortman, 1960). Thus the A1 cells appear to be the source of LTH. The early differentiation of these cells in larvae of *Xenopus* (Kerr, 1966), *R. temporaria* (Doerr-Schott, 1968*b*), *Bufo bufo* (van Oordt, 1966; Mira-Moser, 1969*a*) and *Necto-phrynoides* (Zuber-Vogeli and Bihouès-Louis, 1971) again identifies them as lactotropes, the A2 cells always differentiating later. It is interesting in view of the anti-metamorphic properties of LTH that the A1 cells undergo a temporary regression before the metamorphic climax in *B. bufo* (van Oordt, 1966).

Larval growth has been investigated less in the urodeles, and there is some evidence that early larval growth in some urodeles may be relatively independent of the pituitary (see Licht, Cohen and Bern, 1972). LTH enhances growth in early larvae of the newt *Taricha torosa*, but has no action in late and metamorphosing larvae; STH is effective at both stages, but in the early larva it is particularly effective in promoting trunk growth while LTH is particularly active in promoting tail growth (Cohen *et al.* 1972; Licht, Cohen and Bern, 1972). It may be that LTH is a larval growth-promoting agent in urodeles, as in anurans. The A1 cells are the only acidophils in the larval pars distalis in *Triturus viridescens* and *Pleurodeles*, the A2 cells appearing later, after metamorphosis (Copeland, 1943; Dent and Gupta, 1967; Pasteels, 1960), so that if LTH is a larval growth-factor in these urodeles it must be secreted by the A1 cells.

There is fortunately more conclusive evidence that the urodele A1 cells are lactotropes. The water drive of the terrestrial red-eft stage of *Triturus viridescens* is an LTH-dependent physiological process (Bern and Nicoll, 1968), which seems to be brought about by a reversal of the low LTH–high thyroid condition of the terrestrial eft to the high LTH–low thyroid state of the aquatic adult (Gona, Pearlman and Etkin, 1970). At the onset of the water drive LTH secretion probably increases (Gona, Pearlman and Etkin, 1970). The water drive is associated with a large increase in the size and activity of the A1 cells, detectable with both light and electron microscopes (Copeland, 1943; Dent and Gupta, 1967). The A1 cells of this newt are persistent and very active in ectopic pituitary transplants that secrete LTH (Masur, 1969). A similar water drive occurs annually in the European newt *T. cristatus carnifex*, and is LTH-dependent (see Mazzi, 1969). The A1 cells in this species respond to injections of LTH in the same way as the mammalian lactotropes, becoming enlarged, engorged with secretory granules, while the nuclei become contracted and inactive, effects most probably mediated by the exogenous LTH suppressing the secretion of hypothalamic LTH-inhibiting factor (Meites, 1972), which has been experimentally demonstrated in this newt (Mazzi, 1970). Furthermore, partial hypophysectomy of *T. cristatus*, which removed all A2 cells but left some A1 cells *in situ*, resulted in partial maintenance of tail-height, an LTH-dependent character, again pointing to the A1 cell as the lactotrope (Mazzi, 1971).

The LTH cells in other vertebrates are generally erythrosinophils rather than orangeophils, but the A1 cells of amphibians, like the A1 cells in reptiles (chapter 13) may be either erythrosinophils or orangeophils. However, the mainly rostral location of the A1 cells is in agreement with the rostral location of lactotropes in fishes and birds.

Somatotropin (STH, growth hormone)

Although LTH seems to be the larval growth factor in anurans, this is not true of the adult, in which a distinct STH seems to be secreted. In *Bufo* spp. treatment of young adults with bovine or ovine STH enhanced body growth and produced characteristic metabolic changes, while ovine LTH produced similar but less pronounced effects (Zipser, Licht and Bern, 1969). More significantly, hypophysectomised adult *Rana pipiens* grow in response to STH, but not in response to large doses of LTH (Brown and Frye, 1969b). In this frog, the A1 cells (lactotropes) are present in the larva, but the A2 cells appear only after metamorphosis, which indicates that they are the source of STH (Ortman, 1961; Ortman and Etkin, 1963). In other anurans, in which the mechanisms controlling adult and larval growth have not been investigated, the A2 cells always appear later in the life history than the A1 cell, often not until metamorphosis or even later (van Oordt, 1966; Kerr, 1966; Zuber-Vogeli and Bihouès-Louis, 1971), suggesting that the A2 cell may be the source of adult STH. Both STH and LTH are certainly detectable in adult anuran pituitary glands (Nicoll and Licht, 1971; Nicoll and Nichols, 1971).

Less information is available for urodeles. In *Pleurodeles* the A1 cells appear in the larva, but the A2 cells only after metamorphosis (Pasteels, 1960). *Triturus viridescens* grows rapidly after metamorphosis, coincident with the differentiation and continued secretory activity of the A2 cells (Copeland, 1943; Dent and Gupta, 1967). Both STH and LTH stimulate growth in the intact aquatic adult of this newt (Brown and Brown, 1971), but since the A1 cells are rather well-established as the source of LTH, the A2 cells most probably secrete a distinct growth-promoting factor, STH. However, it is difficult at present to be certain that LTH and STH exist independently in urodeles, despite the presence of both A1 and A2 cells in the adult pituitary, because although both STH and LTH can be detected in the glands of adult anurans, only LTH has so far been found by disc electrophoresis and bioassay in adult *Ambystoma tigrinum* (tiger salamander) and *Triturus cristatus* as well as in the neotenous axolotl *Siredon mexicanum* (Nicoll and Licht, 1971; Nicoll and Nichols, 1971; Mazzi, Vellano and Colucci, 1971).

Thyroid-stimulating hormone (TSH, Thyrotropin)

Studies attempting to allocate TSH secretion to one of the morphological cell-types have led to a sharp division of opinion between those who identify the B1 cell as the thyrotrope and those who allocate TSH to the B3 cell. It now seems possible that the controversy might be resolved by recent evidence that the B3 cells secrete ACTH, since experimental alterations in thyroid activity seem to entail alterations in ACTH secretion in many vertebrates, and workers studying natural changes in the thyroid and pituitary have not usually taken account of the possibility that the adrenal cortex might undergo changes in parallel to the thyroid.

Evidence that the B1 cell is the thyrotrope

Part of the difficulty in identifying the thyrotropes stems from the fact that the B1 cells are often difficult to distinguish in normal adult amphibians. *Xenopus laevis* is one of the species in which the B1 cells are exceptionally large and easy to identify, and all workers agree that these are thyrotropes in this amphibian. It is this cell which is activated selectively after chemical and surgical thyroidectomy, often becoming vacuolated and enlarged as the typical 'thyroidectomy cell' (Kerr, 1965; van Oordt, 1968), and the activity of the B1 cell is reduced by thyroxine treatment, which converts it to a small cell, with only a thin ring of basophilic material around the nucleus (Kerr, 1965), a condition in which it resembles the B1 cell in many normal urodeles (p. 245). Furthermore, the activity of the B1 cells correlates with thyroid changes during the life history: these are the first cells to differentiate in larval *Xenopus*, and they display increased activity during metamorphosis, parallel to the increased thyroid activity at this time (Kerr, 1966; van Oordt, 1968; Pehlemann and Hemme, 1972). *Rana pipiens* is another amphibian with prominent B1 cells (Ortman, 1961), and again their activity correlates with thyroid activity and metamorphosis (Kaye, 1961; Ortman and Etkin, 1963). Work on adult *R. pipiens* has provided some of the strongest evidence that the B1 cells are thyrotopes. Bioassay showed that trichloracetic acid extracted TSH activity from the gland and also removed basophilic granules, but not the acidophilic granules, which confirms that TSH must be secreted by a basophil. Bioassay of rostral and caudal halves of the pars distalis showed TSH to be distributed evenly throughout the gland, in correlation with the distribution of B1 and B2 cells, but not with B3 cells which are about seven times as abundant in the rostral as in the caudal half. Since the B2 cells appear only in the adult as the gonads develop, but the B1 cells are present during metamorphosis, this led to the conclusion that TSH is secreted by the B1 cells (Ortman and Parker, 1968).

The B1 cells are small and scarce in adult *R. temporaria*, in which thyroid activity is never very high (van Oordt, van Dongen and Lofts, 1968), but their appearance and activity in the larva and during metamorphosis indicates their thyrotropic function (van Oordt, 1963, 1968). Doerr-Schott (1968*b*) also described basophils with granules 150–400 nm in diameter (i.e. the same as in the adult B1 cells; Doerr-Schott, 1968*a*) which appeared in *R. temporaria* larvae and displayed great activity during metamorphic climax. She interpreted these as immature gonadotropes (B2 cells), but from her account they are probably B1 cells.

Amongst bufonids, B1 cells are identified as thyrotropes by their behaviour in relation to metamorphosis in *Bufo* and *Alytes* (van Oordt, 1966; Rémy, 1969), and by their selective response in *Alytes* to chemical thyroidectomy (Rémy, 1969). In *Bufo bufo*, chemical thyroidectomy activates the B1 cells, and they are probably converted to chromophobic 'thyroidectomy cells', although the author (Mira-Moser, 1969*b*, 1972) considered the latter to arise from B3 cells, which also showed activation changes. Surgical thyroidectomy of adult *B. bufo* also produced chromophobic 'thyroidectomy cells', again considered by the author (Mira-Moser, 1969*a*) to arise from B3 cells. However, from her photographs, the thyroidectomy cells appear to arise over a wide area, unlike the distribution of B3 cells, but more like the distribution of the B1 cells.

Urodeles commonly have very small and virtually chromophobic B1 cells, and not surprisingly their identification as thyrotropes in these animals has been difficult. In *Triturus cristatus* the insignificant B1 cells hypertrophy after thyroidectomy and form giant 'thyroidectomy cells', in distribution and appearance very like those in *Bufo bufo* (Mazzi *et al.* 1966). The B1 cells of *Triturus viridescens* are probably widely dispersed chromophobes, but shortly before metamorphosis they become more prominent as scattered signet-ring cells which disappear when the adult stage is attained (Copeland, 1943). EM studies on *T. viridescens* identified B1 cells (granule diameter 180–250 nm) as actively secreting elements before and during metamorphosis (Dent and Gupta, 1967). After chemical or radiological thyroidectomy in this newt, large 'thyroidectomy cells' appeared, numerous and scattered throughout the pars distalis and chromophobic apart from a few PAS+ and AF+ granules (Dent, 1961). Because of their distribution, it is unlikely that these cells arose from the B3 cells, and indeed the region containing the B3 cells ('zone 1') showed no alterations in the published photographs (Dent, 1961); this author thought that 'thyroidectomy cells' arose from the scattered acidophils,

but consideration of these results in relation to other work on this newt
(Copeland, 1943; Cardell, 1964*b*; Dent and Gupta, 1967) and on *T.
cristatus* (Mazzi *et al.* 1966) points to the derivation of these cells from
the chromophobes (= inactive B1 cells) present in the region where the
'thyroidectomy cells' appear (Dent, 1961). A similar argument applies to
Necturus, in which after thyroidectomy many large 'thyroidectomy cells'
appeared, vacuolated and containing acidophilic globules (lysosomes?),
scattered throughout the pars distalis. Some of these could be seen with
certainty to arise from nearly chromophobic scattered small cells, with
only a thin rim of lightly basophilic cytoplasm (i.e. B1 cells), but simultaneous changes in the B3 cells led Aplington (1962) to think that they
gave rise to some 'thyroidectomy' cells. Thus in *T. viridescens* and
Necturus, the 'thyroidectomy cells' are probably modified B1 cells, as
they certainly are in *T. cristatus* (Mazzi *et al.* 1966).

The B3 cell as thyrotrope

The most recent and convincing evidence identifies the B3 cell as the
corticotrope (see p. 258), but several workers have obtained results which
led them to consider them as thyrotropes. These results are explicable if
we accept that thyroidectomy leads to altered adrenocortical function, as
shown for example in *Triturus cristatus* (Mazzi *et al.* 1966) and *Rana
cyanophlyctis* (Sarkar and Rao, 1971), and as discussed by van Kemenade
(1969*b*).

Thyroidectomy was shown to activate B3 cells and subsequently to
produce large active chromophobic cells, some containing lysosomes, in
the antero-ventral pars distalis of *Rana temporaria* (Doerr-Schott, 1966*b*,
1968*a*) and *Bufo bufo* (Mira-Moser, 1969*a*, *b*, 1971, 1972*b*). The investigators emphasised that the response in the B3 cells (degranulation,
hypertrophy of RER and Golgi complex) was not synchronous in all the
cells, and that with the light microscope there was no evidence that the
chromophobes were in fact transformed B3 cells, the two elements simply
existing side by side in the same region. Even with the EM the evidence
for this transformation was not conclusive, since the granule sizes in the
B1 and B3 cells overlap in both amphibians (see Doerr-Schott, 1968*a*),
and in any case very few secretory granules were ever seen in the large
chromophobes. Mira-Moser (1969*a*) described the changes in *B. bufo* as
the transformation of 'a certain number' of B3 cells into large chromophobes, but in fact saw only two examples, and the illustration is not
convincing. For *R. temporaria* (Doerr-Schott, 1966*b*, 1968*a*), the descriptions also suggest that the large chromophobes were few in number and
restricted to the antero-ventral region of the gland, and so not corresponding to the extremely abundant 'thyroidectomy cells' widespread
throughout the pars distalis, in *Triturus* and *Necturus* (see above, p. 255).

It is important to recall that Dent (1961) observed vacuolation and enlargement of the B3 cells in *Triturus viridescens* after thyroidectomy, but found that 'thyroidectomy cells' never developed in the region of the B3 cells but were numerous elsewhere in the gland, a pattern exactly similar to that in *T. cristatus* (Mazzi *et al.* 1966) and *Bufo bufo* (Mira-Moser, 1969*a*), as can be seen by comparing Dent's fig. 4 with fig. 5 of Mazzi *et al.* and fig. 30 of Mira-Moser. It is possible that in their EM studies on thyroidectomised animals, Doerr-Schott (1966*b*, 1968*a*) and Mira-Moser (1971, 1972*b*) were studying the collaterally activated B3 cells (corticotropes) rather than the more numerous 'thyroidectomy cells' (transformed B1 cells). The difficulty of recognising the inactive B1 cells of normal frogs was mentioned on p. 245.

Correlative studies have been made on the pars distalis during larval development and metamorphosis, and in some cases have led workers to relate B3 cells to changes in thyroid activity (Doerr-Schott, 1968*b*; Mira-Moser, 1969*a*, 1972*a*; Zuber-Vogeli and Bihouès-Louis, 1971). However in each species the B1 cells and B3 cells displayed parallel changes in function, although not all these authors identified the larval basophil accompanying the B3 cells as the B1 cell, Doerr-Schott (1968*b*) considering it an immature gonadotrope (B2 cell), and Mira-Moser (1972*a*) an 'intermediate' basophil. van Oordt (1966) showed for *Bufo bufo* that the appearance and behaviour of the B1 cells correlated with thyroid activity during the stages pre-metamorphosis to climax, whereas the rostral tip of the pars distalis (site of B3 cells) is composed of small undifferentiated cells until climax, when B3 cells develop in relation to the establishment of the median eminence–portal system; even then, not all specimens display B3 cells, which become a general feature only later after thyroid activity has diminished. Mira-Moser (1969*a*, 1972*a*), however, found that the B3 cells appear in pre-metamorphosis in *B. bufo*, and become more numerous at climax.

Bioassay of rostral and caudal fragments of *Necturus* adenohypophysis showed more TSH per unit weight in the rostral than in the caudal fragments, which led to the conclusion that TSH must be secreted by the B3 cells (Aplington and Tedrow, 1968). These data were distorted, however, by the inclusion of the pars intermedia ('basophilic bed') in the caudal fragments. If the pars intermedia had been excluded, then these results would have shown a more even distribution of TSH throughout the pars distalis, which would correlate better with the distribution of the nearly chromophobic B1 cells than with the B3 cells. After thyroidectomy the decrease in rostral TSH and increase in caudal TSH is explicable in these terms by the fact that degranulated 'thyroidectomy cells' (which would contain little TSH) differentiate from anterior to posterior, and hence would be more strongly represented in the rostral than in the caudal fragments (Aplington and Tedrow, 1968).

It will be seen that the literature on location of TSH secretion in the amphibian pars distalis is confusing, and it is only because of the recent identification of the B3 cells as corticotropes that some general interpretation can be made. As in the seasonal cycle of *R. temporaria* (van Oordt, van Dongen and Lofts, 1968; van Kemenade *et al.* 1968), TSH and ACTH secretion seem often to run in parallel in a variety of circumstances.

Recently, one of the principal advocates of the view that the B3 cells are thyrotropes has identified them as corticotropes in several amphibians (Doerr-Schott, 1972; Doerr-Schott and Dubois, 1970, 1972).

Adrenocortical stimulating hormone (ACTH, corticotropin)

Identification of the ACTH cells has been difficult in all vertebrates, partly because of the extreme reactivity of the ACTH–adrenocortical system, so that many different stimuli increase ACTH output by acting as non-specific stressors.

For many years, the B3 cells were regarded as being the source of an LH-like gonadotropin (van Oordt, 1968), largely on the basis of correlations between the activity of these cells and the activity of the testicular interstitial cells. The unsatisfactory nature of this evidence has recently become obvious with the demonstration that the activity of the interstitial cells parallels that of the adrenal cortex in both normal and experimental circumstances (see van Kemenade, 1969*b*), and with the realisation that, like fishes and reptiles, the amphibian pituitary may secrete only a single gonadotropin (see van Oordt and De Kort, 1969).

The B3 cells are now identified as corticotropes. Specific activation of the B3 cells in *Rana temporaria* occurred in parallel with pituitary-dependent stimulation of the interrenal (adrenal cortex) by metopirone and aldactone (van Kemenade, 1968*a*, *b*, 1969*b*), and the B3 cells regressed, together with the interrenal, when hibernating frogs were subjected to high temperature (van Kemenade, 1969*a*). Two different bioassays demonstrated that ACTH activity in this frog is largely concentrated in the rostral half of the pars distalis, which correlates with the fact that the B3 cell is the only cell-type preferentially located in the rostral region (van Kemenade, 1971; Larsen, van Kemenade and van Dongen, 1971). Bioassay of rostral and caudal halves of *Xenopus* pars distalis showed that all ACTH activity occurs in the rostral half, again pointing to the rostral B3 cells as corticotropes (Evennett and Larsen, 1971). ACTH activity was shown by bioassay to be entirely located in the rostral half of *Necturus* pars distalis, in correlation with the location of all the B3 cells in this part of the gland (Aplington and Vernikos-Danellis, 1968).

The B3 cells of *Rana esculenta* have been identified as corticotropes in experiments in which the interrenal was surgically removed (Dupont, 1967; Doerr-Schott, 1972) or blocked by metopirone (Dupont, 1968), or in which ACTH secretion was stimulated by injection of lysine vasopressin (Dupont and Peltier, 1970) or by unilateral interrenalectomy (Dupont and Gaudray, 1969). Changes in the interrenal and B3 cells after ectopic pituitary transplantation also identified these cells as corticotropes (Dupont, 1971). It will be recalled that Dupont regards the B3 cells of *R. esculenta* as acidophils, but more recent work shows them to be PAS+, though AB−, and AF+, and blue-violet after Aliz BT (Doerr-Schott, 1972; Doerr-Schott and Dubois, 1972).

The use of a fluorescent antibody to synthetic β 1–24 ACTH has identified the B3 cells as corticotropes in *Rana temporaria*, *R. esculenta*, *Bufo bufo* and *Xenopus laevis* (Doerr-Schott, 1972; Doerr-Schott and Dubois, 1972).

Amongst urodeles, partial hypophysectomy showed the B3 cells to be corticotropes in *Triturus cristatus* (Mazzi, 1971), and the fluorescent anti-ACTH technique led to the same identification in *T. marmoratus* (Doerr-Schott and Dubois, 1970, 1972).

Earlier workers tended to allocate ACTH secretion to acidophils. Certainly, the A2 cells of *T. cristatus*, for example, react strongly to metopirone or corticosteroid treatment (Mazzi *et al.* 1966), but these must be collateral responses, as in other species (see van Oordt, 1968; van Kemenade, 1969*b*). However, work involving ectopic autotransplantation of the pars distalis in *Pleurodeles* showed that all cell types except the A1 cells became involuted, and that the interrenal remained normal by histological criteria, findings which led Pasteels (1960) to identify the A1 cells as corticotropes. Clearly this work needs to be repeated in view of the recent evidence that ACTH is secreted by the B3 cells.

Gonadotropin

It is uncertain whether the amphibian pituitary secretes two gonadotropins, FSH and LH, as in birds (Hartree and Cunningham, 1969) and mammals (chapter 3), or whether the gland secretes a single gonadotropin with both FSH- and LH-like properties, as seems to be the case in teleosts (chapter 10) and reptiles (chapter 13). Until recently, the 'two gonadotropins' view was widespread, largely because differential responses to mammalian gonadotropins and to various experimental manipulations are shown in *Rana temporaria* by the spermatogenic tissue (FSH-target) and the testicular interstitial cells and secondary sexual characters (LH-targets) (see van Oordt, 1968). However, similar responses in reptiles are not incompatible with the 'one-gonadotropin' hypothesis (chapter 13), and it now seems possible that amphibians may produce only a single gonadotropin (van Oordt and De Kort, 1969).

Extensive work involving studies of the pituitary during the annual sexual cycle, and during gonad development in juvenile animals, has shown that the B2 cells are gonadotropes. These are also the cells that respond most profoundly to gonadectomy and treatment with gonadal hormones, and regression of the gonads after ectopic pituitary transplantation is always accompanied by atrophy of the B2 cells (Pasteels, 1960; Mazzi *et al.* 1966; van Oordt, 1968; van Oordt, van Dongen and Lofts, 1968; Zuber-Vogeli, 1968; Rastogi and Chieffi, 1970*a, b*; Rastogi, Chieffi and Marmorino, 1972; Zuber-Vogeli and Xavier, 1972). Bioassay of fragments of *R. temporaria* pars distalis showed that total (FSH + LH-like) gonadotropic activity is distributed evenly through the pars distalis, in correlation with the B2 cells (but not the B3 cells) (van Kemenade, 1972). Similar results have been obtained for *Xenopus*, the activity under assay being in this case LH-like, distributed throughout the gland, and arising in the young toad some months after metamorphosis (Evennett and Thornton, 1971), which correlates with the development and distribution of the B2 cells, but not with the B3 cells (Kerr, 1965, 1966).

The evidence, then, points to the B2 cell as the source of a GtH. For many years, on the basis of correlated changes in the interstitial cells and the B3 cells in natural and experimental conditions, the B3 cells were thought to secrete an LH-like gonadotropin (van Oordt, 1963, 1968), although their early development in the larva did not support this idea (e.g. Copeland, 1943; Pasteels, 1957, 1960; Rémy, 1969; Zuber-Vogeli and Bihouès-Louis, 1971; Mira-Moser, 1972*a*). More recently the concept has developed that cyclical changes in the testis, which show lack of correlation between interstitial cell activity and spermatogenesis, can be explained on present evidence on the basis of one gonadotropin, with seasonal variations in the sensitivity of the interstitial cells and germinal tissue towards this single controlling hormone. These variations are probably due to the effects of temperature on the responsiveness of the two components, effects which have been experimentally demonstrated (van Oordt and De Kort, 1969). Thus, with the identification of the B3 cells as corticotropes, the B2 cells are left as the source of a single gonadotropin with both FSH- and LH-like properties. In support of this hypothesis is the observation that LH-type activity is first detectable after metamorphosis in *Xenopus laevis*, long after the appearance of the B3 cells but coincident with the differentiation of the gametogenic B2 cells (Evennett and Thornton, 1971).

HYPOTHALAMIC CONTROL OF
PARS DISTALIS FUNCTIONS

The nature of the control of the pars distalis by the hypothalamus, involving the median eminence and portal system, has been widely investigated during the past decade. Summaries of the field were given by Jørgensen (1968) and Dodd, Follett and Sharp (1971), and the following account attempts to survey the present information.

CONTROL OF LTH

The available information indicates that hypothalamic control of LTH secretion is primarily inhibitory. Ectopic pituitary transplants in *Triturus viridescens* induce precocious water drive, an LTH-dependent phenomenon (Masur, 1969). Similar transplants also induce water drive in *T. cristatus*, and increase the LTH-dependent tail height, and the transplanted glands secrete more LTH than normal glands when excised and incubated *in vitro* (Peyrot *et al.* 1969). Transplants maintain growth in *Pelobates*, *Rana esculenta* and *R. pipiens* tadpoles, and in the last species transplants also inhibit metamorphosis and result in gigantic tadpoles (Jørgensen, 1968; Etkin and Lehrer, 1960; Etkin, Derby and Gona, 1969). The pars distalis of both *Necturus* and *Bufo* secrete LTH autonomously *in vitro*, the latter at a rate comparable to many mammals (Bern and Nicoll, 1968; Nicoll, 1971). Measurements of plasma concentrations of LTH in the toad *Bufo bufo* showed that ectopic transplants of the pars distalis secrete increased amounts of the hormone (McKeown, 1972). Thus, in both anurans (Etkin, 1970) and urodeles (Mazzi, 1970) the hypothalamus probably secretes an LTH-inhibiting factor.

CONTROL OF STH

There is little information about STH control. Adult *Triturus cristatus* grow more rapidly than normal after autotransplantation of the pituitary (Jørgensen, 1968), and the autotransplanted gland maintains growth in adult *Pleurodeles* (Pasteels, 1960). These observations suggest autonomy of STH secretion in these newts, but interpretation is uncertain because of the lack of information about the roles of STH and LTH in controlling growth in adult urodeles (see p. 252), and because only A1 cells (putative lactotropes) persisted in the *Pleurodeles* transplants (Pasteels, 1960).

More definite information is available for *Bufo bufo*, in which the measurement of plasma STH levels, by radioimmunoassay, showed that the ectopically transplanted pars distalis secreted very little of the hormone, indicating that STH is under predominantly stimulatory hypothalamic control (McKeown, 1972).

CONTROL OF TSH

The results of a great deal of work on control of TSH seem to indicate differences between urodeles and anurans, and possibly between larva and adult.

In *adult urodeles*, TSH secretion may be largely independent of the hypothalamus. Animals bearing an ectopic pituitary autotransplant display normal or nearly normal moulting, which depends on thyroid hormone (*Pleurodeles waltlii*; metamorphosed *Siredon* (*Ambystoma*) *mexicanum*; *Triturus* spp: Jørgensen, 1968; Mazzi, 1970; Dodd, Follett and Sharp, 1971). TSH cells in the autotransplanted pituitary become hypertrophied in response to thiouracil and are converted into 'thyroidectomy cells' which secrete excess TSH (*T. cristatus*, Mazzi, 1970; *T. viridescens*, Compher and Dent, 1970). In untreated *T. viridescens* the TSH cells in the ectopic pituitary remain active (Masur, 1969). In *T. cristatus* bearing chronic hypothalamic lesions, moulting was normal and the thyroid gland remained active and responsive to thiourea (Mazzi, 1970). Radio-iodine uptake by the thyroid after ectopic pituitary transplantation is normal (*S. mexicanum*, Jørgensen, 1968; *T. viridescens*, Compher and Dent, 1970) or higher than normal (*T. cristatus*, Mazzi, 1970). However, detailed studies of thyroidal metabolism after pituitary ectopic transplantation in the newt *T. cristatus* indicate temporary changes in intermediate synthetic steps, and a permanent reduction in the rate of thyroxine synthesis (Peyrot *et al.* 1972), and newts in which the median eminence was separated by a collodium plate from the pars distalis showed identical deficiencies in thyroid function, which were corrected by even partial regeneration of the portal vessels (Peyrot, 1969). Thus, although TSH secretion in these urodeles is obviously highly autonomous, hypothalamic stimulation is probably necessary for completely normal secretory rates (see Vellano and Peyrot, 1970). A further illustration of this hypothalamic modulation is that moulting continued after pituitary transplantation in *Pleurodeles*, but the thyroid nevertheless displayed some histological regression (Pasteels, 1960).

Adult anurans display more obvious dependence of TSH secretion on the hypothalamus. Using thyroidal uptake of radio-iodine as a criterion, it seems in *Rana temporaria* and *Bufo bufo* that normal TSH secretion is possible only when the connections between hypothalamus and pars distalis are intact (Jørgensen, 1968; Dodd, Follett and Sharp, 1971). Anurans seem to vary greatly in the dependence of TSH on hypothalamic stimulation, with *B. bufo* showing the greatest dependence among the species studied; additionally, for *B. bufo* and some other anurans, a hypothalamic TSH-inhibitory mechanism is indicated, and it may be that species differ in the balance normally operative between TRF and an inhibitory mechanism (Rosenkilde, 1972).

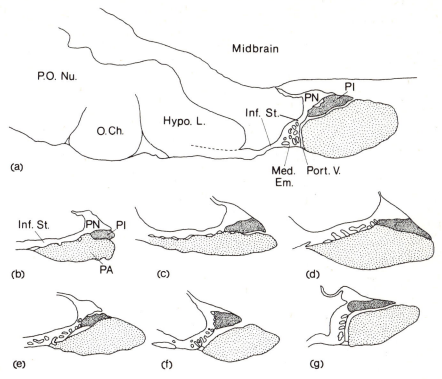

Fig. 12.7. *Rana pipiens*. Development of the median eminence during larval growth and metamorphosis. Line drawings of sagittal sections through the pituitary region, anterior to left. (*a*) Adult, (*b*) premetamorphosis, (*c*) early prometamorphosis, (*d*) late prometamorphosis, (*e*) beginning of metamorphic climax, (*f*) mid-climax, (*g*) post-climax. PA, pars distalis; PI, pars intermedia; PN, neural lobe; Port. V, portal vein; Med. Em., median eminence showing primary capillary bed; Inf. St., infundibular stem; Hypo. L., hypothalamic lobe or posterior hypothalamus; O. Ch., optic chiasma; PO Nu., preoptic nucleus. Note the increasing thickness and vascularity of the median eminence towards climax. From Etkin (1970).

The control of TSH secretion in *larval amphibians* has attracted considerable attention, because metamorphosis to the adult is dependent upon TSH and thyroid hormone. The subject provides a good example of interplay between structure and function in the hypothalamo-adeno-hypophysial complex, and is worth considering in some detail.

TSH and metamorphosis

It appears that portal connections between hypothalamus and pars distalis must be intact if anuran metamorphosis is to proceed to completion beyond climax, even though TSH secretion in the tadpole may be virtually autonomous for a time (Jørgensen, 1968; Dodd, Follett and

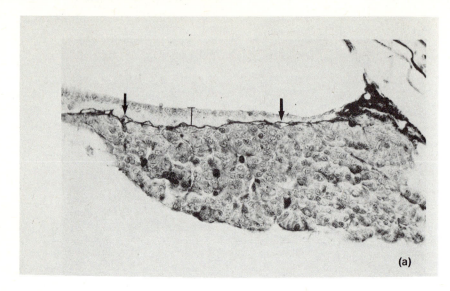

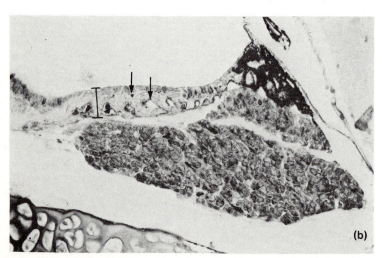

Fig. 12.8. *Rana pipiens*. Median sagittal sections of the pituitary region, to illustrate the effect of thyroid hormone on the differentiation of the median eminence. (*a*) Pituitary and hypothalamic floor in large thyroidectomised tadpole, showing failure of the median eminence to differentiate. (*b*) Similar section in an animal brought to midclimax by exogenous thyroxine, showing increased thickness of median eminence, and elaboration of its capillary bed (arrows). From Etkin (1970).

Sharp, 1971). Etkin (1970) has developed a model for the control of anuran metamorphosis according to which the TSH–thyroid axis operates at a low level in the tadpole, and hypothalamic control of TSH (by TSH releasing factor, TRF) is absent or minimal. Not surprisingly, the isolated

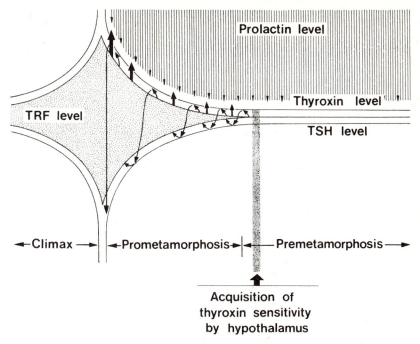

Prolactin level

Thyroxin level

TRF level

TSH level

←Climax→ ←Prometamorphosis→ ←Premetamorphosis→

Acquisition of
thyroxin sensitivity
by hypothalamus

Fig. 12.9. Theoretical representation of the interrelations of thyroid, thyrotropic hormone (TSH) and thyrotropin releasing factor (TRF) and prolactin levels in the life history of the anuran tadpole. Increased activity is indicated by deviation from the midline either above or below. Thin arrows indicate positive feedback relations, heavy arrows indicate inhibition. From Etkin (1970).

pars distalis secretes more-or-less normal amounts of TSH in this stage, the only important controlling factor being negative feedback of thyroid hormone on the TSH cells. The onset of pre-metamorphosis is signalled by the beginning of effective operation of the hypothalamic TRF mechanism, the hypothalamus now becoming for the first time sensitive to thyroid hormone. Details are disputed (see discussion of Etkin's 1970 paper), but in essence thyroid hormone is believed to stimulate the structural development of the median eminence and the portal system, which up to this stage is rudimentary, and which only attains its full adult complexity after metamorphic climax (fig. 12.7). It is certain that differentiation of the median eminence depends on thyroid hormone (fig. 12.8). Starting from the beginning of pre-metamorphosis thyroid hormone increases the operative efficiency of the hypothalamic TRF system, and increases its morphological complexity, the hypothalamic TRF secreting cells becoming more numerous, so that although sensitive to negative feedback by thyroid hormone (Goos, 1969*b*), the output of TRF rises and its delivery to the pituitary is progressively facilitated by development of the median eminence under the influence of thyroid hormone (fig. 12.7). As a result, the levels of TRF, TSH and thyroid hormone build up to the peak necessary for metamorphic climax (fig. 12.9), in a crescendo depending largely on the morphometric actions of thyroid hormone. Beyond metamorphic climax in anurans thyroid activity falls, for reasons not entirely clear but presumably related to the negative feedback of thyroid hormone on TRF secretion and the TSH cells, the whole system having been re-set at a lower level by the completion of development of the hypothalamus and median eminence during climax (Smoller, 1966; Goos, 1969*b*). Etkin (1970) also accommodates LTH in his model. LTH, we have seen, is the pituitary growth-promoting factor in the anuran tadpole, and it also inhibits the metamorphic responses of the tissues to thyroid hormone and is goitrogenic; thus it acts as an anti-metamorphic agent, a kind of juvenile hormone. Etkin (1970) suggests that LTH is secreted freely in the larva, before the median eminence becomes differentiated, but that with the increasing development of the median eminence during metamorphosis (fig. 12.7) LTH is progressively inhibited by hypothalamic LTH inhibiting factor (see p. 261). The falling LTH levels then permit the full tissue responses to thyroid hormone, resulting in metamorphosis (fig. 12.9).

The endocrinology of metamorphosis in urodeles probably differs in details. It is not such a severe change, and probably is equivalent only to the climax phase of the more protracted and extreme process in anurans; another difference is that high levels of thyroid activity continue into the adult stage (Etkin, 1970). Exogenous LTH, which is goitrogenic in high doses in anurans, appears to stimulate TSH release in *Triturus cristatus* (Peyrot *et al.* 1971). Indeed, the idea that LTH is in all circumstances goitrogenic in anuran tadpoles needs qualification in the light of demonstrations that LTH *stimulates* TSH secretion in *Bufo bufo* tadpoles at certain stages (see Peyrot *et al.* 1971). Nevertheless, LTH does prevent metamorphic responses to TSH in the larva of the tiger salamander (*Ambystoma tigrinum*), evidence that LTH–TSH antagonism may operate in the urodele larva as well as in anurans (Gona and Etkin, 1970). This antagonism also operates in the adult newt *Triturus* (*Diemictylus*) *viridescens*, in that high doses of thyroxine inhibit the LTH-dependent water drive (Gona, Pearlman and Etkin, 1970).

To summarise, hypothalamic stimulation of TSH in amphibians is reasonably well-established. TRF is probably always needed for completion of metamorphosis. The relatively low TSH secretion in the early larva may be autonomous. In the adult TSH secretion is largely autonomous in urodeles, but is more generally dependent on hypothalamic TRF in anurans, in which a hypothalamic inhibitory mechanism may also operate.

The hypothalamic TSH controlling centre

Some workers have attempted to locate the hypothalamic neurons which synthesise TRF. Evidence from adult *Bufo bufo* suggests that these neurons are located posterior to the PON, and that their secretion is not transmitted along the AF+ PON-neurohypophysial tract (Jørgensen, 1968). In larval anurans, however, several workers have located the site of TRF secretion in or close to the PON (see Dodd, Follett and Sharp, 1971). In *Xenopus laevis* larvae the TRF cells are located in the dorsal part of the PON, and their product is AF+ and positive to pseudo-isocyanine (PIC). These dorsal cells resemble the magnocellular components of the PON in adult *Xenopus*, and they develop during larval life in close correlation with the TSH cells and the thyroid; more ventrally, cells resembling the parvocellular elements of the adult PON do not develop before metamorphic climax (Goos, Zwanenbeek and van Oordt, 1968). The secretory activity of the TRF cells is depressed by thyroxine, but thyroxine also causes them to differentiate and multiply at metamorphosis, in parallel to the development of the median eminence (Goos, 1969*b*). A fine lesion placed immediately posterior to the PON in *Xenopus* tadpoles at the start of metamorphic climax blocks further metamorphic changes, presumably by severance of the fibre tracts which normally deliver TRF to the median eminence (Dodd, Follett and Sharp, 1971).

Direct action of thyroid hormone on the pars distalis

Abundant evidence indicates that in addition to the negative feedback of thyroid hormone on TRF secretion, thyroxine also acts directly on the pituitary TSH cells and inhibits their activity (see Jørgensen, 1968; Goos, 1969*b*; Etkin, 1970; Dodd, Follett and Sharp, 1971).

CONTROL OF ACTH

Earlier work on anurans indicated that the hypothalamus stimulates ACTH secretion, although interrenal histology suggested some slight ACTH secretion by ectopic pituitary transplants in *Bufo* and *Rana* (Jørgensen, 1968). More recent work has confirmed the failure of ACTH secretion in ectopic transplants in *Rana esculenta*, the failure being partial or total according to the distance of the graft from the hypothalamus, which suggests the intervention of a hypothalamic factor reaching the transplanted ACTH cells via the general circulation (Dupont, 1971). Measurement of plasma corticosterone levels in *Bufo bufo* demonstrated the reduction of ACTH secretion by pituitary grafts on an eye muscle, and transections of the hypothalamus located a region at the level of the optic chiasma (caudal to the PON) which appears to be concerned in ACTH control (Büchmann, Spies and Vijayakumar, 1972). Neural disconnection of the pars distalis by lesions in the hypothalamus also located an ACTH controlling region in *Rana temporaria*, in the region of the optic chiasma or further rostral, in essential agreement with the work on *Bufo* (Dierickx and Goossens, 1970). This region is presumed to secrete a corticotropin releasing factor (CRF). The nature of this factor is not known, but it is noteworthy that as in mammals and a teleost (see Ball *et al.* 1972), neurohypophysial octapeptides can release ACTH from pituitary transplants in *Bufo bufo*, arginine vasopressin being the most potent of those tested (Jørgensen and Larsen, 1963). Thus these neurohypophysial factors can mimic amphibian CRF, as well as the CRF of mammals and teleosts.

Most of the data on urodeles indicate that ACTH continues to be secreted at normal rates by the ectopic pituitary (see Jørgensen, 1968; Dodd, Follett and Sharp, 1971), pointing to greater autonomy of this function than in anurans. Nearly all the earlier work depended on indirect and possibly non-specific criteria of ACTH secretion, and a more recent study of interrenal histology and general hydromineral regulation in *Triturus cristatus* indicates some degree of failure of ACTH output from ectopic transplants (Mazzi, 1970). However, interrenal histology remained normal after pituitary transplantation in *Pleurodeles* (Pasteels, 1960), so it is possible that different urodeles vary in the extent to which the hypothalamus is necessary for ACTH secretion, though it is likely that ACTH secretion is more autonomous in urodeles as a group than in anurans.

CONTROL OF GONADOTROPIN

This subject has attracted a great deal of attention, resulting in a voluminous literature which has been reviewed by Jørgensen (1968), Mazzi (1970) and Dodd, Follett and Sharp (1971). In anurans, ectopic transplantation of the pars distalis or removal of the posterior hypothalamus leads to a reduction in GtH secretion. The GtH cells appear to have a certain autonomous activity, but to depend upon connection with the hypothalamic gonadotropin centre for completely normal function (see reviews, and Vijayakumar, Jørgensen and Kjaer, 1971). The work of Dierickx (1966, 1967*a*, *b*) has located the gonadotropic centre of *Rana temporaria* in the basal hypothalamus, the *pars ventralis tuberis*; the centre appears to be spread rather widely through this region, starting near to the median eminence and passing rostrally close to the anteroventral sloping floor of the infundibular recess (fig. 12.10; Dierickx, 1967*a*). This area is topographically comparable to the hypophysiotropic area of the mammalian hypothalamus (chapter 6). If isolated surgically

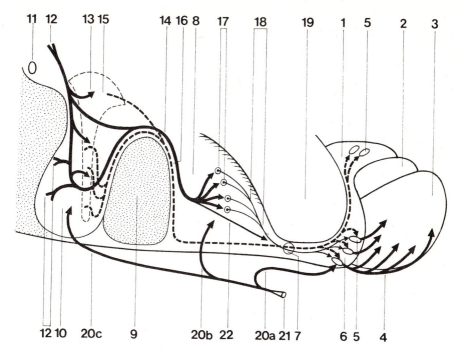

Fig. 12.10. The gonadotropic centre of the hypothalamus of *Rana temporaria*. Diagrammatic mid-sagittal section of the hypothalamo-hypophysial region, anterior to left. 1, neural lobe; 2, pars intermedia; 3, pars distalis; 4, portal vessels to pars distalis; 5, blood capillaries; 6, median eminence; 7, hypothalamo-hypophysial tract; 8, pars ventralis tuberis; 9, optic chiasma; 10, preoptic recess; 11, foramen of Monro; 12, AF− nerve fibre tracts of unknown origin, for higher neural control; 13, higher neural control of the magnocellular preoptic nucleus; 14, higher neural control of the gonadotropic centre of the pars ventralis tuberis; 15, magnocellular neurosecretory preoptic nucleus; 16, AF+ neurosecretory nerve fibres to the median eminence and to the neural lobe; 17, nerve cell bodies of the gonadotropic centre located in the area periventricularis of the pars ventralis tuberis cinerei; 18, AF− axons of the gonadotropic centre running to the blood capillaries of the median eminence; 19, saccus infundibuli; afferent blood vessels, to the median eminence (20*a*), to the pars ventralis tuberis (20*b*) and to the preoptic region of the hypothalamus (20*c*); 21, humoral factors influencing the functions of the pars distalis, of the pars ventralis tuberis and of the preoptic hypothalamus; 22, hypothetical X-fibres to the external zone of the median eminence. From Dierickx (1967*a*).

from all other parts of the brain, the gonadotropic centre reveals a partial autonomy, in that it can stimulate sufficient secretion of GtH by the pituitary to maintain testicular function in *R. temporaria* and *Bufo bufo* and to allow seasonal development of the ovary in *R. temporaria* (Dierickx, 1967*a*; Jørgensen, 1968; Dodd, Follett and Sharp, 1971). Female *B. bufo* apparently require higher levels of gonadotropin for oocyte development than female *Rana*, since the surgically isolated gonadotropic centre in *B. bufo* is unable to support normal oocyte growth after spawning (Jørgensen, 1968). The gonadotropic centre is the source of some AF−axons which terminate in the median eminence (Dierickx, 1966), probably the type B fibres identified as originating in the posterior hypothalamus by Budtz (1970) and presumably the route by which a gonadotropin releasing factor (GRF) reaches the median eminence. Like the hypophysiotropic area of mammals, the amphibian gonadotropic centre is subject to higher control. One indication of this is the failure of the isolated centre to maintain vitellogenesis in *B. bufo* (Jørgensen, 1968). In addition, connections with anterior regions of the brain are necessary for the centre to stimulate ovulation, as was shown by transections of the hypothalamus just behind the optic chiasma in frogs and toads with completely mature ovaries and oviducts (fig. 12.10; Dierickx, 1967*b*; Jørgensen, 1968). The identity of the more anterior region necessary for the induction of ovulation by the gonadotropic centre is uncertain. Some evidence suggests that the PON is necessary for ovulation and spermiation (see Dierickx, 1966, 1967*a*, *b*; Dodd, Follett and Sharp, 1971) but this is not conclusive, and it remains possible that some part of the anterior hypothalamus other than the PON may be the essential anterior component of the ovulation-inducing system (fig. 12.10).

Much less information is available for urodeles. Isolation of the pars distalis from the hypothalamus reduces GtH secretion in both sexes (Pasteels, 1960; Jørgensen, 1968). Lesions of the preoptic region, permanent transection of the median eminence and portal vessels, and ectopic pituitary autotransplantation, all result in testicular atrophy in *Triturus cristatus*, and all these operations largely prevent the re-activation of spermatogenesis that normally follows exposure to high temperature (Mazzi, 1970). Since lesions in the hypothalamic floor in front of the median eminence have a strong and lasting antigonadal effect in this newt, and since electrical stimulation of the PON region evokes ovulation (Mazzi, 1970), it may be that the full stimulation of gonadotropin secretion in *T. cristatus* requires connections between anterior hypothalamus and median eminence, not only for ovulation, as in anurans, but also for the tonic secretion of gonadotropin that maintains gametogenesis. Whatever the details, the hypothalamic gonadotropic control mechanism seems to be broadly similar in both anurans and urodeles.

HISTOPHYSIOLOGY OF THE PARS INTERMEDIA

The cells of the pars intermedia are usually spherical or cuboidal, but they may be columnar with a basal nucleus when they border blood capillaries. In some urodeles A2 cells from the pars distalis may invade the pars intermedia (Aplington, 1942; van Oordt, 1968). Most authorities believe that there is only a single pars intermedia cell-type, PAS+, strongly positive to both AF and AB without oxidation, less reactive following permanganic oxidation (Doerr-Schott, 1968*a*; van Oordt, 1968; Gabe, 1972, for apodans). The pars intermedia cells were shown to be PbH+ in *Xenopus laevis* and *B. bufo* (van Oordt, 1968). In addition to fine secretory granules, the cells often contain large globular bodies, up to *c.* 5 μm in diameter and in light microscope observation usually seeming to lie between the cells. These bodies, which are usually said to be more common when the pars intermedia is most active, contain lipids, phospholipids, and mucoproteins or mucopolysaccharides (van Oordt, 1968). According to Hopkins (1970) these or similar lipid bodies appear as intracellular irregular structures in EM observations on *Xenopus*, and are present in the peripheral cytoplasm no matter what the state of activity of the cell. Imai (1969), however, found them to be present only in *Xenopus* adapted to a black background, with maximal rate of MSH secretion. In other amphibians, the globular bodies may be identical with spherical electron-dense bodies within the spaces of the RER (Saland, 1968; Doerr-Schott and Follénius, 1970*a*; Castel, 1972).

Some workers have described more than one intermedia cell-type. *Xenopus* and *Bufo bufo* are said to have light cells (weakly-staining) and dark cells (strongly-staining), with different distributions, and three cell-types with different locations have been described in an EM study of the pars intermedia of *Bufo arenarum* (see van Oordt, 1968). It is possible, however, that these are but different stages in the secretory cycles of a single cell-type, since intermediate conditions can be found (Doerr-Schott, 1968*a*; Hopkins, 1970; Doerr-Schott and Follénius, 1970*a*). In *Rana esculenta* and other anurans cells containing the globular bodies ('globular cells') occur in the internal zone of the pars intermedia, close to the neuro-intermedia boundary. The external zone is composed of normal secretory cells without the globules, and transitional morphological stages are found (Doerr-Schott and Follénius, 1970*a*). *Xenopus laevis* shows two kinds of granule within a single cell, the first small (150–250 nm in diameter), dense, and confined to the releasing face of the Golgi complex, the second large (250–275 nm in diameter), flocculent or fibrous, and scattered generally in the cells. Animals adapted to a white background (low rate of MSH secretion) contained few small granules but many large ones, but animals placed on a black background (high rate of MSH secretion) developed increased numbers of small granules, while the large ones were progressively lost (probably by exocytosis from the cell) until only a few remained. It is likely that the small granules represent newly-packaged MSH, the large granules being older storage sites (Hopkins, 1970).

In addition to the endocrine cells, stellate cells are present. These form a thin envelope around the pars intermedia, and give rise to long thin

processes which form a network beneath the endothelium of the superficial capillaries, and also penetrate the intercellular spaces throughout
the gland, with occasional desmosomes between the processes (Hopkins,
1970). A similar stellate cell system occurs in the pars distalis (p. 249),
and other workers have mentioned this more briefly in the pars intermedia (Nakai and Gorbman, 1969; Doerr-Schott and Follénius, 1970*a*).
In addition, glia-like supporting cells accompany the nerve fibres throughout the pars intermedia (Saland, 1968; Hopkins, 1971), and may phagocytose moribund nerve fibres (Hopkins, 1971). It is not certain how
the glial cells are related to stellate cells (cf. Nakai and Gorbman,
1969).

President evidence identifies the pars intermedia as the source of a
single hormone, MSH (Gorbman, 1964), which may exist in at least three
different forms (Burgers, 1963). It seems that the hormone is located in
the membrane-bound granules which are secreted by exocytosis (Hopkins,
1970), although not all MSH occurs in granular form (Weatherhead and
Whur, 1972). There is also some evidence that MSH may occur in the
globular bodies within expansions of the RER, possibly as a reserve store
of the hormone (see Doerr-Schott and Follénius, 1970*a*), or perhaps as a
transient form of MSH for rapid release (Castel, 1972). As with the pars
intermedia in other vertebrates, it is surprising that granules containing
simple peptide hormone should be PAS+. In *Rana pipiens*, some of the
PAS+ material is glycogen, but some is glycoprotein, possibly a carrier
for MSH (see van Oordt, 1968). The minor localisation of fluorescent
antibody to β 1–24 ACTH in the pars intermedia cells of several amphibians presumably reflects the structural overlap between ACTH and
MSH (Doerr-Schott and Dubois, 1970, 1972). Antibodies to α and β-
MSH localise specifically in the pars intermedia cells in various amphibians
(Doerr-Schott and Dubois, 1972).

HYPOTHALAMIC CONTROL OF THE
PARS INTERMEDIA

Evidence accumulated over many years indicates that the hypothalamus
exerts a predominantly inhibitory control over secretion of MSH in
amphibians. For example, destruction of connections between hypothalamus and pars intermedia, by whatever means, causes increased
secretion of MSH (e.g. Hopkins, 1970; Castel, 1972). The pars intermedia
is only poorly and indirectly vascularised, capillaries being confined to
the neuro-intermedia boundary and the edge of the gland (p. 286), and
these capillaries receive little if any blood from the median eminence.
Since the pars intermedia is richly innervated, and since transection of
the infundibular stem (fig. 12.2*a*), leaving the portal vessels undisturbed,
leads to excessive MSH secretion, it seems that hypothalamic control is

exerted by direct innervation rather than by a neurovascular route (see Dodd, Follett and Sharp, 1971).

In some amphibians the pars intermedia receives AF+ axons, as well as AF− fibres (Dodd, Follett and Sharp, 1971; Rodríguez, La Pointe and Dellman, 1971). However, it seems unlikely that the pars intermedia is inhibited by AF+ neurosecretory fibres, since ablation of the PON in *Rana temporaria*, which led to the complete loss of AF+ NSM from the neuro-intermedia, did not result in increased MSH secretion, the operated animals being in fact rather paler than the controls (Dierickx, 1967a). Nevertheless, since hypothalamic extracts have been shown to inhibit MSH secretion, the inhibitory control is thought to be by a hypothalamic neurosecretory substance, presumably AF−, and called MSH inhibiting factor (MIF). The mammalian MIF appears to be a small peptidic molecule (Dodd, Follett and Sharp, 1971). Most of the data indicate that the amphibian MIF is a monoamine (Iturriza, 1969; Peute and Goos, 1970; Dodd, Follett and Sharp, 1971), although there is some contradictory evidence (see Jørgensen, 1968). Some slight evidence also indicates the existence of a hypothalamic MSH releasing factor (MRF) (Jørgensen, 1968; Oshima and Gorbman, 1969). Physiological work, then, points to the existence of AF− hypothalamic neurosecretory neurons with direct axonal connections to the pars intermedia, and secreting MIF, which may be a monoamine.

Morphological studies on the amphibian pars intermedia have clarified and elaborated this concept. Type A (i.e. AF+) fibres from the neural lobe cross the neuro-intermedia septum and innervate the intermedia. Several workers (Smoller, 1966; Saland, 1968; Nakai and Gorbman, 1969; Doerr-Schott and Follénius, 1970a; Hopkins, 1971; Rodríguez, La Pointe and Dellman, 1971; Castel, 1972) have emphasised that AF+ material and type A fibres are virtually confined to the internal zone of the pars intermedia, the region close to the neuro-intermedia septum which in *R. esculenta* and other amphibians contains the 'globular' endocrine cells, possibly storage cells (Doerr-Schott and Follénius 1970a). Apart from *type A* fibres, with secretory granules 100–200 nm in diameter (Saland, 1968; Nakai and Gorbman, 1969; Doerr-Schott and Follénius, 1970a; Hopkins, 1971; Rodríguez, La Pointe and Dellman, 1971; Castel, 1972), there are present throughout the pars intermedia many *type B* fibres, with granules 55–100 nm in diameter (Smoller, 1966; Saland, 1968; Nakai and Gorbman, 1969; Imai, 1969; Doerr-Schott and Follénius, 1970a, 1972; Ito, 1971; Rodríguez, La Pointe and Dellman, 1971; Castel, 1972). Both types of fibres contain clear 'synaptic' vesicles, 20–50 nm in diameter, in addition to the secretory granules. Some workers have described a third kind of axonal termination, *type C*, containing 'synaptic' vesicles with few or no secretory granules. These may be cholinergic endings, but it is still uncertain that they form a separate category

(Saland, 1968; Nakai and Gorbman, 1969; Doerr-Schott and Follénius, 1970*a*).

Type B fibres have been shown to be aminergic (Doerr-Schott and Follénius, 1970*a*; Hopkins, 1971; Rodríguez, La Pointe and Dellman, 1971; Rodríguez, 1972), and the newt and toad pars intermedia contains fibres rich in monoamine oxidase (Urano, 1972). In *Rana esculenta* the 'synaptic' vesicles of type B fibres are possibly very active in the turnover of noradrenaline (Doerr-Schott and Follénius, 1970*a*), and adrenaline is sequestered by these structures in *Xenopus* (Hopkins, 1971). In both anurans, labelled catecholamines were located along the course of the axons (associated with small clear vesicles amongst neurofibrils in *R. esculenta*), as well as in the terminal 'synaptic' vesicles. Type C fibres, though containing many 'synaptic' vesicles, do not sequester adrenaline, an indication of the heterogeneous nature of the vesicles (Doerr-Schott and Follénius, 1970*a*).

Both type A and type B fibres synapse with the pars intermedia endocrine cells, but type A contacts are rare and confined to the 'globular' cells of the internal zone (Nakai and Gorbman, 1969; Doerr-Schott and Follénius, 1970*a*; Hopkins, 1971; Rodríguez, La Pointe and Dellman, 1971; Castel, 1972). Double innervation of a single endocrine cell by type A and type B fibres has been seen once (Nakai and Gorbman, 1969). This double innervation by both fibre types may be a commoner feature of the internal zone than this single observation suggests, because of the technical improbability of both endings appearing in the same electron micrograph. Double innervation of an endocrine cell by two type B fibres, or by a type B and a type C fibre, is probably common throughout the gland (Nakai and Gorbman, 1969; Doerr-Schott and Follénius, 1970*a*), and may be the rule, although some workers believe that each cell is innervated by only one type B fibre (Saland, 1968; Ito, 1971).

Some type A fibres terminate on glial cells, and some type B fibres on the vessels of the plexus intermedius (Doerr-Schott and Follénius, 1970*a*). Axo-axonal terminations also occur, especially of type A fibres (the nature of the post-synaptic fibre is uncertain), and a single type A fibre may end both on an endocrine cell and on another axon (Nakai and Gorbman, 1969; Hopkins, 1971).

The morphological evidence of double innervation of the intermedia cells has to be considered in relation to neurophysiological work on the frog (*Rana pipiens*). Illumination of the retina rapidly evokes electrical activity in the pars intermedia (Dawson and Ralph, 1971). Furthermore, it seems that there are two types of *spontaneously* active electrical units in the intermedia, which were shown by lesion experiments to be neuronal fibres that travel separately grouped in the infundibular floor (Oshima and Gorbman, 1969). One type of neuron is indifferent to changes in illumination, and this was considered by the investigators to correspond to type B aminergic fibres, inhibiting MSH secretion. This type travels lateral in the infundibular floor. The second type is inhibited by light acting via the pineal, and it probably stimulates MSH release when its electrical activity is maximal, i.e. in conditions of minimal illumination. This second type of fibre travels medially in the infundibular floor (Oshima and Gorbman, 1969). The ultrastructural equivalent of this second (stimulatory) unit is not identifiable with certainty. The work of Dierickx (1967) previously quoted (p. 273) argues for AF+ type A fibres in this role, but their limited distribution in the gland argues against it. It is more probable that the stimulatory unit is represented by either a second kind of type B fibre, morphologically identical with the inhibitory type B fibre, or by the type C fibres; the paired nerve endings observed on the endocrine cells would allow either hypothesis. If control were by two sets of type B fibres, they could be of the opposed α- and β-aminergic types (Oshima and Gorbman, 1969).

The *central origin* of the nerve fibres of the pars intermedia has been intensively sought. Transection of the hypothalamo-neurohypophysial tract, by extirpating the median eminence, led in *Rana nigromaculata* to degeneration of type B endings in the pars intermedia, ultrastructural signs of activation of the endocrine cells, depletion of stored MSH and increased secretion of MSH. Starting about two weeks post-operatively, MSH secretion declined, the endocrine cells became less active, and type B fibres re-appeared in the pars intermedia, evidence of regeneration of these inhibitory fibres from their hypothalamic origin (Ito, 1969, 1971). In *Rana catesbiana* tadpoles, isolation of the pars intermedia from the hypothalamus resulted in hypersecretion of MSH, degranulation of the intermedia cells, hypertrophy of the RER and Golgi complex, and a rapid loss of neurosecretory granules from the type B fibres. The spherical globules virtually disappeared from the cisternae of the RER, and colloidal material appeared between the cells, possibly representing released MSH, though this is speculative (Castel, 1972). Rodríguez, La Pointe and Dellman (1971) showed by transection experiments that both type A and type B fibres travel through the infundibular stem of *Rana pipiens*. The type B (adrenergic) fibres appear to originate in the posterior hypothalamus, in a pair of elongated curved nuclei containing AF− adrenergic neurons, in larval *Xenopus* and adult *R. temporaria*, *Triturus cristatus* and *B. bufo* (Peute and Goos, 1970; Fasolo and Franzoni, 1971*b*; Rodríguez, 1972). These nuclei lie in part in the region which contains the gonadotropic centre (p. 269), and the rostral tip of each nucleus in *Xenopus* larvae includes the paraventricular organ, the nuclei running caudally alongside the infundibular recess. The neurons have protrusions into the third ventricle. The pathway of type B fibres from these nuclei is difficult to follow, but under certain experimental conditions they can be seen to run in a tract passing close to the median eminence and then into the pars intermedia (Peute and Goos, 1970; Rodríguez, La Pointe and Dellman, 1971; Rodríguez, 1972). They travel together with PON type A fibres through the internal zone of the median eminence, and divide opposite the rostral tip of the pars intermedia. One division terminates on the wall of capillaries which pass from the primary portal plexus to the plexus intermedius (p. 286), and the other division penetrates the neuro-intermedia septum, where some type B fibres end on capillaries, but most pass on into the pars intermedia itself (Doerr-Schott and Follénius, 1970*a*; Rodríguez, 1972). Recent evidence shows that the curved nuclei of the posterior hypothalamus are the site of synthesis of an MSH-inhibiting monoamine (Peute and Goos, 1970).

It appears that all the pars intermedia type B fibres originate in the curved nuclei of the posterior hypothalamus, but nothing is known about the origin and exact role of the possibly cholinergic type C fibres.

THE PARS TUBERALIS

The paired pars tuberalis is usually said to contain chromophobic cells, weakly basophilic and without secretory granules, together with a few intrusive cells from the pars distalis (van Oordt, 1968; Gabe, 1972). Almost nothing is known of possible endocrine functions of this region. In *Rana esculenta* its volume decreases during growth, and decreases after hypophysectomy (Burlet and Legait, 1967). In *Triturus viridescens*, the pars tuberalis, originally small in the aquatic larva, increases in size during the immature adult phase (the red eft), then diminishes during the change to the sexually mature aquatic adult phase. Its cells are weakly basophilic or chromophobic, and their function unknown (Copeland, 1943). Neurosecretory fibres have been described in the pars tuberalis of various amphibians, but most of these probably end on marginal capillaries (Legait and Burlet, 1966).

A recent EM study of the pars tuberalis in *Rana temporaria* has shown that apart from chromophobic 'reserve' cells, there is also a single distinctive glandular cell-type, PAS+ and showing signs of strong secretory activity. Nerve fibres and terminations were not identified with any certainty, but a possibility of contacts between neurosecretory fibres and prolongations of the secretory cells requires further study (Doerr-Schott, 1971).

THE HYPOTHALAMUS AND NEUROHYPOPHYSIS

The neurohypophysis is invariably differentiated into neural lobe and median eminence, the latter varying greatly in its complexity. Both regions are innervated by axonal fibres from hypothalamic neurons. No hypothalamic fibres pass directly into the pars distalis, but as we have seen the pars intermedia is directly innervated.

The origins of the various neurosecretory fibres in the hypothalamus have been sought by many workers, not always successfully, and the literature is confused and sometimes contradictory. The main hypothalamic nuclei known at present are as follows.

The *preoptic nuclei* (PON) lie on either side in the anterior hypothalamus and selective lesioning in *Bufo* has shown the PON to be bipartite. A ventral region, lying in the walls of the preoptic recess, gives rise to the PON-neurohypophysial tract, AF+ and PAS+, and is involved in water balance. A dorsal region, lying higher in the walls of the third ventricle, gives rise to AF+ and PAS− axons terminating in the median eminence which are related to release of sperm from the testis (spermiation). Thus the PON gives rise to two distinct tracts, the ventral PON-neurohypophysial tract, with AF+, PAS+ type A fibres, and the dorsal PON-median eminence tract, with AF+, PAS− type A fibres (Rodríguez, 1966; Rodríguez, La Pointe and Dellman, 1970). There is strong evidence that all AF+ hypothalamic fibres originate in the PON (Dierickx, 1967a).

The *infundibular nucleus* ('periventricular nucleus') lies in the basal hypothalamus, and gives rise to type B fibres running to the median eminence. This nucleus is probably aminergic, and may be homologous with the infundibular nucleus of reptiles and birds and the arcuate of mammals (Zambrano and De Robertis, 1968).

The *gonadotropic centre* is located in the basal hypothalamus, the pars ventralis tuberis, and is presumed to be represented by unidentified AF− parvocellular nuclei in this area, sending type B fibres to the median eminence (Dierickx, 1966, 1967a, b). It is possible that the infundibular nucleus might be part of this centre.

The *caudal aminergic nuclei* that control the pars intermedia are described on p. 275. They are known to occur in *Xenopus laevis* tadpoles, and in adult *Triturus cristatus* and *Bufo* spp. (Goos, 1969a; Fasolo and Franzoni, 1971b; Rodríguez, 1972).

Apart from these regions, it is likely that there are scattered parvocellular nuclei in the hypothalamus, corresponding to the diffuse nuclei of the mammalian hypophysiotropic area (chapter 6).

The cell bodies of the PON, infundibular nucleus and caudal aminergic nuclei are bipolar, sending processes containing their characteristic reactive material through the neighbouring ependyma into the third ventricle (Zambrano and De Robertis, 1968; Goos, 1969a; Gabe, 1972). The PON neurons in *Triturus viridescens*, however, are said to be unipolar (Richerson and deRoos, 1971).

MEDIAN EMINENCE

When fully developed, as in anurans, the amphibian median eminence displays the elaborate structure seen in its mammalian equivalent (chapter 5). The *ependymal layer* lines the floor of the infundibular recess, and its cells bear microvilli and cilia on their free surfaces and are joined laterally by desmosomes. The bases of some of the ependymal cells are prolonged ventrally, and some of these prolongations contact the pericapillary spaces of the primary capillary bed in the zona externa (Rodríguez, 1969, 1972; Doerr-Schott, 1970).

The *zona interna* lies ventral to the ependymal layer, and contains glial cells but is largely occupied by nerve fibres. Bulking large are the fibres of the PON-neurohypophysial tract, which runs through the zona interna on its way to the neuro-intermedia. This tract carries both AF+ and AF− fibres. Some of the AF+ fibres, and most of the AF− ones, leave the tract and pass down to end on the median eminence capillaries (Doerr-Schott, 1970). The EM shows that there are two kinds of type A fibres in the tract, corresponding to the two type A fibres in the neural lobe and originating in the PON (Doerr-Schott, 1970; Rodríguez, 1971). The aminergic type B fibres which pass on in the tract and end in the pars intermedia probably come from the caudal aminergic nuclei (p. 277), and have been found in *Rana*, *Bufo* and *Triturus* (Doerr-Schott, 1970; Rodríguez, 1971; Fasolo and Franzoni, 1971a, b; Rodríguez, 1972).

The *zona externa* carries the superficial primary portal capillaries on its ventral surface, and these give rise to capillary loops in the median eminence (Doerr-Schott, 1970). It has an elaborate structure which has been described in detail for the toad *Bufo* by Rodríguez (1969). Apart from the loops of the portal capillaries, this zone has the usual palisade arrangement, and contains glial cells and nerve fibres (mainly non-myelinated). The primary portal capillaries are elaborated into long and short capillary loops. The *long capillary loops* (fig. 12.11) extend dorsally as far as the ependymal layer, and their most dorsal pericapillary basement membrane interdigitates with the basal prolongations of the ependymal cells. Longer ependymal cell processes terminate more ventrally, on the pericapillary membrane of both long and short capillary loops. The ependymal cells appear to transport materials (possibly monoamines) from the cerebrospinal fluid into the capillaries (Rodríguez, 1969, 1972). Nerve endings are found on both ascending and descending limbs of the long capillary loops, against the outer membrane of the usual kind of collagen-filled pericapillary space. The *short capillary loops* (fig. 12.11) are more numerous, and form the main site for endings of nerve fibres. The structural relation between the capillaries and nerve endings is peculiar. The pericapillary membrane is usually single, only rarely containing a space, and it bears enormously elaborate projections which

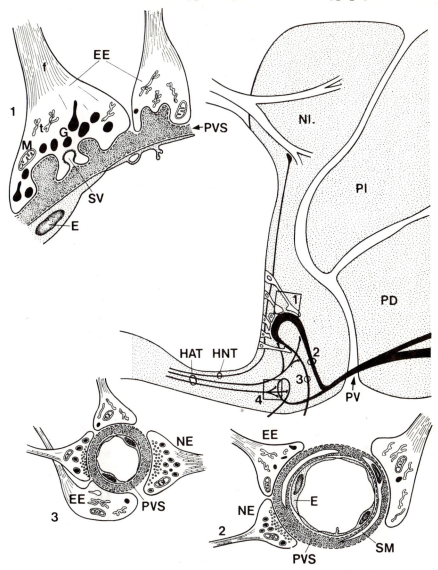

Fig. 12.11. Diagram to show the interrelationships between the ependyma of the toad (*Bufo*) median eminence, the short and long capillary loops of the hypothalamo-adenohypophysial portal system and the nerve tracts entering the hypophysial region. HNT, hypothalamo-neurohypophysial tract; HAT, hypothalamo-adeno-hypophysial tract; NL, neural lobe; PI, pars intermedia; PD, pars distalis; PV, portal vein. The ultrastructure of the areas indicated in square 1 and circles 2 and 3 is sketched in schemes 1, 2 and 3 respectively. A drawing of the area framed in square 4 is shown in fig. 12.12. EE, ependymal ending; NE, nerve ending; M, mitochondrion; G, granule; SV, spinous-surfaced vesicles; PVS, perivascular space; E, endothelium; SM, smooth muscle cell?; f, filaments; t, tubules. From Rodríguez (1972).

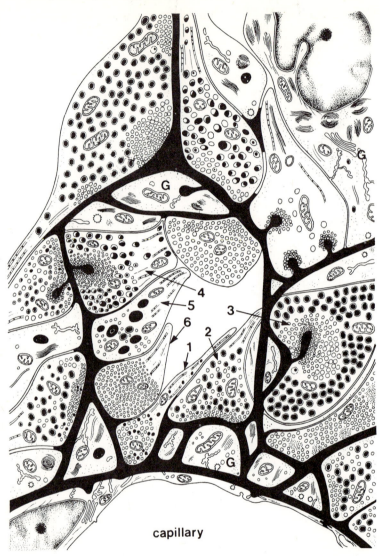

Fig. 12.12. *Bufo*. Semi-schematic representation of the interrelationships between a short loop of the toad median eminence and the surrounding nerve elements. 1, 2, 3, 4, 5 and 6 are different types of nerve terminals. The perivascular basement membrane and its processes are shown in black. G, glial cells. From Rodríguez (1972).

form a three-dimensional PAS+ connective tissue network around the capillary (fig. 12.12). This remarkable arrangement obviously greatly increases the surface area available for nerve terminations in relation to the capillary, and the network presumably acts as a system of connective tissue channels, transporting material from the nerve endings to the capillary. Because of this pericapillary network, nerve fibres may terminate as much as 10 nm away from the capillary itself (Rodríguez, 1969, 1972). An identical arrangement was described earlier in the bufonid tree 'frog', *Hyla* (Smoller, 1966). This elaborate pericapillary network seemingly does not occur in *Rana esculenta* (Doerr-Schott, 1970), and it may be a bufonid specialisation. Glial cells contact the pericapillary membranes in *Rana* (Doerr-Schott, 1970) and *Bufo* (fig. 12.12).

The *types of nerve endings* in the median eminence have been analysed in *Bufo*, *Rana* and *Triturus* (Rodríguez, 1969, 1972; Budtz, 1970; Doerr-Schott, 1970; Doerr-Schott and Follénius, 1972; Fasolo and Franzoni, 1971a). Most, if not all, axons contain neurotubules and small clear 'synaptic' vesicles. There is quite good general agreement in the accounts. It seems that there may be two kinds of type A fibres, though Budtz (1970) found only one kind in *Bufo*. These are probably AF+ and CAH+ but PAS− (Rodríguez, 1966), and are thought to originate in the dorsal PON (Rodríguez, 1966; Rodríguez, La Pointe and Dellman, 1970). Aminergic fibres occur around the median eminence capillaries (Urano, 1972), corresponding to some or all of the several kinds of type B terminations. In *Rana esculenta*, the type B fibre with the smaller secretory granules is certainly aminergic (Doerr-Schott and Follénius, 1970b), as in *Triturus marmoratus* (Doerr-Schott and Follénius, 1972). Four kinds of type B fibres have been described in *T. cristatus* median eminence, one of which (secretory granules 70–100 nm in diameter) is aminergic and is abundant in the zona externa, with terminations on the pericapillary spaces and on ependymal cells more dorsally (Fasolo and Franzoni, 1971a; Fasolo *et al.* 1972). Type B endings have been described in the median eminence of *Hyla*, but were not categorised (Smoller, 1966). The origin of the median eminence type B fibres is not certain, but some may come from the caudal aminergic nuclei (p. 277). The type B fibres with the larger granules in *Bufo* were shown by lesioning experiments to originate in the caudal hypothalamus, possibly in the gonadotropic centre or the infundibular nuclei (Budtz, 1970), and some AF− fibres in the median eminence of *Rana temporaria* originate in the gonadotropic centre (Dierickx, 1966, 1967a). In *Bufo*, the single type A fibre and the type B fibre with smaller granules appear to originate in the PON, or close to it (Budtz, 1970). Rodríguez (1969) has attempted to associate the different kinds of fibres in the toad median eminence with control of the different pars distalis functions, but this is perhaps premature.

In addition to the type A and type B fibres, all workers have reported the presence of fibres containing no dense granules, but only 'synaptic' vesicles. Whether these *type C* fibres are a distinct category, and whether the clear vesicles are truly synaptic, or are empty membranes of discharged granules, are unresolved questions (see p. 85).

Apart from neurosecretory endings in the median eminence, another anatomical link from hypothalamus to the primary portal capillaries has been described. In *Bufo*, silver impregnation revealed bipolar cell bodies in or below the ependymal layer of the infundibular recess, with short processes into the cavity of the recess and long processes extending laterally to end on the portal capillaries in the zona externa; it is not known whether these are neurons, ependymal cells, or some other element (Rodríguez, 1972).

The primary capillary plexus is supplied by branches of the hypophysial arteries, which display elaborate pre-portal tortuosities and loops, possibly retarding blood flow to facilitate neurohaemal exchange in the median eminence (Green, 1947; Rodríguez and Piezzi, 1967; Doerr-Schott, 1970).

The above account applies mainly to anurans. From the little information available, it seems that the urodele median eminence is less well-differentiated. In *Triturus* (*Notophthalmus*) *viridescens*, the infundibular floor is hardly thickened in the median eminence region. In the adult, but not in the larva, there is a primary capillary plexus embedded in superficial connective tissue and indented into the zona externa, where the capillaries presumably receive neurosecretory endings. These capillaries are directly continuous with the vascular bed of the pars distalis, with no portal vessels intervening, an arrangement very like that in some ganoid fishes and in the anterior part of the elasmobranch median eminence. As far as is known, most urodeles conform to this pattern (Richerson and deRoos, 1971).

NEURAL LOBE

The size of the neural lobe is usually said to vary with habitat, being larger in the more terrestrial amphibians (Dodd, Follett and Sharp, 1971). The neural lobe and pars intermedia are clearly separated by a fairly flat connective tissue septum, containing the usual plexus intermedius, except in the aquatic neotenous urodeles *Necturus* and *Amphiuma* in which, as in Dipnoi, the neural lobe sends hollow projections into the intermedia (Wingstrand, 1966a).

The neurohypophysial hormones mesotocin and arginine vasotocin (AVT) physiologically influence water retention in anurans by actions on kidney, skin and urinary bladder, but in urodeles the action is confined to the kidney as far as is known. The more terrestrial the amphibian, the greater is its response to neurohypophysial hormones, and the same rule applies to aquatic and terrestrial phases within the life history (Jørgensen, Rosenkilde and Wingstrand, 1969; Richerson and deRoos, 1971). Histological studies on the neural lobe have yielded interesting structural correlates of these functional aspects. For example, the terrestrial young adult stage (the eft) of *Triturus viridescens* contains more AF + NSM than the aquatic larva. The mature aquatic adult showed an intermediate condition, but increased its content of neural lobe NSM if forced experimentally to stay out of water. It seems that the stainable NSM represents the secretion and storage of the antidiuretic hormone, AVT, varying according to habitat (Richerson and deRoos, 1971).

The neural lobe includes numerous nerve fibres, capillaries, and rather few pituicytes. The nerve fibres are mainly AF + axons from the PON. The ependyma of the infundibular recess contains a few cells apparently specialised for transport, with their bases contacting subependymal capillaries and displaying pinocytotic vesicles towards the pericapillary space, and with similar vesicles at the free apical surface (Rodríguez, 1971). The neural lobe capillaries are surrounded by AF + nerve endings, and occasional processes of pituicytes (Rodríguez and Dellman, 1970; Rodríguez, 1971). This contact of pituicytes and pericapillary space presumably has some functional significance. It has been suggested that phagocytosis may be a normal function of pituicytes, relating to the disposal of neurohypophysial carrier proteins and granule membranes after release of the neurohypophysial octapeptides from nerve endings; it is known that under experimental conditions the pituicytes may hypertrophy and phagocytose the axons themselves (Dellman and Owsley, 1969).

At least two different kinds of type A fibre terminations have been detected on the perivascular spaces of the neural lobe, containing neurotubules and 'synaptic' vesicles (Doerr-Schott, 1970). Rodríguez (1971) described five kinds of fibres in the neural lobe of *Bufo*. There is a type C fibre, containing only 'synaptic' vesicles, and a type B fibre, both rare. Of the type A fibres, A1, with the largest (250 nm) granules, was very rare; type A2 (granules moderately electron-dense, 150–180 nm in diameter) and type A3 (granules denser and smaller, 130 nm) were common, and may correspond to the two known amphibian octapeptides, AVT (type A2) and mesotocin (type A3). Similar A2 and A3 fibres occur in *Rana pipiens* (Rodríguez, 1971). *Rana temporaria* has two kinds of neural-lobe type A fibres, with granules only slightly larger than the A2 and A3 granules of *Bufo* (Doerr-Schott, 1970). It should be said that granule size may vary not only with species but with technique; for example, working on the same toad as Rodríguez (1971), other workers (Zambrano and De Robertis, 1968) distinguished A2 and A3 fibres, but with granules *c.* 210 nm in type A2 fibres, and *c.* 180 nm in type A3. Although the size of the secretory granules probably increases as they pass along the axons (Zambrano and De Robertis, 1969), several workers have shown that the granule sizes in the PON-neurohypophysial tract are essentially the same as those in the neural lobe fibres (for examples see Doerr-Schott, 1970; Fasolo and Franzoni, 1971*a*; Rodríguez, 1969, 1971, 1972).

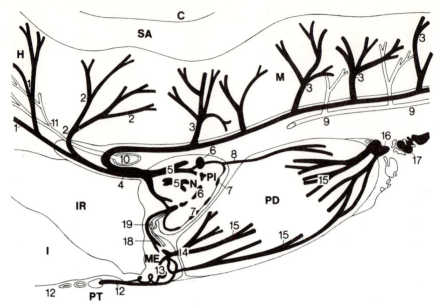

Fig. 12.13. *Bufo*. Semi-schematic representation of the vascularisation of the hypophysial region of the toad, anterior to left. C, cerebellum; SA, aqueduct of Sylvius; M, mesencephalon; H, hypothalamus; IR, infundibular recess; I, infundibulum; PT, pars tuberalis; ME, median eminence; N, neural lobe; PI, pars intermedia; PD, pars distalis. The solid (black) vessels are portal, the empty linear ones are arteries. *Vessels*: 1, hypothalamic group of the primary plexus of the encephalo-posthypophysial portal system; 2, anterior mesencephalic group; 3, posterior mesencephalic and bulbar group; 4, common venous stem; 5, capillarisation in the neural lobe; 6, large capillaries of the plexus intermedius; 7, superficial capillaries of the pars intermedia; 8, pars intermedia–pars distalis connecting vessel; 9, basilar artery communicating branch; 10, retroinfundibular communicating artery; 11, hypothalamic branch of the retroinfundibular communicating artery; 12, hypophysial artery; 13, median eminence capillary loops; 14, hypothalamo-adeno-hypophysial portal veins; 15, sinusoidal capillaries of the pars distalis; 16, pars distalis collecting veins; 17, endolymphatic sac plexus; 18, communicating capillaries between median eminence and pars intermedia; 19, direct branch of the hypophysial artery giving off a branch to the median eminence and another to the large capillaries of the plexus intermedius. From Rodríguez and Piezzi (1967).

Most workers on the neural lobe have described type C fibres, containing only 'synaptic' vesicles, as in the median eminence and pars intermedia. The nature of these vesicles has been debated for years. Vollrath (1970) has recently discussed them, and presented evidence from the rat that they form a heterogeneous structural group (see also Smoller, 1966), the majority of them arising in various ways from neurotubules.

Little is known about the fine structure of the urodele neural lobe. A single type A fibre category has been described in *Triturus viridescens* and *T. cristatus* (Dent and Gupta, 1967; Fasolo and Franzoni, 1971*a*). Type C fibres also occur in the former species, apparently forming synaptoid contacts with the neuro-intermedia septum (Dent and Gupta, 1967).

Type A fibres in anurans terminate on pericapillary spaces in the neural lobe, without the interposition of glial processes (Smoller, 1966; Doerr-Schott, 1970). The terminations are synaptoid, and some fibres also end on other axons, or on pituicytes (Doerr-Schott, 1970).

The rare type B fibres in *Rana esculenta* have been found to terminate close to the neuro-intermedia septum, and to be aminergic (Doerr-Schott, 1970). Fibres containing monoamine oxidase are numerous around the capillaries of the neural lobe in both toad and newt, and have been interpreted as aminergic and in some way concerned in the regulation of the release of neurohypophysial hormones into the capillaries (Urano, 1972). However, some workers report type B endings as being rare or absent in the neural lobe (Doerr-Schott, 1970; Hopkins, 1971: Doerr-Schott and Follénius, 1972), the type B fibres running across the neuro-intermedia septum to innervate the endocrine cells of the pars intermedia (Smoller, 1966; Doerr-Schott, 1970; Doerr-Schott and Follénius, 1972).

The possible role of pituicytes in neural lobe function has long been the object of speculation. Recently, Nakai (1970) has distinguished two kinds of pituicytes in the neural lobe of *Rana pipiens*, both with long processes amongst the nerve fibres, some of which terminate on a pericapillary space. He distinguished three kinds of nerve endings making synaptoid contact with the cell bodies and processes of the pituicytes, type A, type B and type C, and concluded that the pituicytes in some way play a part in controlling the release of neurohypophysial hormones.

BLOOD SUPPLY OF THE AMPHIBIAN PITUITARY

The blood supply of the gland follows the usual tetrapod pattern, with one significant exception in that the supply to the neuro-intermedia is almost entirely portal. This feature has been largely overlooked, most workers having accepted older accounts which described the neuro-intermedia as being directly vascularised by a branch of the basilar artery. This aspect has been investigated in detail by Rodríguez and Piezzi (1967), and the following account is based on their findings in *Bufo*, which follow earlier descriptions for *Bufo* and *Leptodactylus*. It cannot be said at present how generally this account can be extended to other amphibians, but it seems likely to be valid at least for anurans.

The system is illustrated in fig. 12.13. The hypophysial artery (12) gives off branches supplying the capillaries of the primary portal plexus in the median eminence (13), and these pass into the portal veins (14), or capillaries in urodeles, which supply the elaborate system of the secondary plexus in the pars distalis (15). In addition, the hypophysial artery gives off a branch (19) which directly supplies the large capillaries of the plexus intermedius (6).

Some of the median eminence primary capillaries pass along the infundibular floor (18) and end in the plexus intermedius (6); the direction of flow in these vessels is not certain, but is presumed to be towards the neuro-intermedia, because if the pars distalis is removed, blood from the median eminence engorges the neuro-intermedia capillaries.

An extraordinary feature is the presence of a very well-developed second portal system, the *encephalo-neurohypophysial portal system* (fig. 12.13). The primary plexus of this system is spread widely in the mesencephalon (2, 3) and in the region of the hypothalamus close to the PON (1). It is supplied from the basilar (9) and retroinfundibular (10) arteries. Blood flows downwards, a point confirmed in living specimens, and is collected in one or two very large vessels (4) in the roof of the infundibular recess. These pass into the neural lobe, and branch to form the intrinsic capillaries of the lobe (5) and to supply the plexus intermedius (6). The latter receives blood from three sources: the median eminence (18), the hypophysial artery (19) and the encephalo-neurohypophysial portal system (4), the last being quantitatively by far the most important. From the plexus intermedius blood passes to the smaller capillaries at the periphery of the pars intermedia (7), and also some small vessels (direction of flow not known) pass to the dorso-caudal part of the pars distalis (8).

Blood drains from the neural lobe directly into the hypophysial vein (not shown in fig. 12.13), a direct route for conveying neurohypophysial octapeptides to the systemic circulation, and presumably of great importance to amphibians such as *Bufo* with water-conservation problems (see Jørgensen, Rosenkilde and Wingstrand, 1969). Separate vessels collect blood from the plexus intermedius and convey it to the hypophysial vein. Blood from the pars distalis passes into posterior collecting veins (16), and thence into the hypophysial veins, either directly or through the plexus of the endolymphatic sacs (17).

It should be emphasised that all the blood reaching the pars intermedia has first passed through the neural lobe (5) by way of the plexus intermedius (6), and may therefore contain neurohypophysial octapeptides in high concentrations. This is true also of fishes, reptiles and mammals. In addition to this 'neural lobe' blood, the intermedia also receives blood from the median eminence (18), directly from the general circulation (19) and from wide areas of the hypothalamus and mesencephalon (4). In sharp contrast, the pars distalis receives blood only from the median eminence (14), apart possibly from a small contribution posteriorly from the neuro-intermedia (8).

It would be interesting to know more about the functional significance of the anatomical features outlined in the preceding paragraph. The central position of the plexus intermedius is striking, and so is the fact that in amphibians such as bufonids, with marked regional localisation of cell-types in the pars distalis, it is the A2 cells which are most likely to be exposed to blood from the plexus intermedius (8).

There is little intrinsic vascularisation of the pars intermedia parenchyma, a common feature throughout the vertebrates (Wingstrand, 1966*b*), and in consequence MSH must be transported relatively long distances from the endocrine cells to the nearest capillaries. This contrasts with the richly vascularised pars distalis, where all the secretory cells are close to capillaries.

13

THE PITUITARY GLAND IN REPTILES

___

The class Reptilia occupies a central position in the evolution of the tetrapods, and there are reasons for thinking that certain living reptiles (*Sphenodon*, turtles) are closer than living amphibians to the ancestral tetrapods (fig. 12.1). Modern reptiles are fairly abundant in the tropics, but unimportant in the temperate-zone fauna. This distribution is related to their exothermic mode of temperature control, which necessitates hibernation in temperate zones and keeps them out of really cold areas entirely. The relatively few modern forms are in fact but sparse remnants of the great variety of reptiles which once dominated life on land, and which were also important elements in the marine and freshwater faunas.

In essence, the reptiles started their evolution as primitive amphibians which developed the cleidoic (closed) egg, and thereby eliminated the vulnerable aquatic larval stage. This major event is thought to have taken place in the Carboniferous, and by the end of that period the reptiles had already diversified in several directions. One line eventually was to lead to the mammals, and was already distinct from the main stock in the Carboniferous, and a later branch was to give rise to the birds. Meanwhile, the central reptile stock (the 'stem reptiles') radiated in several directions. An early offshoot, retaining perhaps some genuinely primitive features alongside its obvious specialisations, led to the turtles and tortoises (Chelonia). Another line gave rise first to the Rhynchocephalia, represented today by *Sphenodon* of New Zealand, then to the lizards (Lacertilia) and then to the snakes (Ophidia); a closely-related evolutionary line diverged to produce the dinosaurs and their living relatives the crocodiles and alligators (Crocodilia). The ancestors of the birds are thought to have been related to the dinosaurs, so that crocodilians are the nearest living relatives of the birds. In their rather isolated phylogenetic position, the chelonians are the closest living relatives of the mammals.

The reptilian pituitary has been somewhat neglected by cytologists and physiologists, but has had its fair share of attention from comparative anatomists. In general the gland resembles quite strongly the amphibian pituitary on the one hand and the avian pituitary on the other, a most gratifying state of affairs considering the phylogenetic position of the Reptilia.

[288]

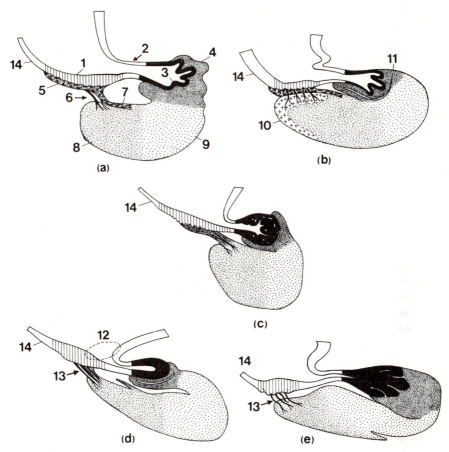

Fig. 13.1. Reptiles, general structure of the pituitary. Diagrammatic median sections of the pituitaries of (*a*) *Sphenodon*; (*b*) a chelonian (*Testudo*); (*c*) a crocodilian (*Alligator*); (*d*) a lizard (*Lacerta*); (*e*) a snake (*Python*). 1, Median eminence; 2, infundibular stem; 3, neural lobe; 4, pars intermedia; 5, juxta-neural pars tuberalis; 6, porto-tuberal tract with portal vessels; 7, pars tuberalis interna; 8, cephalic lobe of pars distalis; 9, caudal lobe of pars distalis; 10 (in *b*), 'zona tuberalis'; 11, hypophysial cavity; 12 (in *d*), the situation of the pars tuberalis plates in *Lacerta*; 13, pars terminalis (connective tissue + portal vessels); 14, pars oralis tuberis (infundibular floor anterior to median eminence). From Wingstrand (1966*a*).

GENERAL ANATOMY OF THE REPTILE PITUITARY

Wingstrand (1966*a*, *b*) has given a full description of the anatomy of the gland, and what follows is mainly based on his account, and on the work of Saint-Girons (1963, 1967, 1970). The most primitive condition is thought to be that in *Sphenodon*, turtles and crocodiles, with a well-developed pars intermedia and pars tuberalis, and a pars distalis fairly distinctly divided into cephalic (rostral) and caudal lobes as in birds. In the lizards the pars tuberalis is reduced or absent, and it is never developed in snakes. In lizards and snakes, the portal vessels pass from the median eminence to the pars distalis in connective tissue and, as in fishes, unaccompanied by any pars tuberalis tissue.

THE PITUITARY OF *Sphenodon* (ORDER RHYNCHOCEPHALIA)

In this primitive lizard-like creature, the tuatara of New Zealand, the pituitary gland is obviously like that of amphibians, but even more strikingly like that of lungfishes; it must be remembered that reptiles, as well as amphibians, were immediate descendants of the osteolepids (crossopterygians) which also gave rise to the lungfishes (chapter 11). The ventral ovoid *pars distalis* is divided histologically into cephalic and caudal lobes (fig. 13.1*a*). It links posteriorly with the pars intermedia, and its anterior region is separated from the infundibular floor by a wide cleft traversed by the median *pars tuberalis* with its associated portal vessels, forming a porto-tuberal tract as in birds (chapter 14). The anterior part of the pars tuberalis is attached to the ventral surface of the median eminence, but it does not invade the eminentia tissue as it does in lizards. Although the adult pars tuberalis is median, it has paired lateral origins in the embryo. The embryonic hypophysial cleft disappears in the adult, and the *pars intermedia* is applied broadly to the caudal pars distalis (fig. 13.1*a*) and consists of a few layers of cells which penetrate into the neural lobe. The *neural lobe*, at the end of a distinct infundibular stem, consists simply of three or four hollow thin-walled lobules on each side, the anlage being bifurcate as usual. The walls of the lobules include an ependymal layer, a fibrous layer and a palisade layer, and contain no pituicytes. The *median eminence* is thin, and has a peculiar structure that is described later (p. 313).

THE PITUITARY OF TURTLES AND TORTOISES (ORDER CHELONIA)

The adenohypophysis is more closely applied to the infundibular floor than in *Sphenodon* (fig. 13.1*b*). The *pars distalis* is only indistinctly divided into cephalic and caudal lobes, and it displays a typically reptilian feature in that posteriorly it has a pronounced dorsal inflection to connect with the pars intermedia (fig. 13.1*b*). Colloid-filled vesicles are said to be common in the chelonian pars distalis, sometimes so large as to give the region a thyroid-like appearance (cf. the potto, chapter 2). The pars tuberalis is usually large and forms a thick layer on the median eminence, linked with the pars distalis by a short porto-tuberal tract;

the portal vessels enter the pars distalis at its rostral tip, where a zona tuberalis is developed, but the pars tuberalis itself attaches more posteriorly to the dorsal surface of the distalis (fig. 13.1*b*). The *pars intermedia* is massive laterally, but medially often consists of only a few layers of cells which penetrate between the lobules of the neural lobe; in *Chelone*, however, a thick cover of intermedia cords and cell plates surrounds the entire neural lobe. The hypophysial cleft persists in some chelonians, with intermedia cells in its ventral as well as its dorsal wall, but in some species it is obliterated. The *neural lobe* is developed at the end of a short (occasionally long) infundibular stem, and has a simple structure, so like that of *Sphenodon* that this may be regarded as the primitive reptile condition. The neural lobe wall has an ependymal layer, a fibrous layer, and an outer palisade layer containing abundant NSM but few or no free glial cells. The wall may be pushed out into a pair of slightly wrinkled sacs, or it may form many separate hollow lobules. The hollow lobulated structure of the neural lobe in so many reptiles contrasts with the solid structure in most amphibians and in birds and mammals, but resembles the hollow neural lobe of many fishes (chapters 9, 11). The *median eminence*, restricted to a small area of the anterior infundibular floor, may be simple or complex, with abundant NSM not only in the deep fibrous layer but also in the superficial palisade layer.

THE PITUITARY OF CROCODILES AND ALLIGATORS (ORDER CROCODILIA OR LORICATA)

Here, the gland is relatively shorter and deeper than in other reptiles (fig. 13.1*c*). The *pars distalis* is sharply divided into cephalic and caudal lobes, as in the avian relatives of these reptiles. The *pars tuberalis* attaches to the median eminence as a thin paired juxta-neural plate, with a portal zone joining to the pars distalis (fig. 13.1*c*). The well-developed *pars intermedia* surrounds the neural lobe and penetrates between its lobules, and the hypophysial cleft is present only in young animals. The *neural lobe*, borne on a long infundibular stem, is deeply folded with small hollow lobules, but its dorsal part may form a single large sac. The walls of the lobules are thick, with many pituicytes, but capillaries are restricted to the septum adjoining the pars intermedia (the plexus intermedius, cf. fishes). The *median eminence*, restricted to the anterior infundibular floor, is very thick and contains many pituicytes, and the primary portal capillaries are deeply folded into its ventral surface.

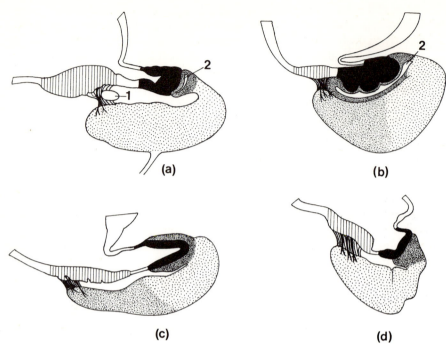

Fig. 13.2. Different types of lizard pituitaries. Diagrammatic median sections of the pituitaries of (*a*) *Uta stansburiana*; (*b*) *Varanus niloticus*; (*c*) *Agama* sp.; (*d*) *Chamaeleo gracilis*. For explanation, see fig. 13.1. In addition, 1, remnants of pars tuberalis; 2, hypophysial cleft. From Wingstrand (1966*a*).

THE PITUITARY OF LIZARDS (ORDER SQUAMATA, SUB-ORDER LACERTILIA OR SAURIA)

Lizards display great variations in many aspects of their biology, and it is not surprising that the pituitary gland varies considerably in its anatomy; the range is illustrated in fig. 13.1*d* and fig. 13.2. The gland is usually symmetrical, but a slight asymmetry is seen in *Varanus exanthematicus*, in which the pars intermedia is much thicker on the right side (Nouhouayi-Besnard, 1966), and in *Xantusia* the gland is strongly asymmetrical, like that of snakes (Miller, 1948).

The *pars distalis* is separated anteriorly from the infundibular floor and median eminence by a cleft filled with connective tissue. The size of the cleft varies greatly (fig. 13.2). Posteriorly the dorsal inflection of the pars distalis to meet the pars intermedia is usually very marked. Since the portal part of the pars tuberalis is always missing, the portal vessels run across the cleft embedded only in connective tissue. The pars distalis is clearly divided into cephalic and caudal lobes, often by a slight constriction; ventrally, an epithelial stalk may persist as a remnant of the stalk of Rathke's pouch (fig. 13.2*a*). The *pars tuberalis* develops in the embryo as typical lateral lobes of the hollow Rathke's pouch, which grow forward and contact the median eminence while still attached to the pars distalis. The portal region disappears later, so that in the adult the pars tuberalis is separated into two structures, the juxta-neural tuberalis plates on the floor of the infundibulum, and the pars tuberalis interna, a pair of processes on the cephalic pars distalis. The juxta-neural pars tuberalis forms a pair of cellular plaques on either side of the median eminence, and they usually undergo a remarkable change in the adult, the basement membrane and pia above them disappearing and the tuberalis cells invading the hypothalamic and median eminence tissues to a greater or lesser degree.

The *pars intermedia* as usual surrounds the neural lobe to a varying extent, as an enclosing cup. It varies greatly in size, being only one or a few cell layers in some lizards (e.g. geckos, *Lacerta*, *Anguis*, *Xantusia*), but forming a massive glandular structure in others (fig. 13.2). It is atrophied in blind burrowing lizards, amphisbaenids and trogonophids. The intermedia is particularly large in iguanids, such as *Anolis*, which have a marked capacity for adaptive colour change controlled by MSH. The hypophysial cleft may or may not be present in the adult, and if present intermedia cells may lie in both dorsal and ventral walls of the cleft, as in chelonians. In *Varanus niloticus*, the large cleft sends diverticuli into the caudal pars distalis, as well as into the pars intermedia, an unusual arrangement recalling that in sturgeons (Nouhouayi-Besnard, 1966).

The *neural lobe* is carried on the end of an infundibular stem which may be short or long (fig. 13.2). It varies from a thin-walled and folded sac to a compact lobulated structure, with only a small lumen and with thick-walled lobules projecting into the pars intermedia. The lacertids (fig. 13.1*d*) have few lobules, often only the original pair of primary branches of the saccus infundibuli, which give rise to the large neural lobe of the adult simply by thickening their walls. The neural lobe is never completely solid, however large, but always contains at least short extensions of the infundibular recess.

The *median eminence* is anterior and discrete, and in smaller lizards may be very thin, with few pituicytes and a smooth ventral surface, but in larger species it is thickened with many pituicytes and with the portal capillaries buried in deep furrows on its ventral surface.

THE PITUITARY OF SNAKES (ORDER SQUAMATA, SUB-ORDER OPHIDIA OR SERPENTES)

Snakes evolved from blind burrowing lizards, perhaps rather like the modern amphisbaenians, but as a group they are not given to burrowing though some primitive snakes (*Typhlops*, *Leptotyphlops*) are blind and burrow like their ancestors. The ophidian pituitary is very like that of lizards, but with certain special features (pronounced dorso-ventral flattening, strong left/right asymmetry) typical of snake anatomy as a whole. The embryonic gland is strictly symmetrical, asymmetry developing just before hatching. In certain primitive snakes, the pituitary in the adult remains symmetrical (*Typhlops*, *Leptotyphlops*), or nearly so (*Python*) and it is symmetrical in the viperid *Bitis* (Wingstrand, 1966a; Saint-Girons, 1967), but in most snakes the pars distalis lies to one side and the neuro-intermedia to the other. The direction of asymmetry is not fixed, since in any one species both 'left-handed' and 'right-handed' glands are found (Wingstrand, 1966a). The entire pituitary being strongly flattened, the caudal end of the asymmetrical pars distalis arches over to the opposite side to fuse with the posterior end of the pars intermedia (fig. 13.3). The pars distalis, though placed to one side, tends to extend rather further ventrally than the neuro-intermedia (fig. 13.3).

The *pars distalis* is clearly divided into cephalic and caudal lobes, the former with a concentration of strongly carminophilic A1 cells. The *pars tuberalis* is completely absent in the adult, and Rathke's pouch produces only traces of lateral lobes in the embryo. The portal vessels pass from the median eminence to the pars distalis (obliquely in asymmetrical glands) embedded in connective tissue (figs. 13.1e, 13.3).

The *pars intermedia* is missing in the burrowing *Typhlops* and *Leptotyphlops*. In these, as in the burrowing lizards with an atrophied pars intermedia, no intermedia cells have been described in the pars distalis, in contrast to the birds and some mammals without a discrete pars intermedia (Saint-Girons, 1963, 1967). In most snakes the pars intermedia is massive, and forms a thick cup around the posterior end of the neural lobe. The *neural lobe* lies at the end of a long infundibular stem, asymmetrical in most snakes (fig. 13.3), and it is always compact with lobules extending into the pars intermedia (fig. 13.1e). The lobules are often solid, with connective tissue septa and numerous pituicytes. The infundibular recess always extends to the base of the neural lobe, but has few and narrow diverticuli into the neural tissue (often only two, corresponding to the paired primary branches of the saccus infundibuli), so that the neural lobe is largely a solid organ. The *median eminence* occupies the anterior infundibular floor, and may be slightly shifted towards the side on which the pars distalis lies. It is always thickened, with portal capillaries deeply embedded in its surface and with numerous free glial cells.

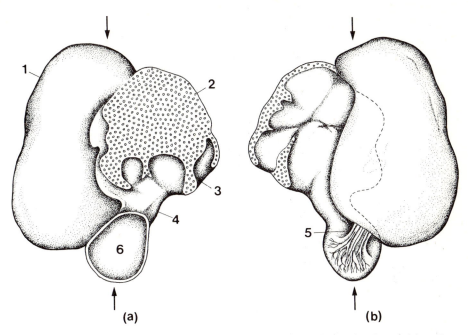

Fig. 13.3. The pituitary of the snake *Vipera berus* seen from the dorsal (*a*) and ventral (*b*) side to show the strong asymmetry. The arrows indicate the median plane. 1, pars distalis; 2, pars intermedia; 3, neural lobe; 4, infundibular stem; 5, pars terminalis (connective tissue and portal vessels); 6, median eminence. From Wingstrand (1966*a*).

The hypophysial cleft is usually obliterated in adult snakes, but persists in the symmetrical gland of *Bitis* (Viperidae), and also in the asymmetrical pituitary of another viperid, *Vipera aspis* (Wingstrand, 1966*a*; Saint-Girons, 1967).

HISTOPHYSIOLOGY OF THE PARS DISTALIS

Many workers have studied the reptile pituitary, some attempting to allocate functions to the different cell-types. Earlier work was reviewed by Saint-Girons (1963) and Grignon (1963). More recently, Saint-Girons (1967, 1970) has given detailed accounts of pituitary structure and histology, Eyeson (1970) has reported experimental studies of the gland in the lizard *Agama*, and an extensive series of investigations by Paul Licht and his collaborators, mainly on the lizard *Anolis carolinensis*, has greatly extended knowledge of the functions of the various cell-types in the pars distalis.

As usual in tetrapods, the pars distalis consists of irregular branching cords of endocrine cells, always narrow and often only two cells thick, interspersed with plentiful capillary vessels which are usually described as sinusoidal (Poris and Charipper, 1938; Saint-Girons, 1967, 1970). In chelonians the cells are often arranged in pseudo-acini (Saint-Girons, 1963, 1970), sometimes containing colloid and resulting in a thyroid-like structure of the entire pars distalis (Wingstrand, 1966a). The division of the pars distalis into cephalic and caudal lobes is usually well-marked, often by a transverse constriction in addition to a differential distribution of cell-types (Saint-Girons, 1967, 1970; Grignon, 1963; Forbes, 1971). This division almost certainly corresponds to that seen in birds (Wingstrand, 1966a). The cephalic lobe (geckonids) or the caudal lobe (some snakes) may be the larger (Saint-Girons, 1967).

Five chromophilic cell-types can be identified in the pars distalis, and in their tinctorial properties these are remarkably similar to the cells of the amphibian pars distalis. For this reason, it is possible to use the same alphabetical nomenclature for the cell-types as in amphibians, given that it is usually possible from the original accounts to assimilate the descriptions to this system. Apart from chromophils, chromophobic cells occur in varying proportions, from rare (e.g. anguid lizards) to abundant (e.g. lacertid and iguanid lizards) (Saint-Girons, 1967, 1970).

ACIDOPHILS TYPE 1

These A1 cells correspond to the X cells of Saint-Girons. They have been described in most detailed accounts as large carminophilic cells, located mainly along capillaries in the cephalic lobe (fig. 13.4). They may be numerous or scarce, well-granulated or sparsely-granulated, depending on species and physiological state. In *Sphenodon* and some lacertids, they tend to be organised in pseudo-follicles (Saint-Girons, 1963, 1965, 1967). The A1 granules are sometimes fine (*Sphenodon*, *Xantusia*, *Agama*), but more usually coarse (Miller, 1948; Saint-Girons, 1965, 1967, 1970; Grignon, 1963; Eyeson, 1970). Like granule-size, the degree of carminophilia seems to vary in different reptiles but is usually strong (Saint-Girons, 1963, 1967; Wingstrand, 1966a; Licht and Nicoll, 1969; Eyeson, 1970). With their rostro-medial distribution, the A1 cells are usually easily distinguished from the caudally-concentrated A2 cells, even when the two have similar staining properties (Saint-Girons, 1967; Licht and Nicoll, 1969). Although only weakly carminophilic in *Agama*, the A1 cells in this lizard are strongly erythrosinophilic, and stain with both Luxol fast blue and OG, appearing yellow or pale green with the combined stains (Eyeson, 1970). In *Anolis* they are strongly carminophilic and azofuchsinophilic (Licht and Nicoll, 1969). They are totally (Eyeson, 1970) or virtually (Saint-Girons, 1965, 1967, 1970) PAS−, and are also negative to AF and AB (Saint-Girons, 1970; Eyeson, 1970). A1 cells are more strongly PAS+ in Chamaelidae than in any other reptiles, and

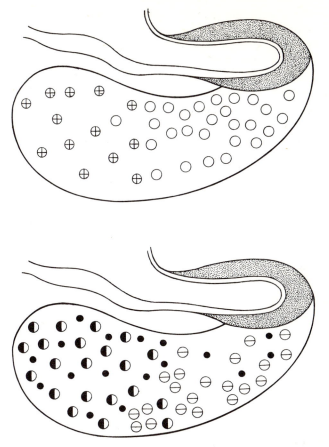

Fig. 13.4. *Agama agama.* Diagrammatic mid-sagittal sections of the pituitary to show the distribution of pars distalis cell-types. Anterior to left. Top diagram: crossed circles, acidophils 1; open circles, acidophils 2. Bottom diagram: circles with horizontal lines, basophils 1; solid circles, basophils 2; half-shaded circles, basophils 3. From Eyeson (1970).

amongst snakes they are notably small and nearly chromophobic in the Viperidae (Saint-Girons, 1963, 1967). Turtles may have poorly-granulated A1 cells, only weakly carminophilic (Licht and Nicoll, 1969), and in chelonians more than in other reptiles these cells may hypertrophy and degranulate totally, though for what reason is not known (Saint-Girons, 1963). Amongst snakes, the A1 cells seem to extend unusually far caudally in *Thamnophis* (see Licht and Nicoll, 1969).

Because of their restricted distribution in most reptiles, it has been possible to allocate function to the A1 cells. By bioassay of cephalic and caudal fragments of the pituitary of a turtle (*Pseudemys*), lizards (*Anolis*, *Dipsosaurus*) and snakes (*Thamnophis*, *Pituophis*), LTH was located in the cephalic lobe (Licht and Nicoll, 1969). With the subsequent allocation of functions to the other cell-types, it was possible to identify the A1 cells as lactotropes (see Licht and Rosenberg, 1969). In *Anolis*, a different bioassay also showed LTH to be located in the anterior cephalic lobe (Sage and Bern, 1972). In its rostral location, the reptile lactotrope recalls the homologous cell-type of fishes, amphibians and birds; in its staining properties it closely resembles the LTH cells in most other vertebrates. Eyeson (1970), however, reported that a weak LTH reaction could be obtained from the caudal lobe of *Agama*, and not from the cephalic lobe, an anomalous finding that requires further investigations.

The LTH cells are highly active and numerous during egg-laying in the tortoise *Testudo* (see Grignon, 1963). They show no changes during the reproductive cycle in either male or female *Agama*, nor any responses to steroid hormones, thyroidectomy, thyroxine and metopirone (Eyeson, 1970).

ACIDOPHILS TYPE 2

The A2 cells are concentrated in the caudal pars distalis (fig. 13.4), and they correspond to the α cells, or classical acidophils of earlier workers (Saint-Girons, 1963; Grignon, 1963). They are often large cells, as in *Agama* and vipers, where they border the dilated capillaries of the caudal pars distalis (Eyeson, 1970; Saint-Girons, 1967) but they may be very small, as in lacertids and many snakes (Saint-Girons, 1967). The granules of the A2 cells are coarser than those of the A1 cells in *Agama* and *Xantusia* (Eyeson, 1970; Miller, 1948), but in many reptiles the A2 granules are the finer (Saint-Girons, 1967, 1970). These cells are usually abundant in the caudal lobe, but their numbers and size vary a great deal with species. Amongst snakes, they are especially abundant and large in Viperidae (Saint-Girons, 1967). Apparently they never show signs of involution, but in the resting stage they are densely packed with granules and when very active become partially degranulated and vacuolated (Saint-Girons, 1963). Commonly the caudal tip of the pars distalis contains a mass of degranulated A2 cells, in many lizards and snakes and in *Sphenodon* (Saint-Girons, 1963, 1965, 1967).

A2 cells take OG rather than erythrosin after Aliz BT, that is they are the orangeophil as opposed to the cephalic erythrosinophil in *Agama* (Eyeson, 1970) and in most reptiles (Saint-Girons, 1963, 1970; Licht and Nicoll, 1969). However, in *Agama* and *Xantusia* they are intensely carminophilic (Eyeson, 1970; Miller, 1948), a rare example of failure of erythrosinophilia and carminophilia to go together. Typical acidophils, they are totally negative to PAS, AF and AB (Eyeson, 1970; Saint-Girons, 1967, 1970). The EM shows the A2 cells of *Lacerta sicula* to contain uniformly rounded granules, 310 nm in diameter and intensely electron-opaque, polarised with the granules concentrated close to a capillary and the Golgi complex near the nucleus (Della Corte, Galgano and Angelini, 1968).

Concerning the function of the A2 cells, Licht and Nicoll (1969) found by disc electrophoresis that while LTH occurred mainly in the cephalic lobe of the turtle *Pseudemys*, the putative STH (later confirmed as STH by bioassay; Licht and Nicoll, 1971) was associated with the caudal lobe, thus pointing to the A2 cells as somatotropes. A purified STH, active in the rat tibia assay, has recently been isolated from turtle pituitary glands (Papkoff and Hayashida, 1972).

The A2 cells tend to enlarge and slightly degranulate during the early stages of vitellogenesis, and to reduce their activity during late vitellogenesis and in sexual inactivity in female *Agama*. In the male, they are regressed and tend towards chromophobia during June to December, presumably the non-breeding period (Eyeson, 1970). There is some correlation between the activity of these cells and interrenal activity in female *Agama*, but none in the male (Eyeson, 1970), and an approximate correlation exists between the A2 cells and interrenal activity in the viper *Vipera* (see Grignon, 1963).

BASOPHILS TYPE 1

The B1 cells (the δ cells of Saint-Girons, 1963) are generally scattered throughout the pars distalis, but show some tendency to concentrate in the caudal lobe, as in *Agama* (fig. 13.4), anguid and helodermatid lizards (Saint-Girons, 1963, 1967; Eyeson, 1970), and *Anolis* (Licht and Rosenberg, 1969). They are generally small cells, though large in some lizards and snakes (Saint-Girons, 1967), and though usually spherical as in *Agama* (Eyeson, 1970) they may be elongated in many snakes, and in anguids and helodermatids they often form a palisade layer around the extremely wide capillary spaces of the caudal lobe (Saint-Girons, 1967). The secretory granules are usually coarse, and strongly PAS +, AF +, AB + and aniline blue +, although in varanid lizards they are unusual in being AF − and AB −. Commonly, and very noticeably in some snakes, the B1 cells contain some larger bodies (lyosomes?) which are erythrosinophilic, OG +, strongly PAS + but AB − (Saint-Girons, 1967; Eyeson, 1970; Forbes, 1971); the secretory granules are moderately PbH + in *Agama* (Eyeson, 1970).

In male *Agama*, the activity of the B1 cells is related to thyroid activity, which varies during the year, and at their most active they degranulate and vacuolate (Eyeson, 1970); they react strongly to thyroidectomy in this lizard, becoming enlarged, vacuolated and degranulated and almost chromophobic, a condition reminiscent of the amphibian thyroidectomy cell (chapter 12). The A2 cells of *Agama* also react slightly, becoming enlarged 35 days after thyroidectomy but later decreasing in size. Thyroxine injections result in regression of the B1 cells, and a simultaneous regression of the A2 cells (Eyeson, 1970). Thyroidectomy also selectively activates the B1 cells of the tortoise *Testudo*, which become regressed after thyroxine or TSH injections (see Grignon, 1963). Thus the B1 cells appear to be thyrotropes, and this identification has been confirmed by partial hypophysectomy and bioassay of cephalic and caudal lobes in *Anolis*. These experiments located TSH in the caudal lobe, in which the B1 cells are concentrated in this lizard (Licht and Rosenberg, 1969). Oestrogen injections caused vacuolation of the B1 cells of *Anolis*, associated with a marked increase in thyroidal activity (Poris, 1941).

With the EM, the B1 cells of *Anolis* are seen to contain ovoid secretory granules, 300–400 nm long and 200–250 nm wide, containing glycoprotein. They show seasonal changes, being inactive during autumn and winter, packed with granules and with little RER and a small Golgi complex; at this time the thyroid gland is also inactive. In spring and summer, the B1 cells enlarge and degranulate, the RER often becoming dilated with electron-dense material, and the thyroid is now active (Forbes, 1971). After thyroidectomy the B1 cells transform into typical enlarged degranulated thyroidectomy cells, with a hypertrophied Golgi complex and dilated RER; eventually the cells are filled by anastomosing RER cisternae packed with PAS+ and AF+ material (Forbes, 1971), these cisternae obviously corresponding to the vacuoles in the active B1 cells of *Agama* (Eyeson, 1970). In *Anolis*, stellate cells are often closely associated with thyroidectomy cells, and may perform some function in the transport of material between the thyroidectomy cell and blood vessels (Forbes, 1971). Putative B1 cells in *Lacerta sicula* contain extremely polymorphous secretory granules, some rounded and very electron-dense (diameter 180–250 nm), others quadrangular or rhomboidal, larger and less electron-dense. After castration, these cells become degranulated, with dilation of the RER (Della Corte, Galgano and Angelini, 1968).

BASOPHILS TYPE 2

These cells, the β cells of Saint-Girons (1963), are generally scattered throughout the gland, fairly evenly in many reptiles (e.g. *Anolis*, *Sphenodon*, many lizards, Boidae amongst the snakes), but concentrated medioventrally in most snakes and some lizards (Iguanidae, Lacertidae, Varanidae) and concentrated in the cephalic lobe in many lizards, including the Agamidae (fig. 13.4; Saint-Girons, 1967; Eyeson, 1970). In chelonians the B1 and B2 cells tend to form a shell around the anterior cephalic lobe (Saint-Girons, 1963). They rarely form homogeneous cords, but are usually scattered among other cell-types (Saint-Girons, 1967). Their secretory granules are usually fine, but are very coarse in the anguid and varanid lizards (Saint-Girons, 1967). The size of the B2 cells varies greatly; they are for example the smallest basophil in *Agama*, and are very small in lacertids, but they are moderately large in most reptiles, and very large in vipers and rattlesnakes (Viperidae, Crotulidae); no doubt their size varies with activity, and even in *Agama* they can become fairly big cells (Saint-Girons, 1967; Eyeson, 1970). In the blind burrowing snake *Typhlops* the B2 cells show spectacular development, with enormous vacuoles and signs of intense activity not encountered in other reptiles (Saint-Girons, 1963, 1970).

The secretory granules of the B2 cells have typical basophil staining properties, PAS+, AF+, AB+, aniline blue+ to various degrees in different species (Saint-Girons, 1963, 1967, 1970; Eyeson, 1970). In *Agama*, they are only slightly PbH+, in contrast to the B1 and B3 cells. In addition to the secretory granules, in *Agama* there occur larger granules, strongly OG+ (Eyeson, 1970); these bodies are present in many reptiles, and are generally erythrosinophilic, strongly PAS+, but only weakly AF+ and AB+, so that after the combined stain PAS–AB they appear red against the blue secretory granules (Saint-Girons, 1963, 1967). These larger granules undoubtedly correspond to the lyosomal R granules of other vertebrates. In *Lacerta sicula* B2 cells have been called type 3 cells, and occur mainly in the cephalic lobe, with small electron-dense granules (150–270 nm in diameter) and enormous globules, 600–800 nm in diameter, of varying shapes and less electron-dense than the secretory granules (Della Corte, Galgano and Angelini, 1968).

All workers agree that the B2 cells are gonadotropes. They usually exhibit marked alterations in structure with activity, varying from a 'storage phase', with many secretory granules and an involuted nucleus, to an 'active phase', showing degranulation, marked vacuolation and large rounded nuclei (Saint-Girons, 1963, 1967). These obvious changes have facilitated the correlation of B2 cell activity with the gonadal cycle, particularly in the male where the correlation with spermatogenesis is especially close; in the female, correlation with vitellogenesis is generally less obvious (Grignon, 1963). On the basis of studies of annual sexual cycles, the B2 cells have been regarded as secreting an FSH-like gonado-tropin. An LH-like gonadotropin has been supposed to originate in the B3 cells, which often display a seasonal cycle correlated with testicular Leydig cell activity in the male, and with the post-ovulatory period in the female (Grignon, 1963; Saint-Girons, 1963, 1967). In *Agama*, for example, B2 cell activity correlates closely with earlier vitellogenesis, while B3 cell activity correlates approximately with later vitellogenesis, during which the cells enlarge and slowly degranulate (Eyeson, 1970).

It now seems likely that in fact the reptile pituitary secretes only one gonadotropin, with both FSH-like and LH-like properties (Licht and Pearson, 1969; Licht and Rosenberg, 1969; Licht, 1970; Licht and Hartree, 1971; Reddy and Prasad, 1970). From experiments in which mammalian or avian FSH and LH were administered to reptiles, this single reptilian gonadotropin appears to resemble FSH rather than LH (Reddy and Prasad, 1970; Licht, 1970), and indeed all the gonadotropic activity measurable in tests on *Anolis* appeared to reside in the β-subunit of ovine FSH (Licht and Papkoff, 1971). Unexpectedly, however, purified turtle (*Pseudemys*) gonadotropin resembles mammalian LH in its biochemical properties but FSH in its biological effects on *Anolis*; furthermore, the turtle hormone had no LH-like actions when tested in mammalian assays (Papkoff and Licht, 1972). Thus a single glycoprotein, biologically resembling mammalian FSH but perhaps chemically more like mammalian LH, may be the only gonadotropin in reptiles, in line with the evidence for teleosts (chapter 10) and amphibians (chapter 12). This being so, it seems that the B2 cell is the only gonadotrope in the reptile pituitary, the B3 cell having some other function (below). In support of this interpretation is the fact that bioassays (using hypophysectomised *Anolis*) of cephalic and caudal lobe of *Anolis* pituitary showed that both FSH-like and LH-like activity occurs throughout the gland, in correspondence to the distribution of the B2 cell in this lizard. There is no evidence of preferential location of LH-like activity in the cephalic lobe, such as would occur if the B3 cells were LH-gonadotropes. Partial hypophysectomy experiments yielded concordant results (Licht and Rosenberg, 1969). Thus the B2 cell, as the only uniformly distributed basophil in *Anolis*, is confirmed as the source of a gonadotropin with both FSH- and LH-like biological properties.

Castration experiments produce predictable changes in the B2 cells, which become enlarged, active, vacuolated and degranulated (Grignon, 1963; Eyeson, 1970). Treatment with testosterone or mammalian gonadotropin caused regression of these cells in *Agama* (Eyeson, 1970), and oestrogens had the same effect in the tortoise *Testudo* (Grignon, 1963). Castration of the lizard *Lacerta sicula* caused an increase in the numbers of poorly granulated cells in the pars distalis, some derived from B1, some from B2 cells; the undoubted B2 cells showed dilation of RER cisternae and loss of secretory granules (Della Corte, Galgano and Angelini, 1968).

BASOPHILS TYPE 3

Like their amphibian counterpart, the B3 cells of reptiles are really amphiphils, and as in amphibians they stain violet or purple with Azan, trichrome or Aliz BT (Saint-Girons, 1963, 1967, 1970; Eyeson, 1970). These are usually large, prismatic or pear-shaped cells, nearly always arranged in palisade along the capillaries of the cephalic lobe, though exceptionally they are scattered in the cephalic lobe of geckonid lizards. In all reptiles they show this restricted cephalic distribution, though they may be rare in geckonid, agamid, iguanid, lacertid and varanid lizards. Only a few intrusive B3 cells may occasionally be found in the caudal lobe (Saint-Girons, 1963, 1967; Eyeson, 1970; fig. 13.4). The nucleus is basal, distal to the capillary pole of the cell. B3 secretory granules vary in size (Saint-Girons, 1967), but they are notably coarse in some lizards (agamids, varanids), and snakes (typhlopids, boids); in colubrid snakes, the granules are coarse, and the B3 cells are unusually numerous (Saint-Girons, 1963, 1967; Eyeson, 1970). As amphiphils, the staining reactions of the B3 cells vary a great deal. They are only weakly PAS+ and AF+ in *Agama* and iguanids, and are usually AB−, though strongly AB+ in many snakes. Alone among the cell-types of *Agama*, they stain with iron haematoxylin and have a very strong affinity for PbH (Eyeson, 1970), and in nearly all reptiles they stain with iron haematoxylin (Saint-Girons, 1963, 1967). *Agama* B3 cells also stain strongly with azocarmine, and weakly with Luxol fast blue and OG (Eyeson, 1970). Their affinity for PAS is strong in many lizards, snakes and crocodiles, weak in many lizards and some snakes, and in varanid lizards they are PAS−. After Azan, they are red (carminophilic) in crocodiles and most snakes, but violet (azocarmine + aniline blue) in most reptiles, including vipers and rattlesnakes, and cyanophilic (aniline blue only) in varanids, trogonophid lizards and leptotyphlid snakes (Saint-Girons, 1963, 1967). The B3 cells are unusual in the lizard *Cnemidophorus* (family Teidae), in being chromophobic, PAS−, OG−, erythrosin−, and only faintly iron haematoxylin+; however, when activated, these cells contain large, sparse granules, OG+, and haematoxylin+, but PAS−: they have the typical rostral location, and are morphologically and tinctorially distinct from the neighbouring A1 cells (Del Conte, 1969).

The B3 cells are said by Saint-Girons (1963) to be the most variable in the pars distalis, displaying strong variations in the annual cycle and often showing spectacular hypertrophy and hyperplasia, frequently accompanied by degranulation. Certain changes in these cells, related in time to changes in the gonads, led earlier workers to identify them as LH-gonadotropes (Grignon, 1963; Saint-Girons, 1963), a matter already discussed in connection with the B2 cells. It now seems that the B3 cells are in fact corticotropes. They are strongly activated in *Cnemidophorus* by metopirone, an inhibitor of the synthesis of adrenocorticosteroids (Del Conte, 1969), and assay of ACTH activity in dissected pars distalis of *Anolis* and *Dipsosaurus* (lizards), a turtle (*Pseudemys*) and a crocodile (*Caiman*) showed ACTH to be restricted to the cephalic lobe. Since only A1 and B3 cells are distributed preferentially in the cephalic lobe, and since the former are lactotropes, this work identified the B3 cells as corticotropes, an identification confirmed by the effects of partial hypophysectomy on the levels of circulating corticosterone in *Anolis* (Licht and Bradshaw, 1969).

Certain earlier observations can now be seen as related to the cortico-tropic function of the B3 cells. They degranulate after castration in *Agama*, and degranulate after testosterone or oestrogen treatment (Eyeson, 1970), all possibly stress responses, or collateral reactions to alteration in blood levels of gonadal steroids. The rough correlation between the annual cycle in these cells and the gonadal cycle, which led workers to identify them as LH cells, might well prove on investigation to relate to seasonal changes in adrenocortical activity, in parallel to the gonadal cycle as in amphibians (chapter 12).

STELLATE CELLS

Chromophobic cells, usually with fine projections between the endocrine cells, are widespread in the vertebrate adenohypophysis (see Vila-Porcile, 1972). They have been described in an EM investigation on the pars distalis of *Anolis* (Forbes, 1972*b*). They are agranular, and possess numerous elongated processes passing between endocrine cells, and they are occasionally linked to each other or to endocrine cells by desmosomes. Their processes approach capillaries, and frequently expand as end-foot processes along the pericapillary membrane, often interposing between the endocrine cells and the pericapillary space. Stellate cells are common in the caudal lobe of *Anolis*, less common in the cephalic lobe (Forbes, 1972*b*). After chemical or surgical thyroidectomy the TSH cells in the caudal lobe were converted into thyroidectomy cells (see above, B1 cells); at the same time, the stellate cells in this region hypertrophied, developing more desmosome contacts with each other and with thyroidectomy cells, and also displaying increased numbers of micropinocytotic vesicles on their end-foot processes against the pericapillary spaces. Injected horse-radish peroxidase was shown to penetrate the intercellular spaces, enter the micropinocytotic vesicles and pass to the interior of the stellate cells. The evidence led Forbes (1972*b*) to suggest that the stellate cells may act as a transport system, conveying material (probably protein) from the blood into the thyroidectomy cells; he did not think it likely that TSH passes out of the thyroidectomy cells by way of the stellate cells, because he could detect no glycoprotein in them. Stellate cells presumably occur in all reptile pituitaries, and have been illustrated in the pars distalis of another lizard, *Lacerta sicula* (Della Corte, Galgano and Angelini, 1968).

HYPOTHALAMIC CONTROL OF PARS DISTALIS FUNCTIONS

Very little is known about the anatomy of the reptilian hypothalamus that relates to hypothalamic control of the adenohypophysis, and very little experimental work has been done to demonstrate the existence of hypothalamic controlling mechanisms. The hypothalamic AF + neuro-secretory system is different from that in lower vertebrates, but resembles that in birds and mammals, in that the original PON has become divided into separate supraoptic and paraventricular nuclei. The median eminence receives AF + fibres, presumably from these nuclei (Dodd, Follett and Sharp, 1971). The *infundibular nucleus* is probably involved in hypo-physiotropic functions, and is considered as homologous with the arcuate nucleus in the hypophysiotropic area of mammals. It lies in the floor of the third ventricle, close to the median eminence, and has recently been studied in lizards and turtles (Vigh-Teichmann and Vigh, 1970). The neurons in the infundibular nucleus have processes projecting into the third ventricle, which are linked by desmosome-like contacts with ependymal cells. Axons from the nucleus run to the median eminence palisade layer and to the pars tuberalis, and all regions of the cells display a strong acetylcholinesterase reaction, suggestive of a cholinergic function. The area of the infundibular nucleus is hypophysiotropic in birds (Dodd, Follett and Sharp, 1971).

Lactotropin (LTH) was secreted by the explanted pituitary of the turtle (*Malaclemys terrapin*) during ten days' incubation, which suggests considerable autonomy on the part of the lactotropes (Bern and Nicoll, 1968). However, more recent data indicate a hypothalamic stimulating influence on LTH secretion in another turtle (*Pseudemys*) and it is possible that both stimulatory and inhibitory factors may be secreted by the hypothalamus (Nicoll and Fiorindo, 1969).

TSH control has received little attention. Seasonal changes in the thyroid and TSH cells have often been reported for reptiles, and these could hardly be explained without assuming some hypothalamic media-tion. The only relevant experimental work has shown that hypothalamic lesions, whether involving the median eminence, antero-medial, posterior or lateral areas, caused a significant *increase* in thyroid weight after seven days in the lizard *Sceloporus cyanogenys* (Callard and Chester Jones, 1970), suggestive of a primarily inhibitory hypothalamic influence on TSH secretion.

That *gonadotropin secretion* is controlled by the hypothalamus is strongly suggested by data showing that temperature and photoperiod interact in complex ways to control seasonal cycles of gonadal activity in many reptiles (see Dodd, Follett and Sharp, 1971). The fact that none of the hypothalamic lesions placed in *Sceloporus* had any effect on testis weight after seven days (Callard and Chester Jones, 1970) does not contradict this evidence, since hypophysectomy did not alter testis weight during the same period, indicating that under the conditions of these experiments seven days is too short a time for the testis to show weight changes in response to alterations in blood gonadotropin levels. However, in the same species Callard and McConnell (1969) found that intrahypothalamic implants of oestradiol suppressed ovulation and reduced oviduct weight without affecting follicular development, results which strongly indicate hypothalamic stimulation of GtH secretion. The dissociation between two gonadotropic functions, induction of ovulation and oestrogen secretion on the one hand, stimulation of follicular development on the other, is reminiscent of the more detailed results concerning the hypothalamic gonadotropin-controlling system in amphibians (chapter 12), and is explicable on the assumption that ovulation requires higher levels of GtH than follicular growth. In another lizard, *Dipsosaurus dorsalis*, implants of testosterone or oestradiol in the median eminence inhibited seasonal gonadal maturation, but implants in the pars distalis or basal hypothalamus were less effective (Lisk, 1967). Thus all the evidence points to a stimulatory hypothalamic control of GtH secretion.

ACTH control has recently been investigated in *Sceloporus cyanogenys*. Implants of betamethasone in the hypothalamus reduced adrenal size over a period of thirty days, and blocked the adrenal enlargement normally produced by metopirone (Callard and Willard, 1969). These findings indicate the presence of a possibly diffuse steroid-sensitive area in the hypothalamus concerned in the stimulation of ACTH secretion. Lesions in the antero-medial hypothalamus (probably involving the infundibular nuclei) reduced adrenal weight within seven days, and blocked adrenal hypertrophy in response to metopirone; but sham-operations and lesions in the cerebral cortex or posterior or lateral hypothalamus resulted in *increased* adrenal weight, possibly a stress-response (Callard and Chester Jones, 1970). These data collectively indicate a hypothalamic stimulatory control of ACTH secretion, sensitive to steroidal feedback.

No information is available concerning hypothalamic *control of STH*.

THE PARS TUBERALIS

The varying development of the pars tuberalis, from the large structure in *Sphenodon*, crocodiles and chelonians to its reduction in lizards and absence in snakes, was noted at the beginning of this chapter. The microscopic anatomy of this region has hardly been studied. Crocodilians display large, virtually chromophobic cells, with peripheral nuclei; chelonians, in addition to chromophobes, have large granulated cells, strongly PAS+, AF+ and AB+, while some snakes, notably the Boidae, have what may be remnants of pars tuberalis tissue in the adult, small involuted chromophobic cells against the lower wall of the infundibular stem (Saint-Girons, 1963, 1970).

THE PARS INTERMEDIA

The size of the pars intermedia is highly variable, and two basic types can be recognised. In the thin type, an internal (dorsal) layer of large cells is separated by part of the hypophysial cleft from an outer (ventral) layer of small flat cells; in the massive pars intermedia, the cells are arranged in irregular cords, and the hypophysial cleft is reduced (Saint-Girons, 1963, 1970). The massive type is found in crocodilians, chelonians and most snakes, and at the other extreme the intermedia is reduced or absent in burrowing snakes and lizards. Amongst the lizards, the intermedia shows an extraordinary range of development. It is reduced or nearly lost in burrowing forms; in most lizards it is of the 'thin' type (e.g. Xantusidae, Gekkonidae, Anguidae, Scincidae), sometimes with the internal layer pseudostratified (Lacertidae, most iguanids); while in other lizards the intermedia proliferates to form a lobulated cellular mass, containing connective tissue septa carrying capillaries. This lobulated intermedia is found in some iguanids (e.g. *Anolis*), agamids (e.g. *Agama, Calotes*) and varanids (e.g. *Varanus*), and, though usually smaller, the snake intermedia is of this type (Saint-Girons, 1963, 1967; Wingstrand, 1966*a, b*; Nayar and Pandalai, 1963; Rodríguez and La Pointe, 1970). Whether the size of the pars intermedia is related to powers of adaptive integumentary colour change is not clear. The intermedia is large in lizards capable of rapid colour change (e.g. *Anolis*, chameleons, *Calotes*, agamids in general, diurnal geckos), but it is also large in some lizards which do not change colour (*Acanthodactylus*, many agamids, nocturnal geckos). Considering the habits of the various lizards, and the fact of its atrophy in burrowing lizards and snakes, Saint-Girons (1967) has suggested that the development of the pars intermedia is related to the amount of direct sunlight experienced by the animal, while emphasising that there are exceptions to this rule: for example the diurnal gecko *Quedenfeldtia* has a pars intermedia less developed than nocturnal geckos. There are indications, as in teleosts, that the pars intermedia may have functions unrelated to colour changes. Nouhouayi-Besnard (1966), for example, has described two species of *Varanus* with different habits, *V. niloticus* being partly aquatic and *V. exanthematicus* entirely terrestrial. The pars intermedia is much larger in *V. exanthematicus*, and in this species it shows changes which appear to relate to aestivation and the problems of survival during the dry season.

Concerning colour changes, despite only limited investigations it seems that the control of the pigment cells differs amongst lizards. *Anolis*, with its massive pars intermedia, displays rapid colour changes in which direct innervation of the melanophores seems to play no part, MSH being the only controlling factor (Hadley and Goldman, 1969). Probably in most lizards, direct innervation plays some role in melanophore control, though MSH is also important (e.g. *Phrynosoma*). Chameleons are exceptional, in that their proverbially rapid colour changes are entirely under nervous control, MSH seemingly playing no part in the process (Hadley and Goldman, 1969; Nayar and Pandalai, 1963). However, the large pars intermedia is clearly not related to physiological colour changes in crocodiles, turtles and snakes.

The single cell-type of the pars intermedia may be basophilic, staining with aniline blue in trichrome techniques (e.g. some lizards and snakes), amphiphilic (most reptiles, including many geckonids) or acidophilic (some lizards and most snakes). In some snakes, islets of intermedia cells may invade the dorsal region of the caudal pars distalis. The acidophilic granules of snake intermedia cells are large (400–600 nm in diameter), and the cells also contain lipoidal osmiophilic bodies, possibly lysosomes. In all reptiles the secretory granules tend to lie in the part of the cell close to a capillary, and the granules are PAS+, AF+ and AB+ to varying degrees (Wingstrand, 1966*b*; Saint-Girons, 1967, 1970).

Most work on the pars intermedia in relation to colour change has been done on *Anolis carolinensis*. Ample evidence shows that MSH is the main controlling factor of melanophores in this lizards, and the pars intermedia contains at least three forms of MSH (Burgers, 1963; Hadley and Goldman, 1969). The gland is well-vascularised by interlobular capillaries, which originate in the plexus intermedius and connect distally with the peripheral venous channels of the pituitary (Meurling and Willstedt, 1970). The cells in the intermedia cords are tall and columnar, and filled with amphiphilic granules, reddish-purple after Masson trichrome (Poris and Charipper, 1938), and these correspond to the light cells revealed by the EM (Forbes, 1972*a*). Mingled with the bases of these are large oval cells with fuchsinophilic granulation and irregular nuclei, the rarer dark cells of Forbes (1972*a*). The cell cords often contain central capillaries. Forbes (1972*a*) showed that the predominant light cells are AF+, with granules varying in size and electron density. The rare dark cells contain OG+ granules, 500–1200 nm in length. Interspersed between the endocrine cells are numerous stellate cells, their processes penetrating extensively between the glandular cells and the cell bodies forming a partial

Fig. 13.5. The neuro-intermediate lobe of the lizard *Klauberina riversiana*. From Rodríguez and La Pointe (1970).

(*a*) Thin section of a portion of the neuro-intermedia. MC, marginal cells; GC, glandular cells of the intermedia; VS, vascular septum, including the plexus intermedius; NL, neural lobe. Hypophysial cleft at the top. The rectangle indicates the approximate area enlarged in (*b*). Toluidine blue–borax, × *c*. 1000.

(*b*) Electron micrograph of an area similar to that shown in the rectangle in (*a*). HC, hypophysial cleft; MC, marginal cell layer; GC, glandular cells of the pars intermedia; VS, vascular septum; NL, neural lobe. A and B refer to the two kinds of intermedia cells that can be recognised (see text, p. 310). III and IV refer to two kinds of nerve endings in the neural lobe. × *c*. 4000.

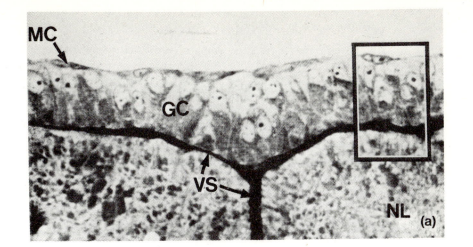

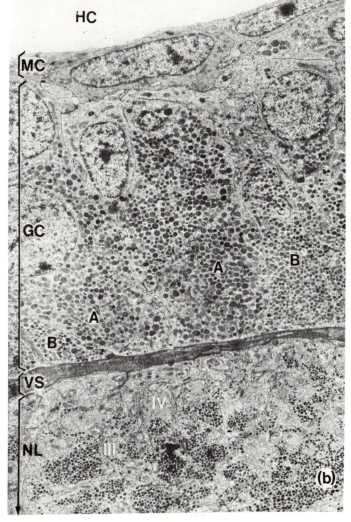

'capsule' round the intermedia; the stellate cells show signs of being involved in the secretory process, like their counterparts in the pars distalis.

In another lizard with a large lobulated pars intermedia, the agamid *Calotes*, the intermedia and neural lobe interdigitate, with the usual thin neuro-intermedia septum containing the plexus intermedius. The plexus gives rise to capillaries which penetrate both neural lobe and pars intermedia, and in the latter these capillaries branch and surround each lobule. The columnar intermedia cells are arranged with their nuclei towards the middle of the cord, and their flattened ends on the interlobular capillaries in a palisade pattern. The secretory granules vary in number, and are acidophilic and carminophilic, as in other agamids, but they are unusual in being AF − (Nayar and Pandalai, 1963).

The single dorsal layer of the thin pars intermedia of the xantusid lizard *Klauberina* has been studied by Rodríguez and La Pointe (1970). All the elongated glandular cells contact the basement membrane of the plexus intermedius, and at their other ends they are bordered by a layer of marginal cells lining the hypophysial cleft. No capillaries penetrate between the cells, their only blood supply being the plexus intermedius (fig. 13.5). As in *Anolis* and *Calotes* (Forbes, 1972a; Nayar and Pandalai, 1963), the secretory granules are concentrated at the end of the cell nearer the capillaries, with the nucleus at the opposite end. The granules in *Klauberina* are strongly PAS +, acidophilic and AF −. Studied with the EM, these cells seem to be of two types, one with granules 200–250 nm in diameter, the other with larger granules, 400–500 nm. The RER and Golgi complex were poorly developed, possibly because the animals were kept illuminated on a pale background, which would reduce the secretion of MSH (Rodríguez and La Pointe, 1970). The EM shows that the marginal cells send processes between the secretory cells which contact the basement membrane of the plexus intermedius and contain granules 100–150 nm in diameter; the cell bodies contain similar granules and also large lipid droplets 400 nm in diameter, and microvilli project from the cells into the hypophysial cleft (Rodríguez and La Pointe, 1970). No doubt the marginal cells of *Klauberina* correspond to the stellate cells of *Anolis*.

The pars intermedia of *Sphenodon* consists of a few layers of cells surrounding the neural lobe. No capillaries penetrate the intermedia from the plexus intermedius, but there are some capillaries on its outer surface. The predominant cell-type, type 1, is oriented with its granulated pole towards the plexus intermedius and the nucleus at the other pole. The other cell-type (type 2) probably corresponds to the stellate cell in other lizards, and lies scattered among the nuclear poles of the type 1 cells. Masses of colloid also occur (Weatherhead, 1971). The EM showed that the type 1 cells elaborate secretory granules which increase in size as they mature (cf. *Xenopus*, chapter 12), starting when distinct and free from the Golgi complex at 100–200 nm in diameter, and eventually reaching 750 nm. The type 2 cells are agranular, and produce long branching processes lying among the type 1 cells and terminating on the basement membrane either of the plexus intermedius or of the superficial capillaries. The processes contain lysosome-like electron-dense bodies, and their terminations on the pericapillary basement membrane expand to form an incomplete barrier between type 1 cells and the pericapillary space. The colloid droplets seen with the light microscope are revealed by the EM to be follicles containing a heterogeneous material and entirely bordered by type 2 cells which shows distinct microvilli towards the follicular lumen (Weatherhead, 1971).

Functional changes in the pars intermedia have been described. In *Calotes* the intermedia cells became more active on a black background, and there was a marked increase in the incidence of colloid droplets, accumulating in the middle of the cell cords and surrounded by a membrane; the amount of colloid decreased when the animals were moved to a white background. On a black background MSH secretion was maximal, as shown by the condition of the melanophores (Nayar and Pandalai, 1963). The light cells showed signs of increased secretory activity in *Anolis* conditioned to maintain rapid MSH secretion, but the dark cells showed no appreciable changes. The light cells decreased in activity in animals conditioned to remain green (low MSH secretion), and the stellate cells had enlarged processes (Forbes, 1972*a*). Whether there are truly two cell-types, and if so, whether the light and dark cells of *Anolis* can be related to the two kinds of granular cells in *Klauberina* is uncertain, but the evidence from *Anolis* points to the light cells as the immediate source of MSH. It may be that as indicated for *Xenopus* and *Sphenodon* the size and appearance of the granules change as they mature within one cell-type, giving the spurious impression of two separate cell-types (cf. Rodríguez and La Pointe, 1970; Weatherhead, 1971). The colloid droplets in *Calotes* have been considered as a hormone store (Nayar and Pandalai, 1963), but this is not certain.

In *Sphenodon* and the lizards investigated, the pars intermedia is apparently not directly innervated; this is indicated both by light microscope studies (Nayar and Pandalai, 1963; Rodríguez and La Pointe, 1970) and by EM work (Rodríguez and La Pointe, 1970; Weatherhead, 1971; Forbes, 1972*a*), and is true of both the thin and the massive types of gland. The massive lobular intermedia is penetrated by blood vessels originating from the plexus intermedius, and is probably very well-vascularised, whereas the thin type of gland is avascular apart from the plexus intermedius and possibly some superficial capillaries (Poris and Charipper, 1938; Nayar and Pandalai, 1963; Sheela and Pandalai, 1966; Wingstrand, 1966*b*; Meurling and Willstedt, 1970; Rodríguez and La

Pointe, 1970; Weatherhead, 1971; Forbes, 1972*a*). This difference in vascularity obviously relates to the volume of intermedia to be supplied, and it seems likely that all hypothalamic control over the lizard pars intermedia is exerted via a neurovascular route, exceptional amongst vertebrates. Nerve fibres, both type A and type B, terminate on the plexus intermedius, the whole arrangement being reminiscent of the hypo-thalamo-median eminence system (Rodríguez, La Pointe and Dellman, 1971) and substances released by these fibres could reach the pars intermedia cells directly in a gland like that of *Klauberina*, in which the intermedia cells contact the pericapillary space of the plexus intermedius, or indirectly, via the stellate cell (type 2 cell) processes in *Sphenodon* or via the plentiful capillaries of the massive glands in *Calotes* and *Anolis*.

In contrast to lizards, it may be that the pars intermedia in other reptiles is more orthodox in being directly innervated. Urano (1972) has described monoamine oxidase not only in the pars intermedia endocrine cells of the turtle (*Clemmys japonica*) but also in fibres between the cells, which he interprets as aminergic fibres and which sometimes were seen to contact the endocrine cells. If this work can be substantiated with the EM, it would be definite evidence of aminergic innervation of the intermedia cells in a reptile. Furthermore, NSM is visible in the massive pars inter-medias of crocodiles and snakes (Wingstrand, 1966*b*), and AF+ material can sometimes be seen passing across the plexus intermedius in snakes (Saint-Girons, 1967). Thus lizards may be unique in lacking direct innervation of the pars intermedia.

Concerning hypothalamic control of MSH secretion, the only evidence comes from work on *Klauberina*. Keeping these lizards on a black background under constant illumination caused degranulation of the intermedia secretory cells. Transection of the infundibulum produced the same effect, and led to slow expansion of the melanophores, suggesting that the hypothalamus may normally inhibit MSH secretion (Rodríguez, La Pointe and Dellman, 1971).

THE HYPOTHALAMUS AND NEUROHYPOPHYSIS

The division of the original preoptic nuclei into two AF+ centres, the supraoptic nuclei (SON) and paraventricular nuclei (PVN) occurred in early reptiles. The distal terminations of the AF+ fibres lie in two clearly separated regions of the neurohypophysis, the median eminence and neural lobe. A system of AF− hypothalamic neurosecretory centres must be present, since it occurs in amphibians, birds and mammals, and must be the source of the AF− (type B) fibres found in the median eminence and neural lobe. The infundibular nuclei belong to this system, and were mentioned on p. 305.

A detailed account of the AF+ nuclei in the snake *Diadophis punctatus* was given by Philibert and Kamemoto (1965). The PVN is the larger, and is located on each side of the third ventricle, anterior and dorsal to the pituitary. Its neurons contain AF+ secretory granules which are also visible in the axons. The main tract from the PVN is distinct at first, but it bends ventrally and merges with the tract from the SON. The latter lie anterior, lateral and ventral to the PVN, and contain larger secretory granules. The mingled axons from the two nuclei pass towards the neural lobe, but some terminate against the capillary bed of the median eminence. Dehydration experiments in this snake (Philibert and Kamemoto, 1965) and in the lizard *Calotes versicolor* (Sheela and Pandalai, 1968) showed that the PVN respond to water shortage, with depletion of NSM in the perikarya, hypothalamo-neurohypophysial tract and neural lobe of the snake, and in the lizard an initial hyperactivity of the PVN cells followed by degeneration. In both animals the SON showed no comparable responses except with the most severe dehydration. Injection of Pitocin and Pitressin in the snake resulted in an increase in NSM in all parts of the system, and an increase in the cell population of the PVN. It appears from these observations that the PVN is involved in salt and water metabolism in these reptiles, which suggests that arginine vasotocin (AVT), the probable physiological antidiuretic hormone of reptiles (Heller, 1969), is secreted by the PVN. AVT also stimulates oviduct contractions in the viviparous lizard *Klauberina* (La Pointe, 1969), and possibly in oviparous forms (Heller, 1969), but it is possible that meso-tocin, the other neurohypophysial factor of reptiles, is actually the physiological agent for stimulation of the oviduct.

The cells of the PVN in *Lacerta* are bipolar, and send swollen ciliated endings into the third ventricle, some containing NSM, others rich in mitochondria; laterally these processes send out branches which synapse with neighbouring processes. Perikarya, branches, and process endings are all rich in acetylcholinesterase (Vigh-Teichmann and Vigh, 1970).

MEDIAN EMINENCE

The median eminence is always distinctly differentiated. Its structure in lizards and snakes is comparable to that of the neural lobe, with ependymal cells next to the infundibular recess, then a thick fibre layer containing pituicytes and NSM, and ventrally a palisade layer, rich in capillaries. Some pars tuberalis cells may invade the palisade layer (Saint-Girons, 1967). The hypothalamo-neurohypophysial tract runs through the fibre layer, just beneath the ependyma (Philibert and Kamemoto, 1965).

Sphenodon has an unusual and perhaps primitive median eminence. The dorsal ependymal layer is normal, and below this is the hypothalamo-neurohypophysial tract carrying only rather sparse NSM. The palisade layer is traversed by ventral processes of the ependymal cells and of dorsally-placed glial cells. The unusual feature is that instead of the primary portal capillaries penetrating into the palisade layer, as for example in snakes, the palisade layer sends projections down into the pars tuberalis. These projections end in swellings, bounded by a thin basement membrane, against which are the endings of axons rich in NSM; the processes also contain pituicytes. The primary portal capillaries run between the cords of tuberalis cells, and abut on the membranes around the median eminence projections, within the pars tuberalis parenchyma. No ultrastructural details are available, but presumably the basement membrane around the median eminence projections contains the perivascular space of the primary capillaries (Gabe and Saint-Girons, 1964).

In other reptiles the primary capillaries either lie on the surface of the median eminence (chelonians, smaller lizards) or are deeply embedded in the palisade layer (crocodilians, larger lizards, snakes) (Wingstrand, 1966a). The chelonian median eminence has been described in some detail in the turtle *Clemmys japonica* (Kobayashi and Matsui, 1969). The fibrous layer contains the hypothalamo-neurohypophysial tract, with NSM and glial cells, and the outer palisade layer is well-developed. The median eminence is divisible into anterior and posterior regions, which may correspond to the divisions of the avian median eminence; there is thus some possibility of a 'point to point' relationship between hypothalamic nuclei and groups of primary portal capillaries in these reptiles, as in birds (cf. Oksche, Zimmermann and Oehmke, 1972). The anterior median eminence in the turtle is rich in AF+ NSM, but little is stored in the posterior region (Kobayashi and Matsui, 1969; Urano, 1972). There are axo-axonal synapses close to the median eminence, in which neurosecretory axons (secretory granules *c.* 120 nm in diameter) contact ordinary nerve fibres. In the palisade layer of the anterior median eminence, three kinds of neurosecretory fibres terminate on the portal capillaries close to the surface, with secretory granules 100, 120 and 150 nm in diameter. The last two (type A fibres) may carry neurohypophysial octapeptides, since similar granules occur in the axons of the neural lobe, and these would account for the strong AF+ reaction of the anterior median eminence. The fibres with the 100 nm granules are probably aminergic (type B), and their hypothalamic origin is not known, though it is possibly the infundibular nucleus. All three axonal endings also contain the usual small clear 'synaptic' vesicles, 50 nm in diameter, and a fourth fibre-type is sometimes found, with only these vesicles and no electron-dense secretory granules: these would correspond to the type C fibres of the amphibian median eminence (chapter 12), with some possibility that they may be cholinergic (Kobayashi and Matsui, 1969). In the posterior median eminence of *Clemmys japonica*, which has not been studied with the EM, numerous monoamine oxidase + fibres (type B?) occur around blood capillaries of the primary plexus, with rather fewer such fibres in the anterior median eminence (Urano, 1972).

NEURAL LOBE

The neural lobe, borne at the end of an infundibular stem, is seen at its most primitive in *Sphenodon*, chelonians and some lizards, in which it is hollow with thin walls consisting simply of ependyma, fibrous layer and palisade layer, and containing few or no pituicytes. A more advanced condition is seen in some lizards (e.g. burrowing forms such as amphisbaenids) and crocodiles, in which the walls of the lobules are thickened and contain many pituicytes, but the lobe still retains at least a narrow cavity continuous with the infundibular recess. The most advanced condition is seen in snakes, in which the large compact neural lobe is invaded by only a few very narrow tubules from the infundibular recess, and solid lobules of neural tissue, containing vascular connective septa and many pituicytes, penetrate into the pars intermedia (Wingstrand, 1966a). The neural lobe is generally packed with NSM in all reptiles, and in the snake *Diadophis* the NSM content is reduced in response to dehydration and increased after injections of neurohypophysial octapeptides (Philibert and Kamemoto, 1965).

In Squamata the general three-layered structure of the infundibular wall as seen in the median eminence is usually preserved in the neural lobe, the middle fibrous layer containing a variable number of pituicytes and the external palisade layer being particularly rich in AF + NSM, where type A fibres usually terminate on the basement membrane of the plexus intermedius. In the compact neural lobes of snakes, and to a lesser extent in some lizards, capillary loops from the plexus intermedius penetrate into the neural tissue, and fibre endings correspondingly occur deeper in the neural lobe. The neural lobe tends to be especially large in burrowing lizards and snakes but otherwise shows no obvious correlation with habits (Saint-Girons, 1967).

The neural lobe of *Sphenodon* has recently been described in detail by Weatherhead (1971). The tuber cinereum merges with the infundibular stem, which expands distally to form the neural lobe, a single hollow sac with two anterior diverticuli projecting forwards on either side of the infundibular stem and surrounded by pars intermedia. The ependymal cells lining the cavity of the neural lobe are conical or flattened, and contain lipoidal bodies which are probably lysosomes. They have long basal processes which may be grouped in bundles and which cross the neural lobe directly or obliquely to the neuro-intermedia septum. On this septum the ependymal processes are produced laterally into ependymal end-feet, which form a discontinuous investment to the neural tissue against the basement membrane of the plexus intermedius; the plexus is supplied by branches of the hypophysial artery, and sends no capillary branches into the neural lobe. The EM shows the apices of the ependymal cells to have irregular processes into the infundibular recess, as well as microvilli. The basal processes contain mitochondria and fine fibrils, and the end-feet form a continuous barrier against the external basement membrane in the infundibular stem, but an incomplete barrier in the neural lobe itself, thus permitting the nerve fibres to make direct contact with the plexus intermedius.

Immediately beneath the ependymal layer is a fibrous layer, containing no pituicytes but with many type A1 fibres (secretory granules, mean diameter 157.5 nm) and type A2 fibres (granules 200 nm, less electron-dense and more irregular). In addition, occasional type B fibres (dense core vesicles, with a space between granule and membrane, mean overall diameter 80 nm) are found, and occasional type C fibres (without electron-dense granules, containing only electron-lucent 'synaptic' vesicles, 50 nm in diameter). Similar 'synaptic' vesicles are found in all the other types of fibres. The most numerous element in the fibrous layer is a non-neuro-secretory fibre-type, containing only neurotubules and neurofilaments.

In the inner palisade layer, the type A fibres predominate, type A1 being the more common, and in the outer palisade layer, between the ependymal end-feet, all four types of fibres occur and make contact with the pericapillary space of the plexus intermedius. The commonest fibre-types here are A1 and B, while the rare type A2 fibre only occasionally contacts the pericapillary space. Type B fibres make synaptoid contact with the ependymal basal processes and end-feet, but these are rare. The pericapillary space is typical, containing numerous collagen fibres and fibroblasts. The endothelium of the plexus intermedius is not apparently fenestrated, but the cytoplasm of the endothelial cells often contains pinocytotic vesicles, RER and mitochondria.

One of the striking features of this primitive reptile is the almost complete cuff formed by the ependymal end-feet between the nerve fibres and the pericapillary space. This does not seem to be typical of reptiles as a group, since Weatherhead (1971) quotes his own observations on a series of reptiles in which the nerve fibres are more directly related to the perivascular membranes, the end-feet (whether of ependymal cells or of pituicytes in the more compact glands) being less important.

In the tuber cinereum of *Sphenodon*, and in the infundibular stem wall, specialised cells lie beneath the ependyma, with clear nuclei, RER and electron-dense granules *c.* 160 nm in diameter. These cells send projections between the ependymal cells into the infundibular recess, and resemble similar AF+ cells in the tortoise, *Emys* (Weatherhead, 1971, 1969). These cells may form part of the 'liquor-contacting neurosecretory system' (Vigh-Teichmann and Vigh, 1970), and may secrete into the infundibular

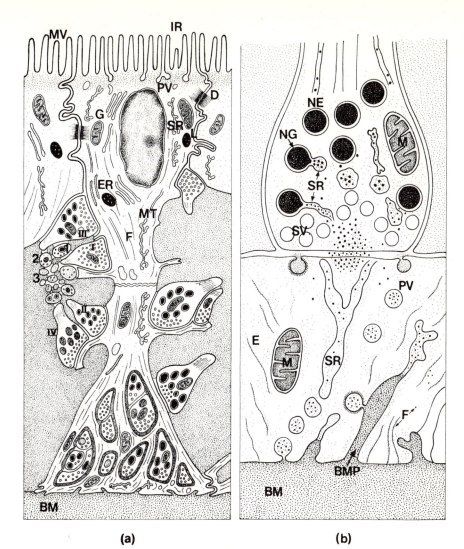

(a)　　　　　　　　　　　　　　**(b)**

Fig. 13.6. Neural lobe of the lizard *Klauberina riversiana*.

(*a*) Diagrammatic section through the wall of the neural lobe showing an ependymal cell and the spatial relationships of primary components to it. The break in the ependymal process indicates that it has been shortened in the diagram for the sake of clarity. IR, infundibular recess; MV, microvilli; PV, pinocytotic vesicles; D, desmosome; G, Golgi apparatus; SR, smooth endoplasmic reticulum; ER, rough endoplasmic reticulum L, lysosome; MT, microtubules; F, filaments; BM, basement membrane; 1, 2 and 3, three kinds of nerve fibres; I, II, III and IV, different kinds of nerve endings.

(*b*) Diagram of the proposed pathway for release of neurosecretory material from the nerve ending (NE) through the ependymal cuff (E) to the basement membrane (BM). The 5 nm particles (represented by solid dots) are shown being released from neurosecretory granules (NG) into either the smooth endoplasmic reticulum (SR) or into the axoplasm. The 5 nm particles congregate in the synaptic region of the nerve ending and in the adjacent intercellular space, suggesting that they are released from the nerve endings. They appear to be transported across the ependymal cuff by means of pinocytotic vesicles (PV) and the smooth endoplasmic reticulum, which in turn opens on to the basement membrane. M, mitochondria; SV, small vesicles; F, filaments; BMP, processes of the basement membrane.

From Rodríguez and La Pointe (1969).

recess. It is clear from Weatherhead's (1972) account of *Sphenodon*, with its thin-walled avascular neural lobe, that all NSM reaching the neural lobe from the hypothalamic centres must be released into the capillaries of the plexus intermedius.

The lizard *Klauberina* has a thin-walled neural lobe very like that of *Sphenodon* (Rodríguez and La Pointe, 1969). It is a simple outpocketing of the infundibular recess, surrounded by pars intermedia and with a typical plexus intermedius which sends occasional capillary loops into the neural tissue, unlike the avascular condition of the lobe in *Sphenodon*. Again, the neural lobe contains the usual three layers. The ependymal cells display basal processes which cross the neural lobe to end on the walls of the plexus intermedius. The fibrous (hilar) layer contains AF + PAS − fibres, and the palisade layer is composed of axonal endings, most of them AF + and only a few PAS + . Pituicytes are rare, and appear to be simply ependymal cells which have sunk into the neural tissue. EM studies showed the ependymal cells to contain lysosomes, as in *Sphenodon*, and their apical surfaces are produced into microvilli, often very long, with abundant pinocytotic vesicles at their bases, and associated dense granular material. Adjacent ependymal cells are joined by projections and desmosomes (fig. 13.6). The basal processes of the ependymal cells branch extensively in the palisade layer, and expand on the basement membrane of the plexus intermedius to form a continuous barrier on the membrane, without the discontinuities seen in *Sphenodon*; these end-feet contain abundant smooth ER, enclosing tiny particles, and occasionally there is evidence of phagocytosis by the end-feet, in the form of large bodies containing inclusions apparently derived from neurosecretory axons. The basement membrane projects into the end-feet, and smooth ER and small vesicles open on to these projections, with pinocytotic vesicles common nearby (fig. 13.6).

As in *Sphenodon*, the neural lobe of *Klauberina* contains four kinds of axonal endings. Using the nomenclature of Weatherhead (1971), the type A1 endings contain dense granules *c.* 150 nm in diameter, the uncommon type A2 endings contain granules about the same size but less dense, type B endings are rare and contain granulated vesicles about 100 nm in diameter, and type C endings contain only clear 'synaptic' vesicles, *c.* 40 nm in diameter. All the granulated endings also contain 'synaptic' vesicles. These fibre terminations are on ependymal cells, a few on the basal processes of the cells as they traverse the fibrous layer, but most in the palisade layer close to the swellings of the ependymal end-feet (fig. 13.6). 'Synaptic' vesicles are especially numerous at the terminations, and tiny particles *c.* 5 nm in diameter occur within the ependymal cells, within the nerve endings, and between the two. These tiny particles resemble the particles seen in the pinocytotic vesicles of the ependymal cells, which occur both at the contact with the pericapillary basement membrane and also in the region of the nerve endings on the ependymal cell (fig. 13.6).

In discussing their findings, Rodríguez and La Pointe (1969) speculate that the more numerous type A1 endings may release AVT, and type A2 endings may release oxytocin or mesotocin or both. Later, however (Rodríguez, 1971), a fifth fibre type (type A3) was distinguished in *Klauberina*, with dense granules about 130 nm in diameter. On the basis of this later finding, and considering the neural lobe granules in vertebrates with different neurohypophysial octapeptides, Rodríguez (1971) speculated that AVT may be released by the type A1 fibres, as before, but that mesotocin probably was released by the new type A3 fibre. The type A2 fibres, with their electron-lucent granules, are now supposed to secrete oxytocin, which may or may not be present in reptiles. Type B fibres are considered aminergic, type C fibres cholinergic (Rodríguez and La Pointe, 1969; Rodríguez, 1971). The pathway for the release of whatever materials are secreted by the various types of fibres in *Klauberina* must obviously be by way of the ependymal cell basal processes. It seems likely that material from the secretory granules is released into the axoplasm, where it appears as the tiny 5 nm particles. These particles are then taken into the ependymal cells by pinocytosis, and pass into the smooth ER of the ependymal cells and from there into the capillaries of the plexus intermedius (fig. 13.6). The role of the ependymal cells in transport of NSM is particularly interesting in view of various lines of evidence that pituicytes (modified ependymal cells) may play a similar role in the more massive neural lobes of birds and mammals (chapters 5 and 14).

Strongly monoamine oxidase positive fibres are distributed around the blood capillaries of the neural lobe in the tortoise *Clemmys japonica* (Urano, 1972), presumably corresponding to type B fibres.

BLOOD SUPPLY OF THE REPTILIAN PITUITARY GLAND

There is some evidence that the details of the blood supply to the gland may show differences, possibly of phyletic significance, in different reptiles. Only a few species have been investigated, but the information already indicates important variations even within the Squamata (Enemar, 1960; Sheela and Pandalai, 1966).

What may be a primitive condition is seen in two lizards, *Lacerta agilis* and *Anguis fragilis*. The sole source of blood is the infundibular arteries. These supply the primary plexus of the median eminence, which is a dense network of vessels on the surface of the median eminence, with no loops penetrating into the tissue. The primary portal plexus on the median eminence is continuous with a plexus (*Lacerta*) or several straight capillaries (*Anguis*) which run backwards on the oral surface of the infundibular stem and supply a superficial capillary network on the surface of the neural lobe. This network is elaborated in the connective tissue septum between the neural lobe and pars intermedia to form the plexus intermedius. In neither genus is there any vascular penetration of either neural lobe or the thin layer of the pars intermedia, the capillaries remaining exclusively superficial. This superficial system also receives blood directly from the infundibular arteries, but a large proportion of their supply is from the median eminence capillaries, a primitive feature (Enemar, 1960).

From the median eminence plexus, four, five or six portal vessels supply the secondary capillary plexus within the cephalic pars distalis, and blood from this region then passes into the caudal pars distalis, where the capillaries tend to be wider, sometimes forming great vascular 'sinusoids' as in the anguid lizards (Saint-Girons, 1967). There is no separate arterial supply to the pars distalis, all blood entering the gland being portal. From the caudal pars distalis and the plexus intermedius, blood drains into the retrohypophysial vein, a dorsal vessel (Enemar, 1960).

The lizard *Calotes versicolor* exhibits some slight differences, possibly representing phyletic advances. Again the infundibular arteries supply the primary capillaries of the median eminence, which is mainly superficial but with some loops penetrating the palisade layer. Only a few capillaries connect the median eminence vascular bed to the neural lobe system, in contrast to the numerous connections in *Lacerta* and *Anguis*. One or two large portal vessels supply the cephalic lobe of the pars distalis, which in turn supplies the caudal lobe. Most blood to the neuro-intermedia comes from neural lobe arteries, branches of the infundibular arteries, which branch and form the plexus intermedius (fig. 13.7). In contrast to the other two lizards, many capillary loops from the plexus intermedius penetrate the neural tissue, and many bundles of capillaries (both inter- and intra-lobular) run through the lobular pars intermedia, some of them connecting with capillaries of the caudal pars distalis (fig. 13.7). All blood from the neural lobe is drained via the intermedia capillaries and thence into the retrohypophysial vein, which also receives the drainage from the caudal pars distalis. There seems to be no independent arterial supply to the pars distalis (Sheela and Pandalai, 1966; Nayar and Pandalai, 1963). *Anolis* is essentially similar, except that capillaries do not penetrate the tissue of the neural lobe, but run between the lobules (Meurling and Willstedt, 1970).

The grass-snake *Natrix natrix* has a hypophysial vascular system which may represent the most advanced condition in the reptiles (Enemar, 1960). The primary plexus is supplied by the infundibular arteries, but it is here more elaborate than in the other forms, very dense and complicated with capillary bundles sinking deep into the palisade layer of the median eminence. A bundle of seven or eight portal vessels passes from the

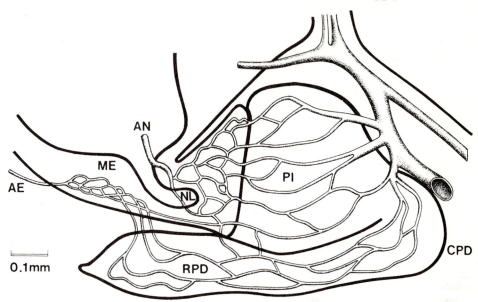

Fig. 13.7. *Anolis carolinensis*. Simplified diagram of the pituitary region in mid-sagittal section, to show the blood supply in this lizard. AE, artery to median eminence; ME, median eminence; AN, artery to neural lobe; NL, neural lobe; PI, pars intermedia; RPD, cephalic lobe of pars distalis; CPD, caudal lobe of pars distalis. See text for details. From Meurling and Willstedt (1970).

primary plexus into the secondary capillaries of the cephalic pars distalis. Only very few capillaries run from the median eminence system to the neural lobe system, the latter now being supplied largely by the hypophysial arteries and also by a branch from the infundibular artery, presumably corresponding to the neural lobe artery of Sheela and Pandalai (1966). The solid lobulated neural lobe contains capillary branches of the plexus intermedius folded into its substance, and the pars intermedia, which to a limited extent interdigitates with the neural lobe, has a superficial plexus supplied from the plexus intermedius. A new feature is the presence of small arteries from the internal carotids which supply the pars distalis independently from the portal system. All venous drainage is into the retrohypophysial veins.

Features of the snake system which may be regarded as advances on *Lacerta* and *Calotes* are: (1) the almost complete separation of the vascular beds of the median eminence and neuro-intermedia; (2) the folding of some primary portal capillaries into the median eminence itself; (3) the direct supply to the neuro-intermedia by the hypophysial arteries, and (4) the direct arterial supply to the pars distalis, which nevertheless is of little functional importance in relation to the much larger volume of blood that reaches the gland from the portal system. It will be seen that *Calotes* and *Anolis* in some ways display intermediate features. The elaborate intrinsic blood vessels in the pars intermedia of these lizards is clearly related to the much greater volume and lobulation of the gland, and to the fact that the lizard intermedia is not directly innervated. The relatively voluminous pars intermedia in *Natrix* has only a superficial capillary vascular plexus, possibly related to the direct neurosecretory innervation of the gland in snakes (Enemar, 1960; Sheela and Pandalai, 1966; cf. Wingstrand, 1966a, b).

It is particularly striking that in these reptiles the separation of the median eminence plexus from the neuro-intermedia plexus, often found in birds and mammals, is not completed, even in *Natrix*.

14

THE PITUITARY GLAND IN BIRDS

The avian pituitary gland, which has been described in a detailed monograph by Wingstrand (1951), differs in several important respects from that of mammals in both its embryological and mature stages. It has the same dual origin as in mammals. Rathke's pouch is an epithelial-lined pocket which extends out from the oral ectoderm and is associated with the saccus infundibuli or neural downgrowth. At an early stage the pouch develops two enlargements, one superiorly where it is in contact with neural tissue, the other inferiorly at the upper end of the now narrowing oral part of the pouch which will give rise to an epithelial stalk (fig. 14.1). The two enlargements, which are joined by a constricted zone of the pouch, form aboral (i.e. juxtaneural) and oral lobes (Wingstrand, 1951).

The aboral lobe remains closely associated with the saccus infundibuli. The cells of the oral lobe proliferate and give rise to an unpaired anterior process which grows upwards and forwards to make contact with the basal hypothalamus in the region of the future median eminence. This gives rise to a part of the pars distalis, and contact with the median eminence is not generally maintained. Meanwhile, also from the oral lobe there arises on each side a lateral outgrowth or lobe which grows upwards towards the median eminence. These develop into the pars tuberalis. As in mammals, the basal parts of the two lateral outgrowths apparently become included in the pars distalis and may form a comparable pars tuberalis interna, which remains histologically distinguishable from the pars distalis derived from the median mass of cells.

In birds the pars tuberalis thus comes to form a bridge between the median eminence and the pars distalis, across which pass the portal vessels – as indeed also occurs in mammals. The difference is, however, that in many avian species the bridge is not closely applied to the neural downgrowth, so that an isolated porto-tuberal tract (so named by Benoit and Assenmacher, 1951) is formed linking neural and glandular regions, but morphologically separated from the derivatives of the saccus infundibuli (fig. 14.2). This has considerable significance from the point of view of experimental studies on function of the avian glands, since it allows the portal vascular system to be interrupted while the neural stem can be left intact.

The pars tuberalis externa usually shows some evidence of its lateral

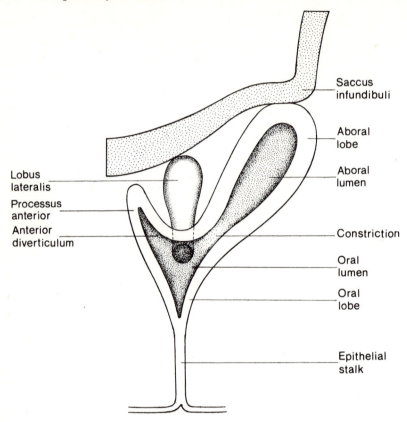

Fig. 14.1. Diagram of Rathke's pouch in amniote vertebrates showing the derivation of the parts of the pituitary gland, notably in birds. From Wingstrand (1951).

origin, fusion of the two outgrowths occurring only in the region of the portal vessels and behind the infundibular stem, so that the latter is enclosed in a collar of tuberalis cells. The pars tuberalis, according to Wingstrand, appears to be always present in birds, although differing in its degree of development. Usually it is one to four cells thick, but Wingstrand illustrates a much more developed structure in *Diomeda melanophris* (his fig. 32), and notes that in this and some other species epithelial cells of the tuberalis lie within the tissue of the median eminence in some areas.

The pars intermedia does not develop in birds. The upper part of the aboral lobe of Rathke's pouch is at an early stage in close contact with the neural downgrowth, but later becomes separated from it by connective tissue, and differentiates to form part of the pars distalis. In the blackcock the membrane between the pars distalis and neural lobe is very thin, and colloid cysts, resembling to some extent those found in the human

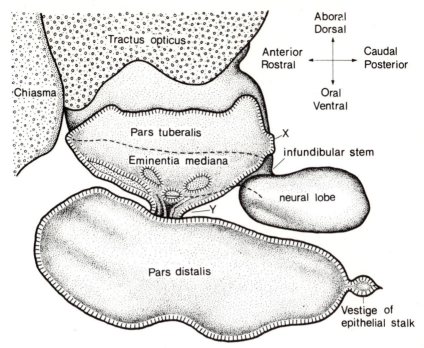

Fig. 14.2. Drawing of the pituitary gland of the goose, to show the relationship of various parts of the gland. X denotes the junction of the pars tuberalis of the left and right sides behind the infundibulum and Y the connection between the pars distalis and the pars tuberalis proper (the portal zone). From Wingstrand (1951).

pituitary, occur along the line of separation. Wingstrand, however, considers that there is no justification for designating any part of the avian pituitary as pars intermedia.

The pars distalis, as already noted, develops from two sources, the oral and aboral divisions of the original Rathke's pouch, which form respectively cephalic and caudal lobes of the fully formed pars distalis (Rahn and Painter, 1941). These two parts, although fused to form a single mass of epithelial cells, can be distinguished histologically (see p. 330). In many species of birds the oral part of the original Rathke's pouch gives rise to an epithelial stalk which persists as a cellular connection between the pars distalis and the oral ectoderm (see Wingstrand, 1951). This stalk is destroyed if the gland is dissected free from the skull, and can only be studied in sections through the whole region.

The separation of the neurohypophysis from the adenohypophysis in birds means that the whole gland often forms less of a single unit than that of mammals. In some species, the pars distalis is elongated and flattened, but as Wingstrand's (1951) drawings show, there is considerable

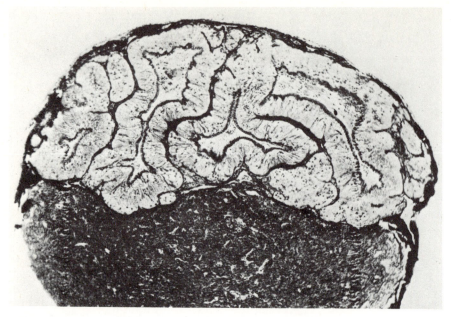

Fig. 14.3. A cross section through the posterior end of the pituitary of the pheasant (*Phasianus colchicus*) to show the sacculated form of the neural process. From Wingstrand (1951).

variation in shape, and also in the spatial relationships between adeno- and neurohypophysial components.

The form of the mature avian infundibular process differs considerably from that of mammals, and varies in different species from a fairly solid mass of tissue to a thin-walled sac. In most it appears as a multilobular complex, each lobule having a lumen and often being enclosed in connective tissue (fig. 14.3). This arrangement is derived directly from its embryogenesis, which is described below based on Wingstrand's detailed descriptions of the development in three species of bird, the chicken (*Gallus gallus*), the gull (*Larus ribibundus*) and the sand martin (*Riparia riparia*).

As already noted, the development of the neurohypophysis in birds resembles that in mammals in that a saccus infundibuli develops from the floor of the diencephalon. In the chick this does not appear until after the formation of Rathke's pouch, to which it is closely related from the first. At this early stage, the optic chiasma limits the neural outgrowth anteriorly. A pair of lateral outgrowths (primary branches) from the saccus next appear and grow latero-caudally; hollow buds sprout from these outgrowths and some also arise from the wall of the saccus between the primary branches.

The saccus gives rise to the infundibular stem and infundibular process (neural lobe). The median eminence is developing at the same time as the saccus, and soon shows the typical three layers, an inner ependymal, a middle fibrous (nerve fibres running parallel to the surface) and an outer 'glandular' layer, which, like the developing saccus infundibuli, is bounded externally by a delicate pial membrane (the intima piae).

The process of proliferation described above (primary budding) apparently plays a part of variable importance in the development of the neural lobe in different specimens, as well as in different species; similarly, a secondary 'outflowing' type of growth also plays a variable part. The beginning of this secondary process is correlated with the arrival of nerve fibres in the neural lobe, via the median eminence and infundibular stem. At this time gaps appear in the bounding pial membrane, through which both ependymal cells and 'colloid' material (the latter, after fixation at any rate, shows a granular component) pass into the surrounding mesenchyme. Delicate nerve fibres, apparently derived from the tractus hypophyseus, also enter the colloid, which Wingstrand suggests may be secreted by them. These fibres, along with ependymal cells and pituicytes, at first lie close to the walls of the capillaries running in the surrounding mesenchyme. Later the cells and fibres withdraw from the vessels, leaving acellular perivascular regions, through which processes of the pituicytes pass to end in expansions on the capillary walls. By this process capillaries come to lie within the tissue of the neural lobe. Wingstrand notes that in parts of the lobe formed by the primary budding process the capillaries remain superficial or lie in the furrows on the surface, while the tissue retains the three-layered structure as found in the median eminence.

The final form of the neural lobe depends on the extent to which each of the two processes, 'budding' and 'outflowing', occur in development. Extreme forms indicate that a predominance of either the primary (budding) or of the secondary methods of growth have occurred. In the pheasant (*Phasianus colchicus*), for example (fig. 14.3), the neural lobe is made up of lobules with obvious lumina derived by a process of budding from the original saccus infundibuli. More solid types of lobe, such as that of the partridge (*Perdix perdix*), indicate a predominance of the secondary type of growth. Wingstrand classifies avian lobes into four types, which relate closely to their mode of development.

The median eminence is in some species thin, in others, such as the goose, thick. It differs from that of the mammal in that the primary capillaries of the portal vascular system lie superficially or in grooves on its surface rather than penetrating to form the often complex vascular formations of mammals. Differences in its microscopic and submicroscopic organisation are also striking (see p. 334). Caudally, the median eminence continues into the infundibular stem and the lumen is usually continued at any rate as far as the neural lobe, so that a compact 'stalk' such as is found in many mammalian pituitaries is often not developed.

CYTOLOGY OF THE PARS DISTALIS

In the 1930s, when a considerable amount of attention was being paid to the cytological features of the mammalian pituitary, the avian gland was relatively neglected. During this period Bissonnette, extending the studies of Rowan (see Bissonnette, 1938, for references), focussed attention on the importance of the pituitary as the link between environmental stimuli and gonadal activity; for birds, the light–dark ratio is a particularly important influence. By the end of this decade, however, cytological studies of the glands of some of the commoner species had been published. Numerous papers dealt with the pituitary of the domestic fowl (Kato and his colleagues in Japan, Payne in the United States – see Matsuo *et al.* 1969, for references) – and Voigt (1939); while Schooley and Riddle (1938) had studied the pituitary of the pigeon. In 1951 Wingstrand's notable monograph appeared, but it was really not until the increasing use of species such as the white-crowned sparrow, the Japanese quail and the duck in experimental studies in the 1960s that the avian pituitary began to be subjected to the same kind of intensive study as that of mammals.

The basic structure in the avian pars distalis resembles that of mammals in so far as the secretory cells, arranged in cords or clumps, are closely related to blood vessels. Although follicular patterns are more common than in many mammalian species and often contain colloid, the occurrence of these is variable, even within species. Wingstrand (1951) suggested that such formations might be associated with age, but found that this was not necessarily always so.

A striking feature of the avian pars distalis is its clear-cut division into two parts, the caudal and the cephalic lobes. Rahn and Painter (1941) found this pattern was consistent in the eighteen different species they examined, and described the cephalic lobe (that is, the more anterior) as containing 'chromophobes, basophils and usually light-staining acidophils', and the caudal lobe as containing 'chromophobes, basophils and deep-staining coarsely granular acidophils'. The two kinds of acidophil were considered to constitute two distinct cell-types, an opinion with which Wingstrand agreed. The subdivision is of particular interest in view of the pattern of the portal blood system in birds (see p. 336).

The evolution of knowledge of the cytology of the avian gland and of the functional implications of this has in general followed the course already described for mammals. Early studies identified only a few types of cell; Schooley and Riddle (1938), for example, described in the pigeon basophils, acidophils and chromophobes, and by correlating the cytological features with the reproductive cycle, ascribed gonadotropic activity to the basophils, and prolactin secretion to the acidophils. In 1963 Wingstrand published a short review based largely on studies of the pituitary gland of the domestic fowl, duck and pigeon. Various techniques had been used by different authors and the terminology was confusing. At that time two major classes of acidophils were described designated A_1 and A_2. The A_1 cells or dark-staining acidophils were reported by some authors as being also PAS +, and stained with azocarmine. Wingstrand, Herlant *et al.* (1960) as well as other authors suggested that these cells were equivalent to the γ cells in other species and were concerned with the secretion of LH. At this time it appeared that a second type of acidophil had also been included in this former class. This, designated the α cell, had only been described in the duck (Herlant *et al.* 1960) and in this species was found only in the caudal lobe. These cells were PAS − and, it was suggested, secreted STH. The third type of acidophil (A_2) appeared to be limited to the cephalic lobe. These cells were said to stain with PAS as well as AF and were correlated with the secretion of prolactin.

Two types of basophil, both PAS +, had been distinguished (Legait and Legait, 1955) in the pituitary of the fowl. Herlant and his colleagues (1960) showed in the duck that with the AB–PAS staining method, red and blue types could be differentiated; the latter were considered to be thyrotropic (δ), the red-stained ones gonadotropic (β).

Recent understanding of functional cytology of the avian gland owes much to the work of Tixier-Vidal who, with various colleagues, has examined the pars distalis of the Pekin duck (Tixier-Vidal and Benoit, 1962), the pigeon (Tixier-Vidal and Assenmacher, 1966) and the Japanese quail (Tixier-Vidal, Follett and Farner, 1967, 1968). Staining techniques used have included Herlant's tetrachrome, AB–PAS–OG, PAS–OG and PAS–PbH. In order to determine the function of the various cell-types, a variety of methods (such as have been widely applied to mammalian studies) were used to bring about known changes in activity of the pars distalis. Thus, changes in the photoperiod and gonadectomy were used to effect changes in activity of the gonadotropic cells and antithyroid drugs and metopirone (which inhibits the synthesis of corticosteroids, and hence results in increased activity of corticotropic cells) were given to influence other types of secretory elements.

In the quail Tixier-Vidal, Follett and Farner (1968), by the comparative study of sections stained by different techniques, were able to distinguish seven distinct types of chromophil cells. Three of these contained glycoprotein and were thus PAS +. The authors designated them as β (PAS +, AB −); δ (PAS +, AB +) and γ (faintly PAS +, deep purple with tetrachrome). Of these types β cells were localised to the cephalic lobe of the pars distalis, γ to the caudal lobe, while δ cells occurred in both lobes. The δ cells became hyperplastic in animals treated with thiourea and diminished in size with the administration of thyroxine, and were considered by the authors to be thyrotropic. As had been observed in the duck, however, these cells were strongly stimulated by castration in birds placed in appropriate long photoperiodic conditions, which also stimulate the gonadotropic (β) cells. Further studies on this problem by Tixier-Vidal, Chandola and Franquelin (1972) led to the conclusion that in the quail both thyrotropes and gonadotropes may be inhibited by thyroid hormones and by gonadal steroids. The γ cells were also thought to be probably gonadotropic in function.

Four types of acidophilic cells were also found: α cells staining orange were found in the caudal lobe; η cells, erythrosinophilic, were located at the periphery of the cephalic lobe; ϵ cells, which were PAS+, took up Orange G and stained fairly weakly with PbH, were found in the cephalic lobe, but only in birds treated with metopirone. The κ cells occurred throughout the pars distalis, and stained intensely black with PbH. The authors considered that η cells secreted prolactin; the ϵ cells ACTH; the κ cells MSH, and the α cells possibly STH. Comparable findings have been reported in other species studied. As with many mammals, problems of course remain. Notably, detailed knowledge of the precise function and nature of the hormones of the avian pituitary is not clear for many species, and Tixier-Vidal and her colleagues in their 1968 paper discussed the question of the two 'gonadotropic' cells. Assays of glands were carried out, but for 'total' gonadotropins. The β cells appear to be concerned with a hormone stimulating spermatogenesis, the γ cells with one stimulating interstitial cells (ICSH). But, as the authors comment, it is not yet certain that separate gonadotropins are present in the quail, and although they have been demonstrated in the chicken (Hartree and Cunningham, 1969) homologies based on staining characteristics may be unreliable. Furthermore, methods using radioimmunoassay (Follett, Scanes and Cunningham, 1971) indicate considerable chemical differences between mammalian and avian gonadotropins.

Despite the lack of a pars intermedia the avian gland does contain MSH, although this is commonly found in the cephalic part of the pars distalis. The cells described above, or at any rate cells resembling them, were first described in the pars distalis of the duck (Mialhe-Voloss and Benoit, 1954). In this species such cells are localised in the cephalic lobe in a region shown to be rich in MSH. The more general distribution of the κ cells in the quail, however, prevented such a correlation between cytology and demonstrable hormone.

The white-crowned sparrow has been used extensively by Farner and his colleagues in studies of effects of photoperiodicity on gonadal activity and in the course of this work many morphological studies of the hypothalamus and pituitary have been made. The description of the cytology of the pars distalis of this species (Matsuo *et al.* 1969) demonstrates that problems of homologies of cell types between different avian species are as considerable as in mammals, particularly when different staining techniques are used. Matsuo *et al.* observed two types of PAS+, AF− basophils, three types of acidophil, located in the caudal lobe, amphiphils showing either acidophilic or basophilic affinities according to the staining techniques used, and chromophobes. The authors, from evidence of seasonal changes, the effects of photoperiodic stimulation and castration, considered that gonadotropic activity could be attributed to basophils, but found no evidence for two distinct gonadotropic functions, in spite of the two types of cells to which such activity was attributed. Homologies between the other types of cell and those described by Tixier-Vidal *et al.* in the quail and by others are considered by the authors, and the problems involved are discussed.

THE PARS TUBERALIS

The general form of the avian pars tuberalis has been noted earlier, together with Wingstrand's (1951) comment that this division of the adenohypophysis is always present, although variable in the degree of development, even in different specimens of the same species. The part of the tuberalis which is closely applied to the surface of the brain lies within pia mater, and cells may penetrate the tissue of the median eminence in some species. Wingstrand also noted that cells of the pars tuberalis extending along the portal vessels and constituting the porto-tuberal tract are orientated along the vessels, and (1963) that in the region where the vessels enter the pars distalis a continuation of tuberalis cells can be seen lying between the cephalic and caudal lobes.

The cells of the pars tuberalis are described as having hyaline or faintly granular cytoplasm, some cells appearing distinctly more heavily granulated, and possibly secretory. Follicular formations and colloid are found.

ULTRASTRUCTURAL STUDIES

Interest in the cytology of the avian pars distalis has naturally led to studies of its fine structure. An early description of the ultrastructure of the gland of the domestic fowl was published by Payne (1946). Recently more detailed reports have been published by various workers who have been concerned with morphological and experimental studies of the avian endocrine system. Tixier-Vidal (1965) described the adenohypophysis of the duck and, with Assenmacher (1966), that of the pigeon. Mikami (1969) wrote on the pituitary of the fowl and white-crowned sparrow; and with co-authors (Mikami, Vitums and Farner, 1969) on the white-crowned sparrow.

Correlations with the types of cell identified by optical microscopy have been made, and functional significance studied by the usual techniques designed to bring about changes in activity and hence in morphology of various categories of secretory cells. Superficially at any rate the resemblance between avian and mammalian secretory cells when shown

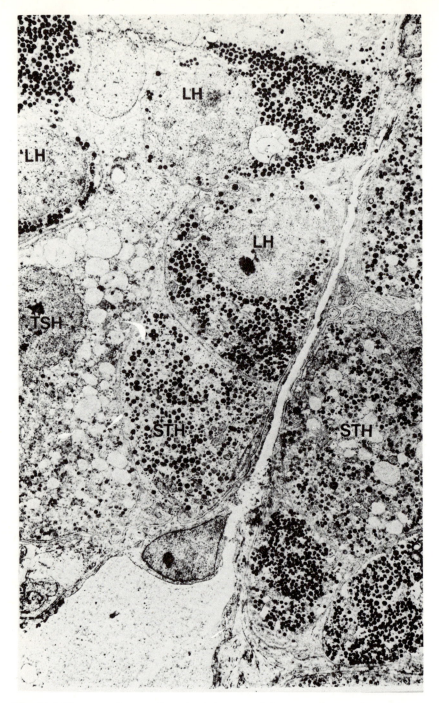

Fig. 14.4. Electron micrograph to show the general electron microscopic appearance of the pars distalis of the duck. The cells thought to secrete the various tropic hormones are lettered appropriately. (See list of abbreviations.) From Tixier-Vidal (1965).

by electron microscopy is close (fig. 14.4), and it is clearly tempting, if unwise, to suggest homologies on morphology alone; but authors have generally been aware of the possible error of such a course.

It may be sufficient in this context to note that the authors cited above consider that they have been able, with a fair degree of certainty, to identify the types of cell concerned with the various hormones. Seven types of cell were distinguished in the gland of the duck, six in that of the pigeon and six in the white-crowned sparrow. Mikami, Vitums and Farner (1969) in their paper dealing with the latter raise interesting problems – notably that they identified two types of gonadotrope, one (designated type A) with granules of about 200 nm in diameter, the other (type B) with granules of more variable size, 150–350 nm. Cells of each of the two types were found in both lobes of the pars distalis, and each showed morphological changes after castration, but on different time scales. Thyrotropic cells were identified by the changes they showed after thyroidectomy and appeared to be limited to the cephalic lobe. Tixier-Vidal, Follett and Farner (1967) had found thyrotropic cells in both lobes, although in another species, the Japanese quail; but in a later paper already referred to, Tixier-Vidal, Chandola and Franquelin (1972) noted that the reaction of presumed thyrotropes to surgical thyroidectomy varied in different parts of the gland, and that thyroidectomy cells developed only at the periphery of the cephalic lobe, while untransformed cells still persisted in both lobes. It may be, as the latter authors suggest, that regional variations in the concentration of hypothalamic releasing factors in different parts of the gland underlie such a differential reaction.

Further understanding of structural and functional aspects of the pars distalis no doubt depends on greater knowledge of the biochemical basis of the various avian adenohypophysial hormones, and of the inter-relationship between them. As in mammals, the authors whose work is discussed above found that interference with a 'single' endocrine system, such as by removal of the thyroid, brings about changes in secretory cells concerned with other tropic hormones – not perhaps surprising, but not easing the interpretation of the functional morphology of the pituitary.

THE MEDIAN EMINENCE

The morphology of the hypothalamic nuclei in birds has been recently reviewed by Dodd, Follett and Sharp (1971). The neurosecretory supra-optic and paraventricular nuclei give rise as in mammals to a supraoptico-hypophysial tract on each side. The tract differs from the mammalian one in two respects – it is generally richer in stainable (AF+) NSM, and it has two main destinations, the infundibular process (neural lobe) and the anterior part of the median eminence, which is also rich in NSM. Typical electron-dense NS granules (*c.* 150–200 nm) are present in supraoptic neurons (Oehmke *et al.* 1969) and although some neurons contain smaller granules (*c.* 100 nm) little trace of monoamines has been found either within these or in the anterior median eminence (see, e.g., Sharp and Follett, 1968).

As in the mammals, considerable interest is now being directed to the ultrastructural features of the avian median eminence in consideration of the hypothalamic control of the pars distalis which, as in the mammals, appears to be mediated by hypothalamic releasing factors. As in the reptiles, the median eminence can be divided into rostral and caudal zones by light microscopy, while passing from its deep (ventricular) to its superficial (pars tuberalis) aspects it has been variously subdivided into layers (see Wingstrand, 1951, and p. 327). An original simple subdivision into a zona interna and a zona externa (or glandular layer) has now given way to one of five layers; ependymal, sub-ependymal and fibrous (z. interna); reticular and palisade (z. externa) (see Oksche, 1962; Calas and Assenmacher, 1970).

There is general agreement that the fibrous layer is made up largely of nerve fibres containing 'typical' large electron-dense neurosecretory granules, destined for the neural lobe. These fibres are crossed at right angles by glial and ependymal processes which pass into the external zone, many ending on the surface. Electron microscopy has shown that the capillaries of the primary plexus of the portal vessels lie separated from the surface of the eminence by basement membrane and perivascular space. Their thin endothelial lining is fenestrated. These capillaries converge to preportal venules lying amid cells of the pars tuberalis, which are surrounded by a wide perivascular space (Mikami *et al.* 1970) which contain irregularly shaped perivascular cells. The portal venules themselves are invested with pericytes or fibroblasts. Direct endings on portal capillaries seem to be rare, and usually the flattened processes of glial and ependymal cells intervene.

The median eminence contains a number of different types of nerve fibres and nerve endings, classified according to the type of inclusion they contain. Published reports, however, differ on how many types of nerve ending occur; this may be due partly to the criteria used in assigning fibres to a given category, but also there appear to be considerable species differences. In the palisade layer of the duck, Calas and Assenmacher (1970) distinguished three types of fibre: I, containing granules measuring from 110 to 160 nm; II, axons with granules of *c.* 100 nm; and III, axons with electron-lucent vesicles (40–60 nm) alone. The latter type of inclusion was also observed within type I fibres. The authors considered that further subdivision might be possible, and that the main difference between rostral and caudal median eminence was in the proportion of the various types of fibre present. Peczely and Calas (1970) described a more elaborate zonation, both in depth and extent, for the median eminence of

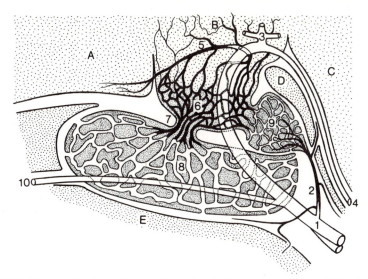

Fig. 14.5. Diagram to show the vessels of the pituitary of the pigeon *Columba livia*. A, Optic chiasma; B, diencephalon; C, medulla oblongata; D, dorsum sellae; E, bony floor of the sella; 1, internal carotid artery; 2, inferior hypophysial artery; 3, anterior branch and 4, posterior branch of the carotid artery; 5, infundibular artery; 6, primary capillary plexus on median eminence; 7, portal vessels; 8, secondary plexus of pars distalis; 9, capillary bed of the neural lobe; 10, internal ophthalamic artery. From Wingstrand (1951).

the pigeon, and reported changes brought about by experimental procedures designed to increase the release of ACTH from the pars distalis. But despite inevitable variations in different reports at this stage, a morphological basis for the complex controlling mechanism for the adenohypophysis seems to be becoming established for birds as for mammals.

THE VASCULAR SYSTEM

The anatomy of the vascular system of the avian pituitary has been described briefly by Green (1951) and in greater detail by Wingstrand (1951). Among other authors, Assenmacher (1952) dealt with the system in the duck, and Sharp and Follett (1969) with that in the quail.

The pattern of the arterial supply resembles in many respects that found in mammals. Thus the primary plexus of the median eminence (see p. 327) is supplied by 'infundibular' arteries (Wingstrand) arising from the internal carotid arteries (fig. 14.5) and drains via portal vessels in the pars distalis and thence to the cavernous sinus. In the duck Assenmacher described the supply to the plexus as being by 'tuberal' arterioles arising from superior hypophysial arteries. Wingstrand noted that the plexus of the median eminence is both largely independent of that of the neural lobe

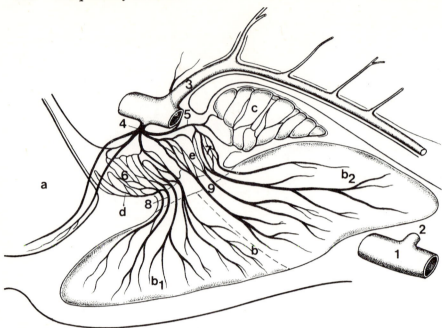

Fig. 14.6. Drawing to show the point-to-point distribution of blood from anterior and posterior median eminence to anterior and posterior parts, respectively, of the pars distalis in the white-crowned sparrow. a, optic chiasma; b_1 and b_2, cephalic and caudal lobes of the pars distalis; c, neural lobe; d, anterior and e, posterior; 1–9, divisions of median eminence vessels. Reproduced from Vitums *et al.* (1964), by permission of the authors and Springer-Verlag.

and also almost entirely isolated from the vascular bed of the rest of the hypothalamus. There is also general agreement that a direct supply to the pars distalis either does not occur, or is very slight and variable.

As noted elsewhere, the portal vessels, usually about 15–30 in number, run from the median eminence in association with cells of the pars tuberalis, the two forming the porto-tuberal tract, which is usually distinct from the infundibular stem. This separation enables the vessels to be divided without interruption of the nerve fibres passing the neural lobe. Benoit and Assenmacher (1953) performed this operation on drakes, and showed that such a lesion was followed by atrophy of the testes, and that the usual testicular response to increased exposure of the birds to light, namely hypertrophy and maturation of the spermatogenic epithelium, did not occur. These findings added to the evidence which pointed to the importance of the vascular link between the median eminence and the pituitary for normal gonadotropic activity.

A further feature of the avian vascular system is that there is good anatomical evidence that in at any rate some species there is a 'point to point' supply between the median eminence and the pars distalis, so that blood from the rostral part of the primary capillary plexus of the median eminence passes to the cephalic lobe of the pars distalis, while blood from the caudal median eminence passes to the caudal lobe (Vitums *et al.* 1964; Sharp and Follett, 1969) (fig. 14.6). Such an arrangement clearly might be of considerable relevance, particularly in view of the differences in cytology of the two lobes, the possible differences in the reaction of a single class of cells to a stimulus (see p. 333) and any variation in structure and function of different parts of the median eminence.

The blood supply to the neural lobe in birds apparently shows considerable variation in different species. Wingstrand described two major sources, the infundibular arteries arising above the pituitary (superior hypophysial arteries of Assenmacher) and inferior hypophysial vessels arising from the region of the inter-carotid anastomotic vessels lying behind the gland. Wingstrand noted that the former are the usual source in passerine birds. As already described the neural lobe and the pars distalis in birds are usually separated by a connective tissue lamina of variable thickness. Hence, it is not surprising that anastomoses between the vascular systems of the two parts are almost always lacking, so that the nerve fibres in the neural lobe are unlikely to influence adenohypophysial function via vascular connections.

It is not the intention to consider in this book the mechanisms concerned in control of the pituitary gland, which involve neural pathways extending well beyond the median eminence. Indeed, any full discussion of the basis for such control should deal both with the environmental factors such as the photoperiod, rainfall, availability of food, the presence of eggs in the nest and many others (see, for example, Marshall, 1964) which influence secretion of the gland, as well as with the way in which such environmental stimuli are transformed into the release or suppression of hypothalamic releasing factors. In effect, one would have to embark on a field of study which is really little understood, where microscopic neuroanatomy, neuropharmacology, and neurophysiology of virtually the whole of the nervous system come together. Problems of technique, of species differences and of interpretation of observed results abound. For birds, some of the studies involving hypothalamic mechanisms have been reviewed in the paper by Dodd, Follett and Sharp (1971) referred to above, and an exploration of this difficult area of investigative studies might well start from such a discussion. It may suffice here to note the opinion of these authors, firstly that the factors which control the release of gonadotropins in birds are probably similar chemically to those occurring in mammals, and that small celled AF— nuclei in the caudal hypothalamus are probably involved. Secondly, that in general the 'classical' neurosecretory system is concerned essentially with the neural lobe hormones and not largely involved in control of adenohypophysial activity.

15

SOME GENERAL CONSIDERATIONS

Much as is now known of the structure, function and mechanisms of control of the pituitary gland, many problems remain to be solved. Its structure, let alone function, has been subjected to detailed study in only a small proportion of the more than 60000 species of vertebrates. Even the pituitary glands of the rat and the frog, to each of which more attention has probably been devoted than to those of any other species, are still incompletely understood. Hence, it seems appropriate to conclude with a brief discussion of a few of the 'areas of uncertainty' which still remain.

PHYLOGENY

All vertebrates possess a pituitary gland, but none is present in any of the protochordates, the soft-bodied non-vertebrate creatures, included in the phylum Chordata. Since a small soft gland or its equally fragile precursor is a poor candidate for fossil immortality, any information in this respect must be gained from the embryology and comparative anatomy of living forms. Not surprisingly, therefore, many workers have attempted to find the homologue of the pituitary complex in some structure in living protochordates.

The lancelet or amphioxus (*Branchiostoma*) is one kind of protochordate. It is a small fish-like marine creature, burrowing in shallow seas and feeding by a complicated system of currents maintained by ciliary action, combined with the secretion of abundant mucus to trap and retain food particles carried by the water current. In the roof of the oral cavity is an asymmetrical diverticulum, *Hatschek's pit*, lined by glandular and ciliated cells and in contact with blood vessels. In the embryonic amphioxus the right pre-oral coelomic cavity opens into Hatschek's pit, a feature that has attracted great interest because in the embryos of a few vertebrates there is some connection between premandibular coelomic cavities and Rathke's pouch. The connection is absent in the majority of vertebrates and tenuous in most of the others, such as the duck, but in at least one elasmobranch (*Torpedo*) there is indeed an open duct between the first pair of embryonic premandibular coelomic cavities and Rathke's pouch. This arrangement is so strikingly reminiscent of the Hatschek's pit complex in the embryo of amphioxus that most authorities now accept the possibility that Hatschek's pit might be the homologue – in some ancestral form, the precursor – of Rathke's pouch, and so of the adenohypophysis.

The function of Hatschek's pit is uncertain; it may be olfactory, and it probably secretes mucus into the oral cavity as part of the feeding mechanism. In the light of this probable function it is interesting to note that in primitive actinopterygians the ventral part of Rathke's pouch persists as the hypophysial duct, and that the cells lining this duct are mucus-secreting and grade into the mucoid cells of the pharyngeal roof (chapters 9 and 10; Olsson, 1967). Furthermore, the basophils of the adenohypophysis of *Myxine* (chapter 7) are more like epidermal mucous cells than endocrine cells, and the secretion of a mucoid colloid into clefts or pseudofollicles occurs widely in the adenohypophysis of different vertebrates. In addition, of course, the glycoprotein pituitary hormones, FSH, LH and TSH, are chemically related to the mucoproteins of mucus. The thyroid gland provides a well-documented example of an endocrine organ derived in evolution from a mucus-secreting pharyngeal structure (the endostyle) which continues to secrete a glycoprotein (thyroglobulin) in its endocrine capacity, and a parallel can be drawn with the postulated derivation of the glycoprotein endocrine cells of the adenohypophysis from mucoid epithelial cells.

If we accept that Hatschek's pit might be the homologue of the adenohypophysis, then what of the neurohypophysis? Hatschek's pit is far removed from the anterior region of the nerve cord, but the hollow tip of the cord contains the so-called infundibular organ which, largely because its cells contain CAH+ granules, has been proposed as the homologue of the neurohypophysis. The infundibular organ, however, secretes Reissner's fibre, and so seems more likely to be homologous with the subcommissural organ and flexural organ of the vertebrate brain.

Related to the more remote ancestors of the vertebrates are the urochordates, sea-squirts and their allies, collectively called tunicates. Like amphioxus, these are marine ciliary-mucus feeders. Tunicates have a *sub-neural gland*, a hollow structure opening by a ciliated funnel into the dorsal roof of the pharynx. Its function is uncertain, but it may in part be chemosensory, responsive to the presence of tunicate eggs and sperm in the water and so perhaps playing a role in the co-ordination of spawning. The gland is in close contact with the ventral surface of the cerebral ganglion, the residual 'brain' of the adult tunicate, and indeed in embryology it is derived from the floor of 'brain vesicle' of the tadpole-like larvae.

The sub-neural gland thus somewhat resembles structurally Hatschek's pit. Embryologically, however, it is reminiscent of the vertebrate saccus infundibuli but in its connection with the pharyngeal cavity it resembles Rathke's pouch. To resolve this dilemma it has been proposed that the dorsal part of the sub-neural gland may represent the neurohypophysis and the ciliated funnel the adenohypophysis. Attempts to demonstrate endocrine activity in the sub-neural gland–cerebral ganglion complex, by testing extracted material in vertebrates, have, however, yielded no conclusive results, and at present we must regretfully accept that the phylogenetic status of this tunicate structure is uncertain. All that can be said in general is that possibly the earliest chordates had a tendency to form a dorsal stomodeal invagination, whether as a sensory structure or as a mucus-secreting feeding device, and that this tendency may be expressed in the vertebrates by Rathke's pouch.

Within the vertebrate groups, the picture is clearer. It is usually accepted that the adenohypophysis evolved from exocrine tissue (probably mucoid) in the stomodeal roof, whatever might be the relationship of this special stomodeal region to Hatschek's pit or sub-neural gland. There are signs that exocrine functions were retained by the earliest adenohypophysis; for example, early fossil fishes sometimes show a parasphenoid foramen, presumably indicative of a persistent hypophysial duct like that in living palaeoniscoid fishes and primitive teleosts (Mellinger, 1969; chapters 9 and 10). In these fossils, as in some of the primitive living actinopterygians, the mucus-secreting cells of the hypophysial duct would still presumably release their secretion into the pharynx (Olsson, 1967). Later, or possibly concurrently with this stage in evolution, as witness the state of the adenohypophysis in *Myxine* and palaeoniscoid fishes, some of the adenohypophysial cells presumably began to secrete directly into the blood. The newly evolved endocrine gland at some stage came under control of the brain, for which purpose the floor of the diencephalon differentiated to form hypophysiotropic neurosecretory centres. Neurosecretion is an ancient property of the central nervous system, and it is not surprising that it should have been selected as the mode of controlling the adenohypophysis. Elaboration of the PON–neural lobe system may well have preceded the differentiation of the hypophysiotropic centres, probably as a development of neurosecretory mechanisms inherited from protochordate ancestors. The widespread occurrence of neurosecretory cells in the brains of invertebrates, and the presence in the tunicate cerebral ganglion of neurosecretory cells which display changing activity correlated with the gonadal cycle (Bouchard-Madrelle and Lender, 1972) in the absence of any adenohypophysis, seem to support this theory. Whatever the details, it seems probable that the neurosecretory hypothalamic–neurohypophysial components of the pituitary complex are phylogenetically older than the endocrine adenohypophysis.

Two views are widely held concerning the more detailed evolution of the stomodeal component to give rise to the adenohypophysis. Many investigators have concluded that the proliferation of the stomodeal roof was such as to form a hollow invaginated gland, with an open duct to the pharynx, like that in primitive actinopterygians. Certainly the presence of a hollow Rathke's pouch in amniote and elasmobranch embryos and the frequent occurrence of clefts and spaces in the otherwise solid adenohypophysis of many fishes and of the apodan embryo is in favour of the idea that the original adenohypophysis was hollow.

On the other hand in most fishes and amphibians the adenohypophysis develops as a solid proliferation from the stomodeal roof; the hypophysial cleft, if present, appears later as a slit in the cell mass. As far as is known the cyclostome adenohypophysis buds from the roof of the nasopharyngeal duct as a solid cord, which proliferates into the discrete adenohypophysis of lampreys or forms the cell clumps or acini of myxinoids. Some workers have concluded on the evidence from the cyclostomes that the primitive adenohypophysis must have taken a form very like that of myxinoids, namely isolated cell clumps which only later in evolution became unified and differentiated as a typical adenohypophysis such as we find in lampreys. This view is usually taken to imply that the hollow Rathke's pouch (as found in elasmobranchs and tetrapods) is a later development, and hence that all speculation about Hatschek's pit and the sub-neural gland is irrelevant. However, this is to ignore the fact that the cell clumps of *Myxine* are commonly hollow, their lumina containing a PAS+ colloid, and that many of the myxinoid adenohypophysial cells are apparently exocrine and mucus-secreting (chapter 7). Thus it remains entirely possible that a hollow stomodeal invagination was the primordial condition, this giving rise either to hollow acini (myxinoids) or to a compact adenohypophysis (lampreys, gnathostomes), but always betraying its origin from a mucoid epithelium by containing cells secreting muco- or glyco-proteins, at first into the pharynx by way of a duct, and later into the bloodstream.

THE MEDIAN EMINENCE

With the development of understanding of the way in which neural control of the adenohypophysis is mediated, the great importance of the median eminence has come to be appreciated. Modified though this is in some vertebrates – in teleosts, for example, it is incorporated as the anterior part of the neural lobe, and in *Sphenodon* extends as finger-like processes into the pars tuberalis – its structure nevertheless shows a striking similarity in many different creatures, even in primitive forms such as the elasmobranchs and actinopterygians (chapter 9). The three-layered structure occurs also in many fishes and in all tetrapods, and at the ultrastructural level the pattern of close association between granule-containing nerve fibres and vessels has striking similarities in widely disparate forms. At less extreme resolutions the overall pattern of the neurovascular complexes does vary. Large and complex vascular spikes (chapter 6, II) occur in larger mammals, smaller ones having simpler capillary loop formations. In mammals the vascular complexes extend deeply into the neural tissue of the eminence, and often of the stalk, but in birds the vessels generally lie superficially and the nerve fibres traverse the eminence to make contact with them. Elaborate capillary loops also penetrate deeply into the median eminence in many fishes and amphibians.

TANYCYTES

During the last few years, during which the idea of hypothalamic releasing factors has become a reality, awareness has been growing of other possible ways in which the central nervous system might influence the activity of the pituitary complex. The portal vascular system clearly plays a dominant role in such control in a wide variety of species. The functional isolation of the portal vascular system has been emphasised, and the absence of any but 'insignificant' capillary anastomoses between the primary plexus in the median eminence and the vascular bed of the rest of the hypothalamus has been repeatedly affirmed. This view is no longer tenable; considerable anastomoses have been repeatedly observed in mammals (see for example Duvernoy, 1972) and although we as yet know little of their functional significance, they may well play an important role in pituitary activity.

Evidence is now accumulating that the CSF may be involved in the functioning of the pituitary complex. In this respect, note should be taken of the close association, in many mammals at any rate, between capillary loops of the primary plexus and the ependymal lining of the infundibular recess and hence their proximity to the CSF. Along with the possibility of such an association enabling the CSF to influence adenohypophysial activity we should also consider another apparent link between the CSF-ependyma and the gland, namely by tanycytes, cells extending across the median eminence from ependyma to either capillaries of the primary plexus or cells of the pars tuberalis (p. 92). Such cells are not limited to the region of the median eminence, but might play a special role there by either secreting into the CSF or absorbing material from it. Changes in the morphology of these cells with different stages of the reproductive cycle strengthen ideas that they may be involved in pituitary activity.

Ependymal cells in amphibia bear microvilli and cilia on their free surfaces and also extend via basal prolongations to end in relation to the pericapillary spaces of the primary plexus, thus resembling tanycytes (chapter 12). A similar ependymal specialisation is also found in relation to the neural lobe. In *Sphenodon*, for example, processes of ependymal cells traverse the lobe to terminate in end-feet on the plexus intermedius.

A different association is found in the lizard *Klauberiana*, in whose neural lobe NS fibres end on basal processes of ependymal cells and probably release their contents into these cells, whence they pass to the plexus intermedius. Such a transport role for ependymal cells has been likened to a similar role for pituicytes in birds and mammals.

A different type of specialisation in relation to CSF involves neurons rather than ependymal elements. These 'liquor-contacting neurons' (LCN) extend processes into the third ventricle. Not described in myxinoids, such cells are found in the PON of petromyzontids (lampreys) (chapter 7), elasmobranchs (chapter 8) and in palaeoniscoid fishes. In the latter the infundibular recess within the hollow neural lobe also contains LCN with ciliated swollen ends projecting into the cavity. In the sturgeon dendrites of neurons of both the NLT and PON pass into the third ventricle. In teleosts, in addition to cells of the PON and NLT, specialised cells lining the infundibular recess appear to send AF+ and PAS+ fibres towards the adenohypophysis: such cells may be homologous with the tanycytes of the mammalian median eminence.

Such LCN are not limited to aquatic vertebrates. They occur in amphibia, where the PON, infundibular nuclei and caudal aminergic nuclei all send processes into the third ventricle. In reptiles the cells of the PVN and infundibular nucleus (equivalent to the arcuate nucleus of mammals) show the same kind of arrangement.

STELLATE CELLS

The function of the specific secretory elements of both the adeno- and neuro-hypophysis is clear for many species but there is uncertainty as to the role played by some other elements found in the gland. Among the latter are the stellate or follicular cells referred to on p. 45. Cells of this type, probably homologous with those described in mammals, have been found in most classes of vertebrates, for example in *Myxine* and in the proximal pars distalis of lampreys. Pericavity cells lining the spaces of the adenohypophysis in elasmobranchs are also probably part of the stellate-follicular cell system, the spaces themselves being equivalent to the hypophysial cleft. In the teleost pars distalis neck cells and interstitial cells appear equivalent to stellate cells. These may form 'pseudofollicles', enclosing extracellular colloid, resembling the follicular cells of the rat; alternatively they may be stellate in shape with processes extending between the secretory cells; in *Gasterosteus* the cell bodies lie at the periphery of the gland (chapter 10).

Typical stellate cells occur in both the pars distalis and pars intermedia of amphibia, associated with the connective tissue capsule either by processes (pars distalis) or by the cell branches (pars intermedia). They occur in the pars distalis of reptiles, where they have been found to

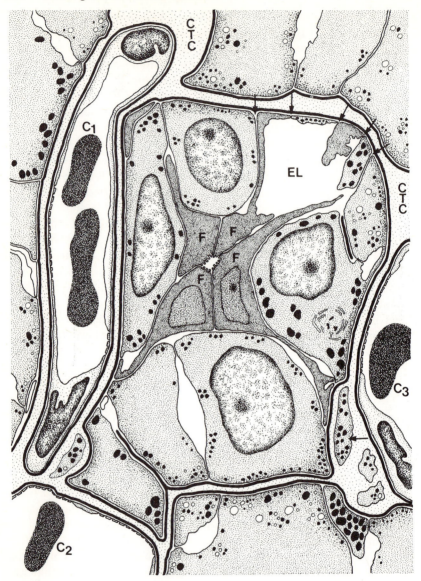

Fig. 15.1. Diagram summarising the relationship between follicular (stellate) cells and components of the rat adenohypophysis. Follicular cells (dark grey, F) lie in the centre of a cellular cord. Note their close association with granular cells, with lacunar spaces (EL) and (by cytoplasmic 'feet') with the basement membrane bounding the 'connective tissue compartment'(CTC) extending between the capillaries (C_1, C_2, and C_3). Reproduced from Vila-Porcile (1972) by permission of the author and Springer-Verlag.

hypertrophy in hypersecretion of TSH; in the pars intermedia they may form a partial capsule around the glandular tissue, processes extending between the glandular cells, as in the pars intermedia of *Anolis*, or in the thin intermedia of *Klauberiana* extending to reach the basement membrane of the plexus intermedius.

In all species in which the stellate elements have been adequately described they appear to be closely related to blood vessels, or at any rate to perivascular channels, by end-feet of cellular processes or by direct cytoplasmic contact with basement membranes (see fig. 15.1). Also they are often seen to be closely related to the granular cells of the adeno-hypophysis, and although liberation of hormone from the secretory cells takes place by exocytosis into the perivascular space, the stellate cells may play a part in some kind of intraglandular transport system, or in the regulation of the metabolism and circulation of the interstitial material as Vila-Porcile (1972) suggests in her extensive review of the topic.

The presence of colloid in the adenohypophysis of many species, including mammals, is interesting, but its function is not clear, and it is not enough to dismiss it as a phylogenetic remnant. It is very variable in its occurrence in different species, and it is sometimes associated with stellate cells. Often in mammals it occurs in the pars intermedia, less commonly, in abundance, in the pars distalis. In the glands of species such as the potto and slender loris, where colloid follicles are particularly abundant, many or even most of the cells which form the follicles are typical granular cells, and both the origin and significance of such colloid poses another problem as yet unsolved.

PITUICYTES

The role of pituicytes has long been an enigma. In general they have been thought of as modified glial cells, and as such assumed to act as 'sheath' cells for the neurohypophysial nerve fibres, and possibly to play a part in their metabolism. At a time before the functional organisation of the neurohypophysis was appreciated, the production of the posterior lobe hormones was attributed to these cells. Difficult to demonstrate satis-factorily by light microscopy, their true relationship to neural elements became apparent from electron microscopical studies. Neurosecretory nerve fibres may be not only closely apposed to pituicytes, but even invaginated into their cytoplasm, in the same way as non-myelinated peripheral nerve fibres in relation to Schwann cells. But, furthermore, neurohypophysial nerve fibres may make synaptoid contacts with pituicytes. In the sturgeon type B nerve fibres have been observed to contact neural-lobe ependymal cells, probably homologous with the pituicytes, while type A fibres end on pituicytes in the eel and other teleosts. Similarly, in Amphibia three different types of nerve fibre, type A

(PON), type B (aminergic) and type C (?cholinergic) have been described ending in such a manner. In Amphibia processes of pituicytes have been described ending on pericapillary spaces, suggesting a similarity to astrocytes.

Derived from the ependymal layer in embryogenesis, pituicytes naturally have affinities with ependymal cells. In the lizard *Klauberiana* they are rare and appear to be simply ependymal cells that have penetrated the neural tissue. In the neural lobe of reptiles, the number of pituicytes varies according to its form. When hollow and thin-walled, they are few in number, but when thick and solid they are numerous, so that there seems to be a kind of inverse ratio between volume and cell content.

Cells classed as pituicytes do not conform to a single morphological type, although the different appearances may simply indicate different functional states (p. 86). Various signs of functional activity have been described. In the eel they apparently secrete PAS + material into tube-like processes of the infundibular recess. In Amphibia as well as mammals there is now some indication that they may exert a phagocytic role, possibly in the disposal of neurophysins and the granule-bounding membranes after liberation of hormone from the neurosecretory nerve fibres (p. 283). Reactions of pituicytes to changes in the level of activity of the neurohypophysis have been described following light microscopic studies, for example increased mitotic activity in these cells, which were long considered not to divide, in dehydrated animals. More recently Kruslovic and Brückner (1969) have shown striking changes in response to dehydration, the cells becoming filled with large granules during the first weeks and then entering a phase of degeneration (p. 87). It is not possible yet to give a dogmatic answer to the question of the role of pituicytes in the functioning of the neurohypophysis, but there can be little doubt that they play an active role rather than a passive 'supportive' one in relation to the secretion of the posterior-lobe hormone.

We have referred here to only some of the topics, centred about the pituitary gland itself, on which further study is needed. In regions beyond the gland – the hypothalamus for example – the uncertainties of correlation of structure and function are even greater. At any rate the pituitary complex as an object of study is unlikely, in the foreseeable future, to lose its fascination for biologists.

ADDENDUM

Cyclostomes (pages 133–5). Ependymal cell processes probably interpose between nerve endings and vascular channels in both dorsal (type A and type B fibres) and ventral (type B fibres only) walls of the neurohypophysis of the hagfish *Eptatretus stouti*. The ependyma may serve to conduct and mediate the release of neurosecretory products into the circulation, and/or the nerve fibres may control ependymal cell functions such as secretion and phagocytosis (Henderson, N. E., 1972. *Acta Zool., Stockh.* **53**, 243–266).

Elasmobranchs (pages 145–6). Immunofluorescence techniques have confirmed in *Torpedo* the locations given here for ACTH and GtH. The ACTH cells are PAS + as described. However, the GtH cells are chromophobic, with rare secretory granules 100–200 nm in diameter. The ventral lobe PAS + cells appear to belong to the pericavity system (Mellinger, J. and Dubois, M. P., 1973. *C. r. hebd. Séanc. Acad. Sci., Paris* D **276**, 1879–1881).

(page 148). Detailed information is now available about the distribution of monoamines in the diencephalon and pituitary of the dogfish (*Scyliorhinus canicula*) (Wilson, J. F. and Dodd, J. M., 1973. *Z. Zellforsch. mikrosk. Anat.* **137**, 451–469).

Ganoid fishes (pages 153–69). The mucinous cells lining the hypophysial duct of *Calamoichthys* and *Polypterus* may be homologous with the adenohypophysial 'follicle boundary cells' of sturgeons, holosteans and some primitive teleosts. In sturgeons, the follicle boundary cells completely line the hypophysial cleft, its tubular extensions and the related closed follicles, including some in the pars intermedia. This arrangement recalls the pericavity cells of elasmobranchs. Chromophobic, often ciliated and apparently homologous with stellate cells (chapter 15), the follicle boundary cells appear to be involved in active exchanges with the colloid in the various spaces. Whereas in sturgeons they form a complete lining to the follicles, in *Amia* these cells are intercalated in the follicle walls between the endocrine cells; while in primitive teleosts such as the eel the follicle boundary cells are almost entirely replaced in the follicular wall by endocrine cells with specialised luminal surfaces which presumably subserve the role of exchanging material with the follicular colloid (Lagios, M. D., 1973. *Gen. comp. Endocr.* **20**, 362–376).

Amphibians (pages 250–60). Immunofluorescence techniques have confirmed the B1 cell as thyrotrope and the B2 cell as gonadotrope in *Xenopus laevis* (Doerr-Schott, J. and Dubois, M. P., 1972. *C. r. hebd. Séanc. Acad. Sci., Paris* D **275**, 1515–1518), and have confirmed the identifications given here of the cells secreting LTH, STH, ACTH, GtH and MSH in *Rana temporaria* (Doerr-Schott, J. and Dubois, M. P., 1973. *C. r. hebd. Séanc. Acad. Sci., Paris* D **276**, 2179–2182).

Reptiles (pages 295–304). Important information has now been published about the ultrastructure of the endocrine and stellate cells of the pars distalis of *Anolis carolinensis* (Pearson, A. K., Licht, P. and Zambrano, D., 1973. *Z. Zellforsch. mikrosk. Anat.* **137**, 293–312).

REFERENCES

Abolins, L. (1952). The visualization, by means of pyronin, of the RNA-system, indicating cytoplasmic protein synthesis in the anterior pituitary of the guinea-pig. *Expl Cell Res.* **3**, 1–9.

Abraham, M. (1971). The ultrastructure of the cell types and of the neurosecretory innervation in the pituitary of *Mugil cephalus* L. from fresh water, the sea, and a hypersaline lagoon. *Gen. comp. Endocrinol.* **17**, 334–350.

Acher, R. (1958). État naturel des principes ocytociques et vasopressiques de la neurohypophyse. In *Zweites Internationales Symposium über Neurosekretion* (Lund, 1957), pp. 71–78. Berlin: Springer-Verlag.

Acher, R., Chauvet, J. and Chauvet, M.-T. (1972). Identification de deux nouvelles hormones neurohypophysaires, la Valitocine (Val^8–ocytocine) et l'Aspartocine (Asn^4–ocytocine) chez un poisson sélacien, l'aiguillat (*Squalus acanthias*). *C. r. hebd. Séanc. Acad. Sci., Paris* D **274**, 313–316.

Acher, R., Chauvet, J. and Olivry, G. (1956). Sur l'existence éventuelle d'une hormone unique neurohypophysaire. Relation entre l'ocytocine, la vasopressine et la protéine de van Dyke extraites de la neurohypophyse du bœuf. *Biochim. biophys. Acta* **22**, 421–427.

Adams, C. W. M. (1956). A stricter interpretation of the ferricyanide reaction with particular reference to the demonstration of protein-bound sulphydryl and disulphide groups. *J. Histochem. Cytochem.* **4**, 23–35.

Adams, C. W. M. and Sloper, J. C. (1956). The hypothalamic elaboration of the posterior pituitary principles in man, the rat and dog. Histochemical evidence derived from performic acid–Alcian blue reaction for cystine. *J. Endocr.* **13**, 221–228.

Adams, C. W. M. and Swettenham, K. V. (1958). The histochemical identification of two types of basophil cell in the normal human adenohypophysis. *J. Path. Bact.* **75**, 95–103.

Adams, J. H., Daniel, P. M. and Prichard, M. M. L. (1963). The volumes of pars distalis, pars intermedia and infundibular process of the pituitary gland of the rat, with special reference to the effect of stalk section. *Q. Jl exp. Physiol.* **48**, 217–254.

Adams, J. H., Daniel, P. M. and Prichard, M. M. L. (1966). Observations on the portal circulation of the pituitary gland. *Neuroendocrinology* **1**, 193–213.

Adams, J. H., Daniel, P. M., Prichard, M. M. L. and Schurr, P. H. (1963). The volume of the infarct in pars distalis of a human pituitary gland, 30 hours after transection of the pituitary stalk. *J. Physiol., Lond.* **166**, 39–41 P.

Adamsons, K., Engel, S. L., Van Dyke, H. B. and Schmidt-Nielsen, B. (1956). The distribution of oxytocin and vasopressin (antidiuretic hormone) in the neurohypophysis of the camel. *Endocrinology* **58**, 272–278.

Addison, W. H. F. (1917). The cell changes in the hypophysis of the albino rat after castration. *J. comp. Neurol.* **28**, 441–461 P.

Aler, G. M. (1970). Prolactin cells: study of the pituitary gland of the roach

(*Leuciscus rutilus*) by immuno-histochemical methods. *Acta zool., Stockh.* **51**, 149–157.

Aler, G. M. (1971*a*). The study of prolactin in the pituitary gland of the Atlantic eel (*Anguilla anguilla*) and the Atlantic salmon (*Salmo salar*) by immuno-fluorescence technique. *Acta zool., Stockh.* **52**, 145–156.

Aler, G. M. (1971*b*). Prolactin-producing cells in *Clupea harengus membras, Polypterus palmas* and *Calamoichthys calabaricus* studied by immuno-histo-chemical methods. *Acta zool., Stockh.* **52**, 275–286.

Aler, G. M., Båge, G. and Fernholm, B. (1971). On the existence of prolactin in cyclostomes. *Gen. comp. Endocr.* **16**, 498–503.

Allanson, M., Foster, C. L. and Menzies, G. (1959). Some observations on the cytology of the adenohypophysis of the non-parous female rabbit. *Q. Jl microsc. Sci.* **100**, 463–482.

Allen, B. M. (1920). Experiments in the transplantation of the hypophysis of adult *Rana pipiens* to tadpoles. *Science, N.Y.* **52**, 274–276.

Alluchon-Gérard, M. J. (1971). Types cellulaires et étapes de la différenciation de l'adénohypophyse chez l'embryon de roussette (*Scyllium canicula, Chondrich-thyens*). Étude au microscope électronique. *Z. Zellforsch. mikrosk. Anat.* **120**, 525–545.

Anand Kumar, T. C. and Knowles, F. (1967). A system linking the third ventricle with the pars tuberalis of the Rhesus monkey. *Nature, Lond.* **215**, 54–55.

Anand, B. K., Malkani, P. K. and Dua, S. (1957). Effect of electrical stimulation of the hypothalamus on menstrual cycle in monkey. *Indian J. med. Res.* **45**, 499–502.

Aoki, K. and Uemura, H. (1970). Cell types in the pituitary of the medaka, *Oryzias latipes. Endocr. jap.* **17**, 45–56.

Aplington, H. W. (1942). Correlative cyclical changes in the hypophysis and gonads of *Necturus maculosus. Am. J. Anat.* **70**, 201–250.

Aplington, H. W. (1962). Cellular changes in the pituitary of *Necturus* following thyroidectomy. *Anat. Rec.* **143**, 133–145.

Aplington, H. W. and Tedrow, B. W. (1968). Distribution of thyrotrophic activity in the hypophysis of *Necturus* before and after thyroidectomy as measured by I[131] bioassay in mice. *Anat. Rec.* **160**, 273–278.

Aplington, H. W. and Vernikos-Danellis, J. (1968). Distribution of ACTH in the hypophysis of *Necturus. Anat. Rec.* **161**, 441–446.

Arey, L. B. (1950). The craniopharyngeal canal reviewed and reinterpreted. *Anat. Rec.* **106**, 1–16.

Arnott, D. G. and Sloper, J. C. (1958). The distribution of ^{35}S in the hypothalamo-neurohypophysial 'neurosecretory' system of the rat following the intracisternal injection of ^{35}S-labelled DL-cysteine. *J. Anat.* **92**, 635–636.

Aschner, B. (1912). Über die Funktion der Hypophyse. *Pflügers Arch. ges. Physiol.* **146**, 1–146.

Assenmacher, I. (1952). La vascularisation du complexe hypophysaire chez le canard domestique. I. La vascularisation du complexe hypophysaire adulte. *Archs Anat. microsc. Morph. exp.* **41**, 69–106.

Atwell, W. J. (1938). The function of the pars tuberalis. In *The pituitary gland. Res. Publs. Ass. Res. nerv. ment. Dis.* **17**, 377–391.

Bachrach, D. (1957). Über einige Probleme der hypothalamischen Neurosekretion. I. Beitrage zur Herkunft des Neurosekrets. *Z. Zellforsch. mikrosk. Anat.* **46**, 457–473.

Bachrach, D. and Köszegi, B. (1957). Über einige Probleme der hypothalamischen Neurosekretion. II. Änderungen der basophilen Substanz (Ribonucleinsäuregehalt) der Ganglienzelle zur Zeit der Abnahme bzw. Bildung der Neurosekrets der Ratte. *Z. Zellforsch. mikrosk. Anat.* **46**, 474–483.

Bailey, P. (1921). Cytological observations on the pars buccalis of the hypophysis cerebri of man, normal and pathological. *J. med. Res.* **42**, 349–381.

Bailey, P. and Davidoff, L. M. (1925). Concerning the microscopic structure of the hypophysis cerebri in acromegaly. *Am. J. Path.* **1**, 185–207.

Baker, B. I. and Ball, J. N. (1970). Background adaptation and the pituitary in teleosts. *J. Endocr.* **48**, xxvi.

Baker, J. R. (1958). *Principles of biological microtechnique.* London: Methuen and Co.

Ball, J. N. (1962). Brood production after hypophysectomy in the viviparous teleost *Mollienesia latipinna* Le Sueur. *Nature, Lond.* **194**, 787.

Ball, J. N. (1969). Prolactin (fish prolactin or paralactin) and growth hormone. In *Fish physiology* (ed. W. S. Hoar and D. J. Randall), vol. ɪɪ, pp. 207–240. New York and London: Academic Press.

Ball, J. N. (1970). Unpublished observations.

Ball, J. N. and Baker, B. I. (1969). The pituitary gland: anatomy and histophysiology. In *Fish physiology* (ed. W. S. Hoar and D. J. Randall), vol. ɪɪ, pp. 1–110. New York and London: Academic Press.

Ball, J. N., Baker, B. I., Olivereau, M. and Peter, R. E. (1972). Investigations on hypothalamic control of adenohypophysial functions in teleost fishes. *Gen. comp. Endocr. Suppl.* **3**, 11–21.

Ball, J. N., Chester Jones, I., Foster, M. E., Hargreaves, G., Hawkins, E. F. and Milne, K. P. (1971). Measurement of plasma cortisol levels in the eel (*Anguilla anguilla*) in relation to osmotic adjustments. *J. Endocr.* **50**, 75–96.

Ball, J. N. and Ingleton, P. M. (1973). Adaptive variations in prolactin secretion in relation to external salinity in the teleost *Poecilia latipinna. Gen. comp. Endocr.* **20**, 312–325.

Ball, J. N. and Olivereau, M. (1966). Experimental identification of the ACTH cells in the pituitary of two teleosts, *Poecilia latipinna* and *Anguilla anguilla*: correlated changes in the interrenal and in the pars distalis resulting from the administration of metopirone (su 4885). *Gen. comp. Endocr.* **6**, 5–18.

Ball, J. N., Olivereau, M., Slicher, A. M. and Kallman, K. D. (1965). Functional capacity of ectopic pituitary transplants in the teleost *Poecilia formosa*, with a comparative discussion on the transplanted pituitary. *Phil. Trans. R. Soc. Ser. B* **249**, 69–99.

Bandaranayake, R. C. (1971). A morphology of the accessory neurosecretory nuclei and of the retrochiasmatic part of the supraoptic nucleus of the rat. *Acta anat.* **80**, 14–22.

Barannikova, I. A. (1949). Localisation of gonadotropic function in the hypophysis of the sturgeon (*Acipenser stellatus*). *Dokl. Akad. Nauk SSSR* **69**, 117–120.

Barannikova, I. A. (1954). Completion of sexual maturation in autumn-running female sturgeons after exclusion of the period of the river spawning migration. *Dokl. Akad. Nauk SSSR* **99**, 641–644.

Barer, R., Heller, H. and Lederis, K. (1963). The isolation, identification and properties of the hormonal granules of the neurohypophysis. *Proc. R. Soc. Ser. B* **158**, 388–416.

Barer, R. and Lederis, K. (1966). Ultrastructure of the rabbit neurohypophysis with special reference to the release of hormones. *Z. Zellforsch. mikrosk. Anat.* **75**, 201–239.

Bargmann, W. (1949). Über die neurosekretorische Verknüpfung von Hypothalamus und Neurohypophyse. *Z. Zellforsch. mikrosk. Anat.* **34**, 610–634.

Bargmann, W. (1951). Zwischenhirn und Neurohypophyse; eine neue Vorstellung über die funktionelle Bedeutung des Hinterlappens. *Med. Mschr. Stuttgart* **5**, 466–470.

Bargmann, W. and von Gaudecker, B. R. (1969). Über die Ultrastruktur neurosekretorischer Elementargranula. *Z. Zellforsch. mikrosk. Anat.* **96**, 495–504.

Bargmann, W. and Scharrer, E. (1951). The site of origin of the hormones of the posterior pituitary. *Am. Scient.* **39**, 255–259.

Bargmann, W. and Scharrer, E. (1970). *Aspects of neuroendocrinology.* Berlin, Heidelberg, New York: Springer-Verlag.

Barnes, B. G. (1962). Electron microscope studies on the secretory cytology of the mouse anterior pituitary. *Endocrinology* **71**, 618–628.

Barrnett, R. J., Ladman, A. J., McAllaster, N. J. and Siperstein, E. (1956). The localisation of glycoprotein hormones in the anterior pituitary glands of rats investigated by differential protein solubilities, histological stains and bio-assays. *Endocrinology* **59**, 398–418.

Barrnett, R. J. and Seligman, A. M. (1954). Histochemical demonstration of sulf-hydryl and disulfide groups of protein. *J. natn. Cancer Inst.* **14**, 769–792.

Barrnett, R. J., Siperstein, E. and Josimovich, J. B. (1956). The localisation of simple protein hormones in the adenohypophysis demonstrated by combined use of differential protein solubilities, histochemical staining and bio-assay. *Anat. Rec.* **124**, 388.

Barry, J. (1960). Recherches sur l'innervation hypothalamique: l'éminence médiane chez le cobaye. *Archs Anat. Histol. Embryol.* **43**, 187–194.

Bartke, A. (1964). Histology of the anterior hypophysis, thyroid and gonads of two types of dwarf mice. *Anat. Rec.* **149**, 225–235.

Baumgarten, H. G., Björklund, A., Holstein, A. F. and Nobin, A. (1972). Organization and ultrastructural identification of the catecholamine nerve terminals in the neural lobe and pars intermedia of the rat pituitary. *Z. Zellforsch. mikrosk. Anat.* **126**, 483–517.

Beato, V. (1935). Über die Pars Intermedia der Hypophyse bei den Haustieren. *Endokrinologie* **15**, 145–152.

Benoit, J. and Assenmacher, I. (1953). Rapport entre la stimulation sexuelle pré-hypophysaire et la neurosécrétion chez l'oiseau. *Archs Anat. microsc. Morph. exp.* **42**, 334–386.

Berkley, H. J. (1894). The finer anatomy of the infundibular region of the cerebrum including the pituitary gland. *Brain* **17**, 515–547.

Bern, H. A. (1967). The hormonogenic properties of neurosecretory cells. In *Neurosecretion* (IVth International Symposium on Neurosecretion (Strasbourg, 25–27 July 1966)), pp. 5–7. Berlin, Heidelberg, New York: Springer-Verlag.

Bern, H. A. and Nicoll, C. S. (1968). The comparative endocrinology of prolactin. *Recent Prog. Horm. Res.* **24**, 681–720.

Bern, H. A., Zambrano, D. and Nishioka, R. S. (1971). Comparison of the innervation of the pituitary of two euryhaline teleosts, *Gillichthys mirabilis* and *Tilapia mossambica*, with special reference to the origin and nature of type 'B' fibres. *Mem. Soc. Endocr.* **19**, 817–822.

Biedermann, G. (1927). Über das farberische Verhalten der Epithelien der mensch-lichen Hypophyse. *Virchows Arch. path. Anat. Physiol.* **264**, 217–223.

Billard, R., Breton, B. and Dubois, M. P. (1971). Immunocytologie et histochimie des cellules gonadotropes et thyréotropes hypophysaires chez la carpe *Cyprinus carpio. C. r. hebd. Séanc. Acad. Sci., Paris* D **272**, 981–983.

Bissonnette, T. H. (1938). The influence of light upon pituitary activity. In *The pituitary gland. Res. Publs Ass. Res. nerv. ment. Dis.* **17**, 361–376.

Blanc-Livni, N. and Abraham, M. (1970). The influence of environmental salinity on the prolactin- and gonadotropin-secreting regions in the pituitary of *Mugil* (Teleostei). *Gen. comp. Endocr.* **14**, 184–197.

Bock (1817). *Beschreibung des fünften Hirnnerven.* Leipzig. (Cited by Romeis, 1940.)

Bodian, D. (1951). Nerve endings, neurosecretory substance and lobular organisation of the neurohypophysis. *Bull. Johns Hopkins Hosp.* **89**, 354–376.

Bodian, D. (1963). Cytological aspects of neurosecretion in opossum neurohypophysis. *Bull. Johns Hopkins Hosp.* **113**, 57–93.

Boeke, J. (1940). *Problems of nervous anatomy.* Oxford University Press.

Boisseau, J. P. (1967). Les régulations hormonales de l'incubation chez un vertébré mâle: recherches sur la réproduction de l'hippocampe. Thesis, Faculty of Science, University of Bordeaux.

Bouchard-Madrelle, C. and Lendron, Th. (1972). Mise en évidence de la neurosécrétion et étude de sa variation chez *Ciona intestinalis* (tunicier), au cours du développement et de la régénération des gonades. *Annls Endocr., Paris* **33**, 129–138.

Boyd, J. D. (1956). Observations on the human pharyngeal hypophysis. *J. Endocr.* **14**, 66–77.

Bradshaw, S. D. and Waring, H. (1969). Comparative studies on the biological activity of melanin-dispersing hormone (MDH). *Colloque Internatl CNRS, Paris* **177**, 135–152.

Brahms, S. (1932). The development of the hypophysis of the cat. *Am. J. Anat.* **50**, 251–283.

Breton, B., Jalabert, B., Billard, R. and Weill, C. (1971). Stimulation *in vitro* de la libération d'hormone gonadotrope hypophysaire par un facteur hypothalamique chez la carpe *Cyprinus carpio* L. *C. r. hebd. Séanc. Acad. Sci., Paris* **D 273**, 2591–2594.

Breton, B., Kann, G., Bursawa-Gérard, E. and Billard, R. (1971). Dosage radioimmunologique d'une hormone gonadotrope de carpe (*Cyprinus carpio* L.). *C. r. hebd. Séanc. Acad. Sci., Paris* **D 272**, 1515–1517.

Breton, B., Weill, C., Jalabert, B. and Billard, R. (1972). Activité réciproque des facteurs hypothalamiques de bélier (*Ovis aries*) et de poissons téléostéens sur la sécrétion *in vitro* des hormones gonadotropes c-HG et LH respectivement par des hypophyses de carpe et de belier. *C. r. hebd. Séanc. Acad. Sci., Paris* **D 274**, 2530–2533.

Briggs, F. N. and Munson, P. L. (1955). Studies on the mechanism of stimulation of ACTH secretion with the aid of morphine as a blocking agent. *Endocrinology* **57**, 205–219.

Brooks, C. McC. and Gersh, I. (1941). Innervation of the hypophysis of the rabbit and rat. *Endocrinology* **28**, 1–5.

Brown, P. S. and Brown, S. C. (1971). Growth and metabolic effects of prolactin and growth hormone in the red-spotted newt, *Notophthalmus viridescens*. *J. exp. Zool.* **178**, 29–34.

Brown, P. S. and Frye, B. E. (1969a). Effects of prolactin and growth hormone on growth and metamorphosis of tadpoles of the frog, *Rana pipiens*. *Gen. comp. Endocr.* **13**, 126–138.

Brown, P. S. and Frye, B. E. (1969b). Effect of hypophysectomy, prolactin and growth hormone on growth of postmetamorphic frogs. *Gen. comp. Endocr.* **13**, 139–145.

Büchmann, N. B., Spies, I. and Vijayakumar, S. (1972). Hypophysial corticotropic function and its hypothalamic control in *Bufo bufo* (L) evaluated by the plasma concentration of corticosterone. *Gen. comp. Endocr.* **18**, 306–314.

Bucy, P. C. (1930). The pars nervosa of the bovine hypophysis. *J. comp. Neurol.* **50**, 505–519.

Budtz, P. E. (1970). Effect of transection at different levels of hypothalamus on the hypothalamo-hypophysial system of the toad *Bufo bufo*, with particular reference to the ultrastructure of the zona externa of the median eminence. *Z. Zellforsch. mikrosk. Anat.* **107**, 210–233.

Bunt, A. H. (1969). Fine structure of the pars distalis and interrenals of *Taricha torosa* after administration of metopirone (SU 4885). *Gen. comp. Endocr.* **12**, 134–147.

Burgers, A. C. J. (1963). Melanophore-stimulating hormones in vertebrates. *Ann. N.Y. Acad. Sci.* **100**, 669–677.

Burlet, A. and Legait, H. (1967). Étude histophysiologique et expérimentale des lobes tubéraux de la grenouille verte *Rana esculenta. Bull. Assoc. Anat.* **52**, 286–291.

Burzawa-Gérard, E. and Fontaine, Y. A. (1972). The gonadotropins of lower vertebrates. *Gen. comp. Endocr. Suppl.* **3**, 715–728.

Cajal, S. Ramon y (1894). Cited in Cajal (1911). *Histologie du système nerveux*, vol. II, pp. 487–491. Paris.

Calas, A. and Assenmacher, I. (1970). Ultrastructure de l'éminence médiane du canard (*Anas platyrhynchos*). *Z. Zellforsch. mikrosk. Anat.* **109**, 64–82.

Callard, I. P. and Chester Jones, I. (1970). The effect of hypothalamic lesions and hypophysectomy on adrenal weight in *Sceloporus cyanogenys. Gen. comp. Endocr.* **17**, 194–202.

Callard, I. P. and McConnell, W. F. (1969). Effects of intra-hypothalamic estrogen implants on ovulation in *Sceloporus cyanogenys. Gen. comp. Endocr.* **13**, 496.

Callard, I. P. and Willard, E. (1969). Hypothalamic steroid implants and adrenal size in male *Sceloporus cyanogenys. Gen. comp. Endocr.* **13**, 496.

Cameron, E. and Foster, C. L. (1972). Some light- and electron-microscopical observations on the pars tuberalis of the pituitary gland of the rabbit. *J. Endocr.* **54**, 505–511.

Campbell, D. J. and Holmes, R. L. (1966). Further observations on the neuro-hypophysis of the hedgehog. *Z. Zellforsch. mikrosk. Anat.* **75**, 35–46.

Campbell, H. J., Feuer, G. and Harris, G. W. (1964). The effect of intrapituitary infusion of median eminence and other brain extracts on anterior pituitary gonadotrophic secretion. *J. Physiol., Lond.* **170**, 474–486.

Cardell, R. R. (1964a). Observations on the cell types of the salamander pituitary gland: an electron microscope study. *J. ultrastruct. Res.* **10**, 317–333.

Cardell, R. R. (1964b). Ultrastructure of the salamander thyroidectomy cell. *J. ultrastruct. Res.* **10**, 515–527.

Cardell, R. R. (1969). The ultrastructure of stellate cells in the pars distalis of the salamander pituitary gland. *Am. J. Anat.* **126**, 429–456.

Castell, M. (1972). Ultrastructure of the anuran pars intermedia following severance of hypothalamic connection. *Z. Zellforsch. mikrosk. Anat.* **131**, 545–557.

Catchpole, H. R. (1947). Cellular distribution of glycoprotein of the anterior lobe of the pituitary gland. *Fedn Proc. Fedn Am. Socs exp. Biol.* **6**, 88.

Catchpole, H. R. (1948). Cell fractionation and gonadotrophin assays of anterior pituitary glands. *Fedn Proc. Fedn Am. Socs exp. Biol.* **7**, 19.

Chester Jones, I., Ball, J. N., Sandor, T., Henderson, I. W. and Baker, B. I. (1973). The endocrinology of fish. In *Chemical zoology* (ed. M. Florkin and B. T. Scheer), vol. 8. New York and London: Academic Press.

Chester Jones, I., Chan, D. K. O., Henderson, I. W. and Ball, J. N. (1969). The adrenal corticosteroids, adrenocorticotropin and the corpuscles of Stannius. In

Fish physiology (ed. W. S. Hoar and D. J. Randall), vol. II, pp. 322–376. New York and London: Academic Press.

Chevins, P. F. D. (1968). The anatomy and physiology of the pituitary complex in the genus *Raia*, Elasmobranchii. Ph.D. Thesis, University of Leeds.

Chevins, P. F. D. (1972). Ultrastructure of the pars intermedia in the skate (genus *Raia, Elasmobranchii*). *Gen. comp. Endocr.* **18**, 582.

Chevins, P. F. D. and Dodd, J. M. (1970). Pituitary innervation and control of colour change in the skates *Raia naevus, R. clavata, R. montagui* and *R. radiata*. *Gen. comp. Endocr.* **15**, 232–241.

Clark, W. E. le Gros. (1938). Morphological aspects of the hypothalamus. In *The hypothalamus* (by W. E. le Gros Clark, J. Beattie, G. Riddock and N. M. Dott), pp. 1–68. Edinburgh and London: Oliver and Boyd.

Clarke, J. R. and Forsyth, I. A. (1964). Seasonal changes in the adenohypophysis of the vole (*Microtus agrestis*). *Gen. comp. Endocr.* **4**, 243–252.

Clauss, R.-O. and Doerr-Schott, J. (1970). Ultrastructure de l'hypophyse distale de *Bombina variegata. C. r. hebd. Séanc. Acad. Sci., Paris* D **271**, 1100–1103.

Clegg, M. T., Santolucito, J. A., Smith, J. D. and Ganong, W. F. (1958). The effect of hypothalamic lesions on sexual behaviour and estrous cycles in the ewe. *Endocrinology* **62**, 790–797.

Clementi, F., Ceccarelli, B., Cerati, E., Demonte, M. L., Felici, M., Motta, M. and Pecile, A. (1970). Subcellular localization of neurotransmitters and releasing factors in the rat median eminence. *J. Endocr.* **48**, 205–213.

Cleveland, R. and Wolfe, J. M. (1932). A differential stain for the anterior lobe of the hypophysis. *Anat. Rec.* **51**, 409–413.

Cohen, D. C., Greenberg, J. A., Licht, P., Bern, H. A. and Zipser, R. D. (1972). Growth and inhibition of metamorphosis in the newt *Taricha torosa* by mammalian hypophysial and placental hormones. *Gen. comp. Endocr.* **18**, 384–390.

Compher, M. K. and Dent. J. N. (1970). Responses to thiourea and to surgical thyroidectomy by the autotransplanted pituitary gland in the red spotted newt. *Gen. comp. Endocr.* **14**, 141–147.

Coons, A. H. (1956). Histochemistry with labelled antibody. *Int. Rev. Cytol.* **5**, 1–23.

Coons, A. H., Creech, H. J., Jones, R. N. and Berliner, E. (1942). The demonstration of pneumococcal antigen in tissues by the use of fluorescent antibody. *J. Immun.* **45**, 159–170.

Copeland, D. E. (1943). Cytology of the pituitary gland in developing and adult *Triturus viridescens. J. Morph.* **72**, 379–409.

Cowdry, E. V. (1922). Anatomy, embryology, comparative anatomy and histology of the hypophysis cerebri. In *Barker's Endocrinology and Metabolism*, vol. I, pp. 704–718. New York: Appleton and Co.

Crighton, D. B. and Schneider, H. P. G. (1969). Localisation of luteinising hormone-releasing factor in the pre-optic area. *J. Reprod. Fert.* **18**, 166.

Croll, M. M. (1928). Nerve fibres in the pituitary of a rabbit. *J. Physiol., Lond.* **66**, 316–322.

Cross, B. A. (1966). Neural control of oxytocin secretion. In *Neuroendocrinology* (ed. L. Martini and W. F. Gangong), vol. 1, pp. 217–259. New York and London: Academic Press.

Cushing, H. (1909). The hypophysis cerebri: clinical aspects of hyperpituitarism and hypopituitarism. *J. Am. med. Ass.* **53**, 249–255.

Cushing, H. (1912). *The pituitary body and its disorders*. Philadelphia and London: Lippincott Co.

Cushing, H. (1932). The basophil adenomas of the pituitary body and their clinical manifestations (pituitary basophilism). *Bull. Johns Hopkins Hosp.* **50**, 137–198.

Dahlström, A. and Fuxe, K. (1966). Monoamines and the pituitary gland. *Acta endocr., Copnh.* **51**, 301–314.

Dandy, W. E. (1913). The nerve supply to the pituitary body. *Am. J. Anat.* **51**, 333–343.

Daniel, A. R. and Lederis, K. (1963). Hormone release from the neurohypophysis *in vitro. Gen. comp. Endocr.* **3**, 693–694.

Daniel, A. R. and Lederis, K. (1966). Effects of ether anaesthesia and haemorrhage on hormone content and ultrastructure of the rat neurohypophysis. *J. Endocr.* **34**, 91–104.

Daniel, P. M. (1966). The blood supply of the hypothalamus and the pituitary gland. *Br. med. Bull.* **22**, 202–208.

Daniel, P. M. and Prichard, M. M. L. (1956). Anterior pituitary necrosis. Infarction of the pars distalis produced experimentally in the rat. *Q. Jl exp. Physiol.* **41**, 215–229.

Daniel, P. M. and Prichard, M. M. L. (1957*a*). The vascular arrangements of the pituitary gland of the sheep. *Q. Jl exp. Physiol.* **42**, 237–248.

Daniel, P. M. and Prichard, M. M. L. (1957*b*). Anterior pituitary necrosis in the sheep produced by section of the pituitary stalk. *Q. Jl exp. Physiol.* **42**, 248–254.

Daniel, P. M. and Prichard, M. M. L. (1958). The effects of pituitary stalk section in the goat. *Am. J. Path.* **34**, 433–469.

Daniel, P. M., Prichard, M. M. L. and Schurr, P. H. (1958). Extent of the infarct in the anterior lobe of the human pituitary gland after stalk section. *Lancet* i, 101–103.

Davidson, J. M. and Sawyer, C. H. (1961). Effects of localized intracerebral implantation of oestrogen on reproductive function in the female rabbit. *Acta endocr., Copnh.* **37**, 385–393.

Dawson, A. B. (1937). The relationships of the epithelial components of the pituitary gland of the rabbit and cat. *Anat. Rec.* **69**, 471–485.

Dawson, A. B. (1938). The epithelial components of the pituitary gland of the opossum. *Anat. Rec.* **72**, 181–193.

Dawson, A. B. (1942). Some morphological aspects of the secretory process. *Fedn Proc. Fedn Am. Socs exp. Biol.* **1**, 233–240.

Dawson, A. B. (1948). The relationship of pars tuberalis to pars distalis in the hypophysis of the rhesus monkey. *Anat. Rec.* **102**, 103–121.

Dawson, A. B. and Friedgood, H. B. (1938). Differentiation of two classes of acidophiles in the anterior pituitary of the female rabbit and cat. *Stain Technol.* **13**, 17–21.

Dawson, D. C. and Ralph, C. L. (1971). Neural control of the amphibian pars intermedia: electrical responses evoked by illumination of the lateral eyes. *Gen. comp. Endocr.* **16**, 611–614.

Del Conte, E. (1969). The corticotroph cells of the anterior pituitary gland of a reptile: *Cnemidophorus l. lemniscatus* (Sauria, Teiidae). *Experientia* **25**, 1330–1332.

Della Corte, F. and Biondi, A. (1964). The localisation of the fluorescent anti-FSH globulin in the pituitary of pig (*Sus scrofa* L. var. *Domestica Gray*). *Riv. Biol.* **57**, 369–376.

Della Corte, F. and Chieffi, G. (1962). Modificazioni dell'ipofisi di *Torpedo marmorata* Risso, durante la gravidaza. *Boll. Zool.* **28**, 219–225.

Della Corte, F., Galgano, M. and Angelini, F. (1968). Ultrastruttura della pars distalis dell'ipofisi di *Lacerta s. sicula* Raf., nei maschi in attivita sessuale ed in quelli castrati. *Z. Zellforsch. mikrosk. Anat.* **90**, 596–615.

Dellman, H.-D. and Owsley, P. A. (1969). Investigations on the hypothalamo-neurophypophysial neurosecretory system of the grass frog (*Rana pipiens*) after transection of the proximal neurohypophysis. II. Light- and electron-microscopic findings in the disconnected distal neurohypophysis with special emphasis on the pituicytes. *Z. Zellforsch. mikrosk. Anat.* **94**, 325–336.

Deminatti, M. (1959). Recherches cytochimiques sur la teneur en acide ribonucléique des différents types cellulaires de la préhypophyse chez le cobaye. *C. r. Séanc. Soc. Biol.* **153**, 320–322.

Deminatti, M. (1961a). Étude comparative histoautoradiographique et histochimique de la préhypophyse, après administration de ^{35}S-SO$_4$Na$_2$, chez le cobaye. *C. r. hebd. Séanc. Acad. Sci., Paris* **253**, 329–330.

Deminatti, M. (1961b), Études histoautoradiographiques de l'incorporation de DL-^{35}S methionine dans la préhypophyse, *in vivo* et *in vitro* chez le cobaye. *C. r. Séanc. Soc. Biol.* **155**, 1076–1078.

Dempsey, E. W. (1939). The relationship between the central nervous system and the reproductive cycle in the female guinea-pig. *Am. J. Physiol.* **126**, 758–765.

Dempsey, E. W. and Wislocki, G. B. (1945). Histochemical reactions associated with basophilia in the placenta and pituitary gland. *Am. J. Anat.* **76**, 277–301.

Dent, J. N. (1961). Cytological response of the newt pituitary gland to thyroidal depression. *Gen. comp. Endocr.* **1**, 218–231.

Dent, J. N. and Gupta, B. L. (1967). Ultrastructural observations on the development of the pituitary gland in the spotted newt. *Gen. comp. Endocr.* **8**, 273–288.

deRoos, R. and deRoos, C. C. (1967). Presence of corticotropin activity in the pituitary gland of chondrichthyean fish. *Gen. comp. Endocr.* **9**, 267–275.

Desclin, L. (1940). Détection de substance pentose nucléique dans les cellules du lobe antérieur de l'hypophyse du rat et du cobaye. *C. r. Séanc. Soc. Biol.* **133**, 457–459.

Dey, F. L. (1943). Evidence of hypothalamic control of hypophyseal gonadotrophic functions in the female guinea-pig. *Endocrinology* **33**, 75–82.

Dhaliwal, G. K. and Prasad, M. R. N. (1965). Cytology and histochemistry of the pituitary gland of the five-striped palm squirrel, *Funambulus pennanti* (Wroghton). *Am. J. Anat.* **117**, 339–352.

Dhariwal, A. P. S., Grosvenor, C. E., Anteunes-Rodriques, J. and McCann, S. M. (1968). Studies on the purification of ovine prolactin-inhibiting factor (PIF). *Endocrinology* **82**, 1236–1240.

Dhariwal, A. P. S., Krulich, L. and McCann, S. M. (1969). Purification of a growth hormone-inhibiting factor (GIF) from sheep hypothalamus. *Neuroendocrinology* **4**, 282–288.

Dharmamba, M. and Nishioka, R. S. (1968). Response of 'prolactin-secreting' cells of *Tilapia mossambica* to environmental salinity. *Gen. comp. Endocr.* **10**, 409–420.

Dicker, S. E. and Tyler, C. (1953a). Estimation of the anti-diuretic vasopressor and oxytocic hormones in the pituitary glands of dogs and puppies. *J. Physiol., Lond.* **120**, 141–145.

Dicker, S. E. and Tyler, C. (1953b). Vasopressor and oxytocic activities of the pituitary glands of rat, guinea-pigs and cats, and of human foetuses. *J. Physiol., Lond.* **121**, 206–214.

Diepen, R. (1962). *Der Hypothalamus. Handbuch der mikroskopischen Anatomie des Menschen*, vol. v, part 7 (ed. W. von Möllendorff). Berlin, Göttingen, Heidelberg: Springer-Verlag.

Dierickx, K. (1966). Experimental identification of a hypothalamic gonadotropic centre. *Z. Zellforsch. mikrosk. Anat.* **74**, 53–79.

Dierickx, K. (1967a). The function of the hypophysis without preoptic neurosecretory control. *Z. Zellforsch. mikrosk. Anat.* **78**, 114–130.

Dierickx, K. (1967*b*). The gonadoptropic centre of the tuber cinereum hypothalami and ovulation. *Z. Zellforsch. mikrosk. Anat.* **77**, 188–203.

Dierickx, K. and Goossens, N. (1970). The residual adrenocorticotropic activity of the hypophysis after its neural disconnection. *Z. Zellforsch. mikrosk. Anat.* **106**, 371–375.

Dodd, J. M., Follett, B. K. and Sharp, P. J. (1971). Hypothalamic control of pituitary function in submammalian vertebrates. In *Advances in comparative physiology and biochemistry* (ed. O. Lowenstein), vol. IV, pp. 113–223. New York and London: Academic Press.

Dodd, J. M. and Kerr, T. (1963). Comparative morphology and histology of the hypothalamo-neurohypophysial system. *Symp. zool. Soc. Lond.* **9**, 5–27.

Doerr-Schott, J. (1966*a*). Étude aux microscopes optique et électronique des différents types de cellules de la *pars distalis* et de la *pars intermedia* de *Triturus marmoratus* Latr. *Ann. Endocr., Paris* **27**, 101–119.

Doerr-Schott, J. (1966*b*). Modifications ultrastructurales des cellules thyréotropes de l'hypophyse de la grenouille rousse après thyroïdectomie. *C. r. hebd. Séanc. Acad. Sci., Paris* **D 262**, 1973–1976.

Doerr-Schott, J. (1968*a*). Cytologie et cytophysiologie de l'adénohypophyse des amphibiens. *Ann. Biol.* **7**, 189–225.

Doerr-Schott, J. (1968*b*). Développement de l'hypophyse de *Rana temporaria* L. Étude au microscope électronique. *Z. Zellforsch. mikrosk. Anat.* **90**, 616–645.

Doerr-Schott, J. (1970). Étude au microscope électronique de la neurohypophyse de *Rana esculenta* L. *Z. Zellforsch. mikrosk. Anat.* **111**, 413–426.

Doerr-Schott, J. (1971). La 'pars tuberalis' de *Rana temporaria* L: cytologie et ultrastructure. *Gen. comp. Endocr.* **16**, 516–523.

Doerr-Schott, J. (1972). Les cellules corticotropes de l'hypophyse d'un amphibien après interrénalectomie. *Z. Zellforsch. mikrosk. Anat.* **132**, 333–346.

Doerr-Schott, J. and Dubois, M. P. (1970). Les cellules corticotropes de l'hypophyse de triton (*Triturus marmoratus* Latr.). Mise en évidence par immunofluorescence d'une sécrétion apparentée à l'hormone corticotrope [$\beta - (1–24)$ corticotropine]. *C. r. hebd. Séanc. Acad. Sci., Paris* **D 271**, 1534–1536.

Doerr-Schott, J. and Dubois, M. P. (1972). Identification par immunofluorescence des cellules corticotropes et mélanotropes de l'hypophyse des amphibiens. *Z. Zellforsch. mikrosk. Anat.* **132**, 323–333.

Doerr-Schott, J. and Follénius, E. (1970*a*). Innervation de l'hypophyse intermédiaire de *Rana esculenta*, et identification des fibres aminergiques par autoradiographie au microscope électronique. *Z. Zellforsch. mikrosk. Anat.* **106**, 99–118.

Doerr-Schott, J. and Follénius, E. (1970*b*). Identification et localisation des fibres aminergiques dans l'éminence médiane de la grenouille verte (*Rana esculenta* L.), par autoradiographie au microscope électronique. *Z. Zellforsch. mikrosk. Anat.* **111**, 427–436.

Doerr-Schott, J. and Follénius, E. (1972). Innervation adrénergique de l'hypophyse de *Triturus alpestris*. *C. r. hebd. Séanc. Acad. Sci., Paris* **D 274**, 2712–2714.

Donovan, B. T. and Harris, G. W. (1954). Effect of pituitary stalk section on light-induced oestrus in the ferret. *Nature, Lond.* **174**, 503–504.

Douglas, W. W. (1963). A possible mechanism of neurosecretion. Release of vasopressin by depolarization and its dependence on calcium. *Nature, Lond.* **197**, 81–82.

Douglas, W. W., Nagasawa, J. and Schultz, R. (1971). Electron microscopic studies on the mechanism of secretion of posterior pituitary hormones and significance of micro-vesicles ('synaptic vesicles'): evidence of secretion by exocytosis and formation of micro-vesicles as a by-product of this process. *Mem. Soc. Endocr.* **19**, 353–377.

Drager, G. A. (1945). The innervation of the hypophysis. *Endocrinology* avian **36**, 124–129.

Drager, G. A. (1947). Innervation of the anterior lobe of the armadillo hypophysis: a comparative discussion. *Tex. Rep. Biol. Med.* **5**, 390–408.

Dubois, M. P. (1972). Localisation cytologique par immunofluorescence des sécrétions corticotropes, α et β melanotropes au niveau de l'adénohypophyse des bovins, ovins et porcins. *Z. Zellforsch. mikrosk. Anat.* **125**, 200–209.

Duchen, L. W. (1962). The effects of ingestion of hypertonic saline on the pituitary gland in the rat: a morphological study of the pars intermedia and posterior lobe. *J. Endocr.* **25**, 161–168.

Duggan, A. W. and Reed, G. W. (1958). Hypothalamus and oxytocin. *Nature, Lond.* **181**, 1278–1279.

Dupont, W. (1967). Effets de la surrénalectomie bilatérale sur la cytologie du lobe distale de l'hypophyse de la grenouille verte (*Rana esculenta*): essai d'identification des cellules responsables de la sécrétion de l'hormone corticotrope. *C. r. Séanc. Soc. Biol.* **161**, 2374–2376.

Dupont, W. (1968). Action de la métopirone sur la cytologie du lobe distale de l'hypophyse de la grenouille verte, *Rana esculenta* (L.). *C. r. Séanc. Soc. Biol.* **162**, 383–385.

Dupont, W. (1971). Évolution de la formation corticotrope chez la grenouille verte, *Rana esculenta* L., après transplantation ectopique du lobe distale de l'hypophyse. *Ann. Endocr.* **32**, 639–652.

Dupont, W. and Gaudray, A. (1969). Modifications cytologiques de l'hypophyse et de la glande interrénale de la grenouille verte, *Rana esculenta*, après surrénalectomie unilatérale. *C. r. Séanc. Soc. Biol.* **163**, 34–37.

Dupont, W. and Peltier, J.-C. (1970). Action d'une substance neurohypophysaire, la lysine-vasopressine, sur la fonction corticotrope chez la grenouille verte, *Rana esculenta* L. *C. r. Séanc. Soc. Biol.* **164**, 2175–2180.

Duvernoy, H. (1958). Contribution à l'étude de la vascularisation de l'hypophyse. Thèse pour le Doctorat en Medicine. Faculté de Medicine, Paris.

Duvernoy, H. (1972). The vascular architecture of the median eminence. In *Brain–endocrine interaction. Median eminence: structure and function* (ed. K. M. Knigge, D. E. Scott and A. Weindl). Basel: Karger.

Eayrs, J. T. and Holmes, R. L. (1964). Effects of neonatal hyperthyroidism on pituitary structure and function in the rat. *J. Endocr.* **29**, 71–81.

Ekengren, B. (1972). The nucleus preopticus and the nucleus lateralis tuberis in the roach, *Leuciscus rutilis. Gen. comp. Endocr.* **18**, 589.

Emmart, E. W. (1969). The localisation of endogenous 'prolactin' in the pituitary gland of the goldfish, *Carassius auratus*, Linnaeus. *Gen. comp. Endocr.* **12**, 519–525.

Emmart, E. W. and Mossakowski, M. J. (1967). The localisation of prolactin in cultured cells of the rostral pars distalis of the pituitary of *Fundulus heteroclitus* (Linnaeus). *Gen. comp. Endocr.* **9**, 391–400.

Emmart, E. W. and Mossakowski, M. J. (1970). The behaviour and appearance in tissue culture of rostral pituitary cells from *Fundulus heteroclitus* Linnaeus. *Gen. comp. Endocr.* **14**, 517–523.

Enemar, A. (1960). The development of the hypophysial vascular system in the lizards *Lacerta a. agilis* (Linnaeus) and *Anguis fragilis* (Linnaeus) and in the snake *Natrix n. natrix* (Linnaeus), with comparative remarks on the Amniota. *Acta. Zool., Stockh.* **41**, 141–237.

Enemar, A. (1961). The structure and development of the hypophysial portal system in the laboratory mouse, with particular regard to the primary plexus. *Ark. Zool. Ser.* 2 **13**, 203–252.

Enemar, A. and Falck, B. (1965). On the presence of adrenergic nerves in the pars intermedia of the frog *Rana temporaria. Gen. comp. Endocr.* **5**, 577–583.

Engelhardt, Fr. (1956). Über die Angioarchitektonik der hypophysär-hypothalamischen Systeme. *Acta neuroveg.* **13**, 129–170.

Ensor, D. M. and Ball, J. N. (1972). Prolactin and osmoregulation in fishes. *Fedn Proc. Fedn Am. Socs exp. Biol.* **31**, 1615–1623.

Etkin, W. (1970). The endocrine mechanism of amphibian metamorphosis, an evolutionary achievement. *Mem. Soc. Endocr.* **18**, 137–155.

Etkin, W., Derby, A. and Gona, A. G. (1969). Prolactin-like antithyroid action of pituitary grafts in tadpoles. *Gen. comp. Endocr. Suppl.* **2**, 253–259.

Etkin, W. and Gona, A. G. (1967). Antagonism between prolactin and thyroid hormone in amphibian development. *J. exp. Zool.* **165**, 249–258.

Etkin, W. and Lehrer, R. (1960). Excess growth in tadpoles after transplantation of the adenohypophysis. *Endocrinology* **67**, 457–466.

Etkin, W. and Ortman, R. (1960). Cellular differentiation in relation to growth-promoting activity of pituitary grafts in tadpoles. *Anat. Rec.* **137**, 353.

Evennett, P. J. (1963). Localization of gonadotropin secretion in the pituitary gland of the lamprey (*Lampetra fluviatilis*). *Gen. comp. Endocr.* **3**, 697–698.

Evennett, P. J. and Larsen, L. O. (1971). Unpublished observations on the localisation of ACTH in *Xenopus* pituitary, quoted by Larsen, van Kemenade and van Dongen (1971).

Evennett, P. J. and Thornton, V. F. (1971). The distribution and development of gonadotropic activity in the pituitary of *Xenopus laevis. Gen. comp. Endocr.* **16**, 606–607.

Eyeson, K. N. (1970). Cell types in the distal lobe of the pituitary of the West African rainbow lizard, *Agama agama* (L.). *Gen. comp. Endocr.* **14**, 357–367.

Falck, B. (1962). Observations on the possibilities of the cellular localisation of monoamines by a fluorescent method. *Acta physiol. scand., Suppl.* **197**, 1–26.

Farquhar, M. G. (1957). 'Corticotrophs' of the rat adenohypophysis as revealed by electron microscopy. *Anat. Rec.* **127**, 291 (abstract).

Farquhar, M. G. (1961). Fine structure and function in capillaries of the anterior pituitary gland. *Angiology* **12**, 270–292.

Farquhar, M. G. (1971). Processing of secretory products by cells of the anterior pituitary gland. *Mem. Soc. Endocr.* **19**, 79–124.

Farquhar, M. G. and Rinehart, J. F. (1954*a*). Electron microscopic studies of the anterior pituitary gland of castrated rats. *Endocrinology* **54**, 516–541.

Farquhar, M. G. and Rinehart, J. F. (1954*b*). Cytologic alterations in the anterior pituitary gland following thyroidectomy; an electron microscope study. *Endocrinology* **55**, 857–876.

Fasolo, A. and Franzoni, M. F. (1971*a*). The neurohypophysis of the crested newt. *Atti Accad. Sci., Torino* **105**, 585–591.

Fasolo, A. and Franzoni, M. F. (1971*b*). On the occurrence of monoamine-containing neurons in the hypothalamus of the newt. *Atti Accad. Sci., Torino* **105**, 681–683.

Fasolo, A., Franzoni, M. F. and Mazzi, V. (1972). Monoaminergic innervation of the median eminence in the crested newt. *Gen. comp. Endocr.* **18**, 590.

Fee, A. R. and Parkes, A. S. (1929). Studies on ovulation. I. The relation of the anterior pituitary body to ovulation in the rabbit. *J. Physiol., Lond.* **67**, 383–388.

Fendler, K. and Endröczi, E. (1965). Changes of adrenal compensatory hypertrophy in the rat after removal of the sympathetic superior cervical ganglia. *Acta. physiol. hung.* **28**, 171–176.

Fernandez-Moran, H. and Luft, R. (1949). Sub-microscopic cytoplasmic granules in the anterior lobe cells of the rat hypophysis as revealed by electron microscopy. *Acta endocr., Copnh.* **2**, 199–211.

Fernholm, B. (1972*a*). The ultrastructure of the adenohypophysis of *Myxine glutinosa*. *Z. Zellforsch. mikrosk. Anat.* **132**, 451–472.

Fernholm, B. (1972*b*). Neurohypophysial-adenohypophysial relations in hagfish (Myxinoidea, Cyclostomata). *Gen. comp. Endocr. Suppl.* **3**, 1–10.

Fernholm, B. and Olsson, R. (1969). A cytopharmacological study of the *Myxine* adenohypophysis. *Gen. comp. Endocr.* **13**, 336–356.

Feyel, T. (1939). Sur les constituants cytoplasmiques et sur l'évolution de la cellule acidophile dans la pars antérieure de l'hypophyse du cobaye. *C. r. Séanc. Soc. Biol.* **131**, 560–562.

Ficq, A. and Flament-Durand, J. (1963). Autoradiography in endocrine research. In *Techniques in endocrine research* (ed. P. Eckstein and F. G. W. Knowles), pp. 73–85. New York and London: Academic Press.

Fink, G. and Harris, G. W. (1970). The luteinizing hormone releasing activity of extracts of blood from the hypophysial portal vessels of rats. *J. Physiol., Lond.* **208**, 221–241.

Fisher, C., Ingram, W. R. and Ranson, S. W. (1938). *Diabetes insipidus and the neuro-hormonal control of water balance: a contribution to the structure and function of the hypothalamico-hypophyseal system.* Ann Arbor: Edwards Bros.

Flament-Durand, J. (1965). Observations on pituitary transplants into the hypothalamus of the rat. *Endocrinology* **77**, 446–454.

Flerkó, B. and Szentágothai, J. (1957). Oestrogen sensitive nervous structure in the hypothalamus. *Acta endocr., Copnh.* **26**, 121–127.

Flesch, M. (1884). Compte rendu des travaux présentés à la 67ᵉ Session de la Société Helvétique des Sciences Naturelles, Réunie à Locano. *Archs Sci. phys. nat.* **112**.

Follénius, E. (1965). Bases structurales et ultrastructurales des corrélations diencéphalo-hypophysaires chez les sélaciens et les téléostéens. *Archs Anat. microsc. Morph. exp.* **54**, 195–216.

Follénius, E. (1968). Analyse de la structure fine des différents types de cellules hypophysaires des poissons téléostéens. *Path.-Biol.* **16**, 619–632.

Follénius, E. (1970*a*). La localisation fine des terminaisons nerveuses fixant la noradrenaline ³H dans les différents lobes de l'adénohypopophyse de l'épinoche (*Gasterosteus aculeatus* L.). In *Aspects of neuroendocrinology* (ed. W. Bargmann and B. Scharrer), pp. 232–244. Berlin, Heidelberg, New York: Springer-Verlag.

Follénius, E. (1970*b*). Mise en évidence, au microscope électronique, de l'innervation de l'hypophyse de *Gasterosteus aculeatus* L. par la technique de Maillet Champy. *C. r. hebd. Séanc. Acad. Sci., Paris* D **271**, 1034–1037.

Follénius, E. (1971). Intégration de la dopamine dans les terminaisons aminergiques de la méta-adénohypophyse de l'épinoche (*Gasterosteus aculeatus* L.). *C. r. hebd. Séanc. Acad. Sci., Paris* D **273**, 1039–1040.

Follénius, E. (1972*a*). Cytologie fine de la dégénérescence des fibres aminergiques intrahypophysaires chez le poisson téléostéen *Gasterosteus aculeatus* après traitement par la 6-hydroxydopamine. *Z. Zellforsch. mikrosk. Anat.* **128**, 69–82.

Follénius, E. (1972*b*). Intégration sélective du GABA H³ dans la neurohypophyse du poisson téléostéen *Gasterosteus aculeatus* L. Étude autoradiographique. *C. r. hebd. Séanc. Acad. Sci., Paris* D **275**, 1435–1438.

Follénius, E. and Porte, A. (1960). Ultrastructure de l'hypophyse des cyprinodontes vivipares. Étude des types cellulaires composant l'adénohypophyse. *C. r. Séanc. Soc. Biol.* **154** 1247–1250.

Follénius, E. and Porte, A. (1961). Étude des différents lobes de l'adénohypophyse de la perche, *Perca fluviatilis*, au microscope électronique. *C. r. Séanc. Soc. Biol.* **155**, 128–131.

Follett, B. K. (1970). Gonadotropin-releasing activity in the quail hypothalamus. *Gen. comp. Endocr.* **15**, 165–179.

Follett, B. K., Scanes, C. G. and Cunningham, F. J. (1971). A radioimmunoassay for avian luteinizing hormone. *J. Endocr.* **51**, v–vi.

Forbes, M. S. (1971). Ultrastructure of the thyrotrophic cell in the pars distalis of the lizard. *Gen. comp. Endocr.* **16**, 452–464.

Forbes, M. S. (1972*a*). Observations on the fine structure of the pars intermedia in the lizard *Anolis carolinensis*. *Gen. comp. Endocr.* **18**, 146–161.

Forbes, M. S. (1972*b*). Fine structure of the stellate cells in the pars distalis of the lizard *Anolis carolinensis*. *J. Morph.* **136**, 227–246.

Ford, E. H., Hirschman, A., Rhines, R. and Zimberg, S. (1961). The rate of uptake and radioautographic localisation of S³⁵ in the central nervous system, pituitary and skeletal muscle of the normal male rat after injection of S³⁵-labelled cystine. *Exp. Neurol.* **4**, 444–459.

Foster, C. L. and Wilson, R. R. (1952). Studies upon the Gram reaction of the basophil cells of the anterior pituitary. Part I. Some preliminary observations upon the basophil cell of the human pituitary. *Q. Jl microsc. Sci.* **93**, 147–155.

Friedgood, H. B. and Dawson, A. B. (1940). Physiological significance and morphology of the carmine cell in the cat's anterior pituitary. *Endocrinology* **26**, 1022–1031.

Frykman, H. M. (1942). A quantitative study of the paraventricular nucleus and its alteration in hypophysectomy. *Endocrinology* **31**, 23–29.

Fumagalli, Z. (1942). La vascolarizzazione dell'ipofisi umana. *Z. Anat. EntwGesch.* **111**, 266–306.

Furth, J. (1955). Experimental pituitary tumours. *Recent Prog. Horm. Res.* **11**, 221–249.

Furth, J. and Clifton, K. H. (1958). Experimental pituitary tumours. *Ciba Fdn Colloq. Endocr.* **12**, 3–17.

Gabe, M. (1972). Contribution à l'histologie du complexe hypothalamo-hypophysaire d'*Ichthyophis glutinosus* L. (Batricien apode). *Acta anat.* **81**, 253–269.

Gabe, M. and Saint-Girons, H. (1964). Le troisième type de contact hypothalamo-hypophysaire proximal: l'éminence médiane de *Sphenodon punctatus. C. r. hebd. Séanc. Acad. Sci., Paris* **259**, 2136–2139.

Gaillard, P. J. (1937). An experimental contribution to the origin of the pars intermedia of the hypophysis. *Acta. neerl. Morph.* **1**, 3–11.

Ganong, W. F., Frederickson, D. S. and Hume, D. M. (1955). The effect of hypothalamic lesions on thyroid function in the dog. *Endocrinology* **57**, 355–362.

Gemelli, A. (1906). Ulteriori osservazioni sulla struttura dell'ipofisi. *Anat. Anz.* **28**, 613–628.

Gersh, I. (1939). The structure and function of the parenchymatous glandular cells in the neurohypophysis of the rat. *Am. J. Anat.* **64**, 407–443.

Ginsburg, M., Jayasena, M. and Thomas, P. J. (1966). Subfractions from porcine neurophysin with different hormone binding properties. *J. Physiol., Lond.* **183**, 45–46.

Girod, M. C. (1966). Contribution à l'étude de la cytologie du lobe antérieur de l'hypophyse. *Rev. lyonn. Méd.* **15**, 91–126.

Godet, R. (1964). Évolution des types de cellules hypophysaires au cours de la période de repos en climat tropical chez les vertébrés sans régulation thermique. *C. r. Séanc. Soc. Biol.* **158**, 1380–1382.

Goldberg, R. C. and Knobil, E. (1957). Structure and function of intraocular hypophyseal grafts in the hypophysectomised male rat. *Endocrinology* **61**, 742–752.

Goldman, H. (1968). The failure of cervical sympathectomy to alter pituitary blood flow. *Endocrinology* **83**, 603–606.

Gomori, G. (1950). Aldehyde-fuchsin: a new stain for elastic tissue. *Am. J. clin. Path.* **20**, 665–666.

Gona, A. G. and Etkin, W. (1970). Inhibition of metamorphosis in *Ambystoma tigrinum* by prolactin. *Gen. comp. Endocr.* **14**, 589–591.

Gona, A. G., Pearlman, T. and Etkin, W. (1970). Prolactin–thyroid interaction in the newt, *Diemictylus viridescens*. *J. Endocr.* **48**, 585–590.

Goos, H. J. T. (1969*a*). Hypothalamic control of the pars intermedia in *Xenopus laevis* tadpoles. *Z. Zellforsch. mikrosk. Anat.* **97**, 118–124.

Goos, H. J. T. (1969*b*). Hypothalamic neurosecretion and metamorphosis in *Xenopus laevis*. IV. The effect of extirpation of the presumed TRF cells and of a subsequent PTU treatment. *Z. Zellforsch. mikrosk. Anat.* **97**, 449–458.

Goos, H. J. T., Zwanenbeek, H. C. M. and van Oordt, P. G. W. J. (1968). Hypothalamic neurosecretion and metamorphosis in *Xenopus laevis*. II. The effect of thyroxine following treatment with propylthiouracil. *Archs Anat. Histol. Embryol.* **51**, 269–274.

Gorbman, A. (1964). Endocrinology of the Amphibia. In *Physiology of the Amphibia* (ed. J. A. Moore), pp. 371–425. New York and London: Academic Press.

Gorbman, A. (1965). Vascular relations between the neurohypophysis and adeno-hypophysis of cyclostomes and the problem of evolution of hypothalamic endo-crine control. *Archs Anat. microsc. Morph. exp.* **54**, 163–194.

Gorbman, A. and Bern, H. A. (1962). *A textbook of comparative endocrinology.* New York: John Wiley and Sons.

Gorbman, A., Kobayashi, H. and Uemura, H. (1963). The vascularisation of the hypophysial structures of the hagfish. *Gen. comp. Endocr.* **3**, 505–514.

Goslar, H. G. and Schultze, B. (1958). Autoradiographische Untersuchungen über den Einbau von S^{35}-Thioaminosäuren im Zwischenhirn von Kaninchen und Ratte. *Z. mikrosk.-anat. Forsch.* **64**, 556–574.

Green, J. D. (1947). Vessels and nerves of amphibian hypophyses. *Anat. Rec.* **99**, 21–45.

Green, J. D. (1948). The histology of the hypophysial stalk and median eminence in man with special reference to blood vessels, nerve fibres and a peculiar neuro-vascular zone in this region. *Anat. Rec.* **100**, 273–295.

Green, J. D. (1951). The comparative anatomy of the hypophysis with special refer-ence to its blood supply and innervation. *Am. J. Anat.* **88**, 225–311.

Green, J. D. (1952). Comparative aspects of the hypophysis, especially of blood supply and innervation. *Ciba Fdn Colloq. Endocr.* **4**, 72–84.

Green, J. D. (1966). The comparative anatomy of the portal vascular system and of the innervation of the hypophysis. In *The pituitary gland* (ed. G. W. Harris and B. T. Donovan), vol. I, pp. 127–146. London: Butterworths.

Green, J. D. and Harris, G. W. (1947). The neurovascular link between the neuro-hypophysis and the adenohypophysis. *J. Endocr.* **5**, 136–146.

Green, J. D. and Harris, G. W. (1949). Observation of the hypophysio-portal vessels of the living rat. *J. Physiol., Lond.* **108**, 359–361.

Green, J. D. and van Breemen, V. L. (1955). Electron microscopy of pituitary and observations on neurosecretion. *Am. J. Anat.* **97**, 177–227.

Greenspan, F. S. and Hargadine, J. R. (1965). The intracellular localisation of pituitary thyrotropic hormone. *J. Cell Biol.* **26**, 177–185.

Greep, R. O. (1936). Functional pituitary grafts in rats. *Proc. Soc. exp. Biol. Med.* **34**, 754–755.

Greving, R. (1926*a*). Beiträge zur Anatomie der Hypophyse und ihrer Funktion.

I. Eine Faserverbindung zwischen Hypophyse und Zwischenhirnbasis (Tr. Supraoptico-hypophysius). *Dt. Z. NervHeilk.* **89**, 179–195.

Greving, R. (1926*b*). Beiträge zur Anatomie der Hypophyse und ihrer Funktion. II. Das nervöse Regulationszentrum des Hypophysenhinterlappens (der Nucleus supraopticus und seine Fasersysteme). *Z. ges. Neurol. Psychiat.* **104**, 466–479.

Greving, R. (1928). Die zentralen Anteile des vegetativen Nervensystems. In *Handbuch der mikroskopischen Anatomie des Menschen* (ed. W. von Mollendorff), vol. iv/1, pp. 917–1060. Berlin, Heidelberg, New York: Springer-Verlag.

Grignon, G. (1963). Cytophysiologie de l'adénohypophyse des reptiles. *Colloq. Internat. CRNS, Paris* **128**, 287–300.

Guillemin, R. (1964). Hypothalamic factors releasing pituitary hormones. *Recent Prog. Horm. Res.* **20**, 89–130.

Guillemin, R., Yamazaki, E., Jutisz, M. and Sakiz, E. (1962). Présence dans un extrait de tissus hypothalamiques d'une substance stimulant la sécrétion de l'hormone hypophysaire thyréotrope (TSH). Première purification par filtration sur gel Sephadex. *C. r. hebd. Séanc. Acad. Sci., Paris* **255**, 1018–1020.

Gurdjian, E. S. (1927). The diencephalon of the albino rat; studies on the brain of the rat. *J. comp. Neurol.* **43**, 1–114.

Hadley, M. E. and Goldman, J. M. (1969). Physiological color changes in reptiles. *Am. Zool.* **9**, 489–504.

Hagen, E. (1954). Zur Frage der afferenten Nervenfasern im Drüsenlappen der Hypophyse. *Z. Zellforsch. mikrosk. Anat.* **41**, 79–88.

Haider, S. and Sathyanesan, A. G. (1972*a*). Comparative study of the hypothalamo-neurohypophysial complex in some Indian freshwater teleosts. *Acta anat.* **81**, 202–224.

Haider, S. and Sathyanesan, A. G. (1972*b*). The nucleus lateralis tuberis of the freshwater teleost *Heteropneustes fossilis* (Bl.). *Acta anat.* **82**, 75–84.

Hair, G. W. (1938). The nerve supply of the hypophysis of the cat. *Anat. Rec.* **71**, 141–160.

Halász, B. and Pupp, L. (1965). Hormone secretion of the anterior pituitary gland after physical interruption of all nervous pathways to the hypophysiotrophic area. *Endocrinology* **77**, 553–562.

Halász, B., Pupp, L. and Uhlarik, S. (1962). Hypophysiotrophic area in the hypothalamus. *J. Endocr.* **25**, 147–154.

Halász, B., Pupp, L., Uhlarik, S. and Tima, L. (1965). Further studies on the hormone secretion of the anterior pituitary transplanted into the hypophysiotrophic area of the rat hypothalamus. *Endocrinology* **77**, 343–355.

Halász, B., Slusher, M. A. and Gorski, R. A. (1967). Adenocorticotrophic hormone secretion in rats after partial or total deafferentation of the medial basal hypothalamus. *Neuroendocrinology* **2**, 43–55.

Hall, S. R. (1938). Possible evidence for a second type of basophile in anterior pituitary of cattle. *Anat. Rec.* **72**, Suppl. 123.

Halmi, N. S. (1950). Two types of basophils in the anterior pituitary of the rat and their respective cytophysiological significance. *Endocrinology* **47**, 289–299.

Halmi, N. S. (1952*a*). Differentiation of two types of basophils in the adenohypophysis of the rat and mouse. *Stain Technol.* **27**, 61–64.

Halmi, N. S. (1952*b*). Two types of basophils in the rat pituitary: 'thyrotrophs' and 'gonadotrophs' vs. beta and delta cells. *Endocrinology* **50**, 140–142.

Hannover, A. (1844). *Recherches microscopiques sur le système nerveux.* Copenhagen: Philipsen.

Hanström, B. (1947). A comparative study of the hypophysis in the polar bear and some Swedish carnivora. *K. svenska VetenskAkad. Handl., Ser. 3* **24**, 1–46.

Hanström, B. (1952*a*). The hypophysis in some South African insectivora, carnivora, hyracoidea, proboscidea, artiodactyla, and primates. *Ark. zool., Ser.* 2 **4**, 187–294.

Hanström, B. (1965). Wulzen's cone, a capriciously occurring lobe in the mammalian hypophysis. *Acta Univ. lund., Sect. II* **11**, 1–15.

Hanström, B. (1966). Gross anatomy of the hypophysis of mammals. In: *The pituitary gland* (ed. G. W. Harris and B. T. Donovan), vol. I, pp. 1–57. London: Butterworths.

Harris, G. W. (1937). The induction of ovulation in the rabbit, by electrical stimulation of the hypothalamo-hypophysial mechanism. *Proc. R. Soc. Ser. B* **122**, 374–394.

Harris, G. W. (1947). The blood vessels of the rabbit's pituitary gland, and the significance of the pars and zona tuberalis. *J. Anat.* **81**, 343–351.

Harris, G. W. (1948). Electrical stimulation of the hypothalamus and the mechanism of neural control of the adenophyophysis. *J. Physiol., Lond.* **107**, 418–429.

Harris, G. W. (1950). Hypothalamo-hypophysial connections in the Cetacea. *J. Physiol., Lond.* **111**, 361–367.

Harris, G. W. (1955). *Neural control of the pituitary gland.* London: Edward Arnold Ltd.

Harris, G. W. (1972). Humours and hormones. *J. Endocr.* **53**, ii–xxiii.

Harris, G. W. and Campbell, H. J. (1966). The regulation of the secretion of luteinising hormone and ovulation. In *The pituitary gland* (ed. G. W. Harris and B. T. Donovan), vol. II, pp. 99–165. London: Butterworths.

Harris, G. W. and Jacobsohn, D. (1952). Functional grafts of the anterior pituitary gland. *Proc. R. Soc. Ser. B* **139**, 263–276.

Harris, G. W. and Ruf, K. B. (1970). Luteinizing hormone releasing factor in rat hypophysial portal blood collected during electrical stimulation of the hypothalamus. *J. Physiol., Lond.* **208**, 243–250.

Harris, I. (1960). The chemistry of intermediate lobe hormones. In *The pituitary gland* (ed. G. W. Harris and B. T. Donovan), vol. III, pp. 33–40. London: Butterworths.

Harrison, R. J. and Young, B. A. (1969). Stellate cells in the delphinid adenohypophysis. *J. Endocr.* **43**, 323–324.

Hartley, M. W., McShan, W. H. and Ris, H. (1960). Isolation of cytoplasmic pituitary granules with gonadotropic activity. *J. biophys. biochem. Cytol.* **7**, 209–218.

Hartmann, J. F. (1944). Seasonal cytological changes in the anterior hypophysis of the garter snake. *Am. J. Anat.* **75**, 121–149.

Hartmann, J. F., Fain, W. R. and Wolfe, J. M. (1946). A cytological study of the anterior hypophysis of the dog, with particular reference to the presence of a fourth cell type. *Anat. Rec.* **95**, 11–27.

Hartree, A. S. and Cunningham, F. J. (1969). Purification of chicken pituitary follicle-stimulating hormone and luteinizing hormone. *J. Endocr.* **43**, 609–616.

Hawkins, E. F. and Ball, J. N. (1973). Current knowledge of the mechanisms involved in the control of ACTH secretion in teleost fishes. In *Brain–pituitary–adrenal interrelationships* (ed. A. Brodish and E. S. Redgate), pp. 293–315. Basel: Karger.

Hayashida, T. (1971). Biological and immunochemical studies with growth hormone in pituitary extracts of holostean and chondrostean fishes. *Gen. comp. Endocr.* **17**, 275–280.

Hayashida, T. and Lagios, M. D. (1969). Fish growth hormone: a biological, immunochemical and ultrastructural study of sturgeon and paddlefish pituitaries. *Gen. comp. Endocr.* **13**, 403–411.

Heller, H. (1969). Class and species specific actions of neurohypophysial hormones. *Coll. Internat. CNRS, Paris* **177**, 35–44.

Heller, H. (1972). The effect of neurohypophysial principles on the female reproductive tract of lower vertebrates. *Gen. comp. Endocr., Suppl.* **3**, 703–714.

Henderson, N. E. (1969). Structural similarities between the neurohypophyses of brook trout and tetrapods. *Gen. comp. Endocr.* **12**, 148–153.

Herlant, M. (1958). L'hypophyse et le système hypothalamo-hypophysaire du pangolin (*Manis tricuspis* et *Manis tetradactyla*). *Archs Anat. microsc. Morph. exp.* **47**, 1–23.

Herlant, M. (1960). Étude critique de deux techniques nouvelles destinées à mettre en évidence les différentes catégories cellulaires présentes dans la glande pituitaire. *Bull. Micr. appl.* **10**, 37–44.

Herlant, M. (1964). The cells of the adenohypophysis and their functional significance. *Int. Rev. Cytol.* **17**, 199–382.

Herlant, M. and Racadot, S. (1957). Lobe antérieur de l'hypophyse de la chatte au cour de la gestation et de la lactation. *Archs. Biol.* **58**, 217–248.

Herlant, M., Benoit, J., Tixier-Vidal, A. and Assenmacher, I. (1960). Modifications hypophysaires au cours du cycle annuel chez le canard Pékin. *C. r. hebd. Séanc. Acad. Sci., Paris* **250**, 2936–2938.

Herring, P. T. (1908). The histological appearances of the mammalian pituitary body. *Jl exp. Physiol.* **1**, 121–159.

Hertz, R. (1959). Growth in the hypophysectomised rat sustained by pituitary grafts. *Endocrinology* **65**, 926–931.

Higgins, K. M. and Ball, J. N. (1972). Failure of ovine prolactin to release TSH in *Poecilia latipinna*. *Gen. comp. Endocr.* **18**, 597.

Higgins, K. M., Ball, J. N. and Wigham, T. (1973). Studies on hypothalamic control of TSH secretion in the teleost *Poecilia latipinna*. *J. comp. Physiol.* (in press).

Hild, W. and Zetler, G. (1951). Über des Vorkommen der Hypophysenhinterlappenhormone im Zwischenhirn. *Arch. exp. Path. Pharmak.* **213**, 139–153.

Hild, W. and Zetler, G. (1953a). Experimenteller Beweis für die Enstehung der sog. Hypophysenhinterlappenwirkstoffe im Hypothalamus. *Pflügers Arch. ges. Physiol.* **257**, 169–201.

Hild, W. and Zetler, G. (1953b). Über die Funktion des Neurosekrets im Zwischenhirn-Neurohypophysensystem als Trägersubstanz für Vasopressin, Adiuretin und Oxytocin. *Z. ges. exp. Med.* **120**, 236–243.

Hillarp, N.-Å. (1949). Studies on the localisation of the hypothalamic centres controlling the gonadotrophic function of the hypophysis. *Acta. endocr., Copnh.* **2**, 11–23.

Hillarp, N.-Å. and Jacobsohn, D. (1943). Über die Innervation der Adenohypophyse und Ihre Beziehungen zur Gonadotropen Hypophysenfunktion. *Acta Univ. lund., N.S.* **54**, No. 7, 1–25.

Hirzel, L. (1824). *Nexus nervi sympathici cum nervis cerebralibus.* Diss. Heidelbergae. (Cited by Romeis, 1940.)

Hoffman, R. A. and Zarrow, M. X. (1958). Seasonal changes in the basophilic cells of the pituitary gland of the ground squirrel (*Citellus tridecemlineatus*). *Anat. Rec.* **131**, 727–735.

Hökfelt, P. and Fuxe, K. (1972). On the morphology and the neuroendocrine role of the hypothalamic catecholamine neurones. In *Brain–endocrine interaction. Median eminence: structure and function* (ed. K. M. Knigge, D. E. Scott and A. Weindl), pp. 181–223. Basel: Karger.

Holder, F.-C. (1969a). Séparation chromatographique et dosage des hormones de type ocytocique (arginine-vasotocine et isotocine) de l'hypophyse et du noyau préoptique de l'anguille européenne (*Anguilla anguilla* L.). Anguilles d'Alsace (Auenheim) et de Loire-Atlantique (Grand-Brière). *C. r. hebd. Séanc. Acad. Sci., Paris* D **269**, 1304–1307.

Holder, F.-C. (1969*b*). Séparation chomatographique et dosage des hormones de type ocytocique (arginine-vasotocine et isotocine) de l'hypophyse et du noyau préoptique de l'anguille européenne (*Anguilla anguilla* L.). Anguilles de Mer Baltique. *C. r. hebd. Séanc. Acad. Sci., Paris* D **269**, 1441–1444.

Holder, F.-C. (1970). Hypophysectomie chez l'anguille européenne (*Anguilla anguilla* L.): étude, par séparation chromatographique et dosage biologique, du devenir des hormones de type ocytocique (arginine-vasotocine et isotocine) le long du tractus préopticohypophysaire. *C. r. hebd. Séanc. Acad. Sci., Paris* D **270**, 2692–2695.

Holmes, R. L. (1960). The pituitary gland of the female ferret. *J. Endocr.* **20**, 48–55.

Holmes, R. L. (1961*a*). Changes in the pituitary gland of the ferret following stalk section. *J. Endocr.* **22**, 7–14.

Holmes, R. L. (1961*b*). Esterases of the hypothalamo-hypophysial system. In *Cytology of nervous tissue. Proc. Anat. Soc. G.B. & I.* pp. 1–4. London: Taylor and Francis.

Holmes, R. L. (1962). The pituitary gland of normal and stalk sectioned monkeys with particular reference to the pars intermedia. *J. Endocr.* **24**, 53–58.

Holmes, R. L. (1963*a*). Gonadotrophic and thyrotrophic cells of the pituitary gland of the ferret. *J. Endocr.* **25**, 495–503.

Holmes, R. L. (1963*b*). The pituitary stalk and water metabolism in the monkey. *J. Endocr.* **28**, 107–118.

Holmes, R. L. (1964*a*). Experimental, histochemical and ultrastructural contributions to our understanding of mammalian pituitary function. *Int. Rev. gen. exp. Zool.* **1**, 187–240.

Holmes, R. L. (1964*b*). Comparative observations on inclusions in nerve fibres of the mammalian neurohypophysis. *Z. Zellforsch. mikrosk. Anat.* **64**, 474–492.

Holmes, R. L. (1965). The fine structure of supraoptic neurons of the hedgehog. *Z. Zellforsch. mikrosk. Anat.* **66**, 685–689.

Holmes, R. L. (1967). The vascular pattern of the median eminence of the hypophysis in the macaque. *Folia primatol.* **7**, 216–230.

Holmes, R. L., Hughes, E. B. and Zuckerman, S. (1959). Section of the pituitary stalk in monkeys. *J. Endocr.* **18**, 305–318.

Holmes, R. L. and Kiernan, J. A. (1964). The fine structure of the infundibular process of the hedgehog. *Z. Zellforsch. mikrosk. Anat.* **61**, 894–912.

Holmes, R. L. and Knowles, F. G. W. (1960). 'Synaptic vesicles' in the neurohypophysis. *Nature, Lond.* **185**, 710–711.

Holmes, R. L. and Mandl, A. M. (1961). A spontaneous pituitary tumour in a rat associated with adrenal hypertrophy. *J. Endocr.* **22**, xxix–xxx.

Holmes, R. L. and Zuckerman, S. (1959). The blood supply of the hypophysis in *Macaca mulatta. J. Anat.* **93**, 1–8.

Holmes, R. L. and Zuckerman, S. (1962). The evolution of ideas on the innervation of the pituitary gland. *Anat. Anz.* **109**, 836–846.

Holtzman, S. and Schreibman, M. P. (1972). Morphological changes in the 'prolactin' cell of the freshwater teleost, *Xiphophorus helleri*, in salt water. *J. exp. Zool.* **180**, 187–196.

Honma, Y. (1969). Some evolutionary aspects of the morphology and role of the adenohypophysis in fishes. *Gunma Symp. Endocr.* **6**, 19–36.

Hopkins, C. R. (1969). The fine structural localisation of acid phosphatase in the prolactin cell of the teleost pituitary following the stimulation and inhibition of secretory activity. *Tissue and Cell* **1**, 653–671.

Hopkins, C. R. (1970). Studies on secretory activity in the pars intermedia of *Xenopus laevis*. *Tissue and Cell* **2**, 59–98.

Hopkins, C. R. (1971). Localisation of adrenergic fibers in the amphibian pars intermedia by electron microscope autoradiography and their selective removal by 6-hydroxydopamine. *Gen. comp. Endocr.* **16**, 112–120.

Hopkins, C. R. and Baker, B. I. (1968). The fine structural localisation of acid phosphatase in the prolactin cell of the eel pituitary. *J. Cell Sci.* **3**, 357–364.

Horstmann, E. (1954). Die Faserglia des Selachiergehirns. *Z. Zellforsch. mikrosk. Anat.* **39**, 588–617.

Houssay, B.-A., Biasotti, A. and Sammartino, R. (1935). Modifications fonctionelles de l'hypophyse après les lésions infundibulo-tubériennes chez le crapaud. *C. r. Séanc. Soc. Biol.* **120**, 725–727.

Howe, A. (1973). The pars intermedia. *J. Endocr.* (in press).

Howell, J. S. and Mandl, A. M. (1961). The mammary glands of senile nulliparous and multiparous rats. *J. Endocr.* **22**, 241–255.

Howell, W. H. (1898). The physiological effects of extract of the hypophysis cerebri and infundibular body. *Am. J. exp. Med.* **3**, 245.

Hymer, W. C. and McShan, W. H. (1962). Isolation of cytoplasmic pituitary granules by column chromatography. *J. Cell Biol.* **13**, 350–354.

Imai, K. (1969). Light and electron microscopic studies on the pars intermedia of the pituitary of *Xenopus laevis* under different experimental conditions. *Gunma Symp. Endocr.* **6**, 89–103.

Ishii, S. (1970). Association of luteinizing hormone-releasing factor with granules separated from equine hypophysial stalk. *Endocrinology* **86**, 207–216.

Ishii, S. (1972). Classification and identification of neurosecretory granules in the median eminence. In *Brain–endocrine interaction. Median eminence: structure and function* (ed. K. M. Knigge, D. E. Scott and A. Weindl), pp. 119–141. Basel: Karger.

Ito, T. (1969). Further studies on the hypothalamic control of the pars intermedia activity of the frog *Rana nigromaculata*. *Gunma Symp. Endocr.* **4**, 492–502.

Ito, T. (1971). Changes in the skin colour and fine structure of the intermediate pituitary gland of the frog *Rana nigromaculata* after extirpation of the median eminence. *Neuroendocrinology* **8**, 180–197.

Iturriza, F. C. (1969). Further evidence for the blocking effect of catecholamines on the secretion of melanocyte-stimulating hormone in toads. *Gen. comp. Endocr.* **12**, 417–426.

Jasinski, A. (1969). Vascularisation of the hypophyseal region in lower vertebrates (cyclostomes and fishes). *Gen. comp. Endocr. Suppl.* **2**, 510–521.

Jasinski, A. and Gorbman, A. (1966). Hypothalamo-hypophysial vascular and neurosecretory links in the ratfish, *Hydrolagus colliei* (Lay and Bennett). *Gen. comp. Endocr.* **6**, 476–490.

Jasinski, A., Gorbman, A. and Hara, T. (1967). Activation of the preoptico-hypophysial neurosecretory system through olfactory afferents in fishes. In *Neurosecretion. IVth Int. Symposium on Neurosecretion* (ed. F. Stutinsky), pp. 106–123. Berlin, Heidelberg, New York: Springer-Verlag.

Jewell, P. A. (1953). The occurrence of vesiculated neurons in the hypothalamus of the dog. *J. Physiol., Lond.* **121**, 167–181.

Jewell, P. A. and Verney, E. B. (1957). An attempt to determine the site of the neurohypophysial osmoreceptors in the dog. *Phil. Trans. R. Soc. Ser. B* **240**, 197–324.

Jørgensen, C. B. (1968). Central nervous control of adenohypophysial functions. In *Perspectives in endocrinology* (ed. E. J. W. Barrington and C. B. Jørgensen), pp. 469–541. New York: Academic Press.

Jørgensen, C. B. and Larsen, L. O. (1963). Neuro-adenohypophysial relationships. *Symp. zool. Soc. Lond.* **9**, 59–82.

Jørgensen, C. B., Rosenkilde, P. and Wingstrand, K. G. (1969). Role of the preoptic-neurohypophysial stystem in the water economy of the toad, *Bufo bufo* L. *Gen. comp. Endocr.* **12**, 91–98.

Jost, A. (1966). Anterior pituitary function in foetal life. In *The pituitary gland* (ed. G. W. Harris and B. T. Donovan), volume II, pp. 299–323. London: Butterworths.

Kása, P. (1963). Sekretomotorische Fasern und Endigungen in der Adenohypophyse. *Experientia* **19**, 589–591.

Kasuga, S. and Takahashi, H. (1971). The preoptico-hypophysial neurosecretory system of the medaka, *Oryzias latipes*, and its changes in relation to the annual reproductive cycle under natural conditions. *Bull. Fac. Fish. Hokkaido Univ.* **21**, 259–268.

Kaye, N. W. (1961). Interrelationships of the thyroid and pituitary in embryonic and premetamorphic stages of the frog, *Rana pipiens. Gen. comp. Endocr.* **1**, 1–19.

van Kemenade, J. A. M. (1968a). Effect of ACTH and hypophysectomy on the interrenal tissue in the common frog, *Rana temporaria. Z. Zellforsch. mikrosk. Anat.* **92**, 549–566.

van Kemenade, J. A. M. (1968b). The effect of metopirone and aldactone on the interrenal tissue of intact and pars distalisectomized common frogs, *Rana temporaria. Z. Zellforsch. mikrosk. Anat.* **92**, 567–582.

van Kemenade, J. A. M. (1969a). Effects of a rise in ambient temperature on the pars distalis of the pituitary, the interrenal gland and the interstitial tissue of the testis in the common frog, *Rana temporaria*, during hibernation. *Z. Zellforsch. mikrosk. Anat.* **95**, 620–630.

van Kemenade, J. A. M. (1969b). The effects of metopirone and aldactone on the pars distalis of the pituitary, the interrenal tissue and the interstitial tissue of the testis in the common frog, *Rana temporaria. Z. Zellforsch. mikrosk. Anat.* **96**, 466–477.

van Kemenade, J. A. M. (1971). The localisation of corticotrophic function in the pars distalis of the pituitary in the common frog, *Rana temporaria. J. Endocr.* **49**, 349–350.

van Kemenade, J. A. M. (1972). The localisation of corticotropic and gonadoptropic function in the distal lobe of the pituitary gland in the frog, *Rana temporaria. Gen. comp. Endocr.* **18**, 627.

van Kemenade, J. A. M., van Dongen, W. J. and van Oordt, P. G. W. J. (1968). Seasonal changes in the endocrine organs of the male common frog, *Rana temporaria*. II. The interrenal tissue. *Z. Zellforsch. mikrosk. Anat.* **91**, 96–111.

Kerr, T. (1949). The pituitaries of *Amia, Lepidosteus* and *Acipenser. Proc. zool. Soc. Lond.* **118**, 973–983.

Kerr, T. (1965). Histology of the distal lobe of the pituitary of *Xenopus laevis* Daudin. *Gen. comp. Endocr.* **5**, 232–240.

Kerr, T. (1966). The development of the pituitary in *Xenopus laevis* Daudin. *Gen. comp. Endocr.* **6**, 303–311.

Kerr, T. (1968). The pituitary in polypterines and its relationship to other fish pituitaries. *J. Morph.* **124**, 23–36.

Kerr, T. and van Oordt, P. G. W. J. (1966). The pituitary of the African lungfish *Psrotopteru* sp. *Gen. comp. Endocr.* **7**, 549–558.

Knigge, K. M. (1971). Pituitary ocular graft function in the rat, with a comparison of the qualitative nature of TSH from normal pituitaries and ocular grafts. *Endocrinology* **68**, 101–114.

Knigge, K. M., Scott, D. E. and Weindl, A. (ed.)(1972). *Brain–endocrine interaction. Median eminence: structure and function.* (Proceedings of International Symposium on Brain–Endocrine Interaction, Munich. 2–3 August 1971). Basel: Karger.

Knowles, F. (1965). Evidence for a dual control, by neurosecretion, of hormone synthesis and hormone release in the pituitary of the dogfish, *Scylliorhinus stellaris. Phil. Trans. R. Soc. Ser. B* **249**, 435–456.

Knowles, F. and Anand Kumar, T. C. (1969). Structural changes related to reproduction, in the hypothalamus and in the pars tuberalis of the Rhesus monkey. *Phil. Trans. R. Soc. Ser. B* **256**, 357–375.

Knowles, F. and Bern, H. A. (1966). The function of neurosecretion in neuroendocrine regulation. *Nature, Lond.* **210**, 271–272.

Knowles, F. and Vollrath, L. (1966a). Neurosecretory innervation of the pituitary of the eels *Anguilla* and *Conger*. I. The structure and ultrastructure of the neuro-intermediate lobe under normal and experimental conditions. *Phil. Trans. R. Soc. Ser. B* **250**, 311–327.

Knowles, F. and Vollrath, L. (1966b). Neurosecretory innervation of the pituitary of the eels *Anguilla* and *Conger*. II. The structure and innervation of the pars distalis at different stages of the life-cycle. *Phil. Trans. R. Soc. Ser. B* **250**, 329–342.

Knowles, F. and Vollrath, L. (1966c). Cell types in the pituitary of the eel, *Anguilla anguilla* L., at different stages in the life-cycle. *Z. Zellforsch. mikrosk. Anat.* **69**, 474–479.

Knowles, F. and Vollrath, L. (1966d). Changes in the pituitary of the migrating European eel during its journey from rivers to sea. *Z. Zellforsch. mikrosk. Anat.* **75**, 317–327.

Knowles, F., Weatherhead, B. and Martin, R. (1970). The ultrastructure of neurosecretory fibre terminals after zinc–iodine–osmium impregnation In *Aspects of neurosecretion* (ed. W. Bargmann and B. Scharrer), pp. 159–165. Berlin, Heidelberg, New York: Springer-Verlag.

Kobayashi, H. (1972). Median eminence of the hagfish and ependymal absorption in higher vertebrates. In *Brain–endocrine interaction. Median eminence: structure and function.* (ed. K. M. Knigge, D. E. Scott and A. Weindl), pp. 67–78. Basel: Karger.

Kobayashi, H. and Matsui, T. (1969). Fine structure of the median eminence and its functional significance. In *Frontiers in neuroendocrinology 1969* (ed. W. F. Ganong and L. Martini), pp. 3–46. Oxford University Press.

Kobayashi, H., Matsui, T. and Ishii, S. (1970). The functional electron microscopy of the hypothalamic median eminence. *Int. Rev. Cytol.* **29**, 281–381.

Kobayashi, H. and Uemura, H. (1972). The neurohypophysis of the hagfish, *Eptatretus burgeri* (Girard). *Gen. comp. Endocr. Suppl.* **3**, 114–124.

Kobayashi, Y. (1964). Functional morphology of the pars intermedia of the rat hypophysis as revealed with the electron microscope. I. Ultrastructural changes after dehydration. *Gunma Symp. Endocr.* **1**, 173–181.

Kobayashi, Y. (1965). Functional morphology of the pars intermedia of the rat hypophysis as revealed with the electron microscope. II. Correlation of the pars intermedia with the hypophyseal-adrenal axis. *Z. Zellforsch. mikrosk. Anat.* **68**, 155–171.

Koelle, G. B. and Geesey, C. (1961). Localisation of acetylcholinesterase in the neurohypophysis and its functional implications. *Proc. Soc. exp. Biol. Med.* **106**, 625–628.

Kojima, M. (1917). Studies on the endocrine glands. II. The relations of the pituitary body with the thyroid and parathyroid and certain other endocrine organs in the rat. *Q. Jl exp. Physiol.* **11**, 319–338.

Koneff, A. A. (1938). Adaptation of the Mallory azan staining method to the anterior pituitary of the rat. *Stain Technol.* **13**, 49–52.

Krause, W. (1876). *Handbuch der menschlichen Anatomie*, Bd 1: *Allgemeine und Mikroskopische Anatomie*, p. 347.

Kreitner, D. and Laget, P. (1971). Étude des activités bioélectriques unitaires du noyau préoptique des salmonidés. *C. r. Séanc. Soc. Biol.* **165**, 547–553.

Krisch, B., Becker, K. and Bargmann, W. (1972). Exocytose im Hinterlappen der Hypophyse. *Z. Zellforsch. mikrosk. Anat.* **123**, 47–54.

Krsulovic, J. and Brückner, G. (1969). Morphological characteristics of pituicytes in different functional stages. *Z. Zellforsch. mikrosk. Anat.* **99**, 210–220.

Kurachi, K. and Suchowsky, G. (1958). Zur Frage der Beziehung des Hypothalamus zur Ovulation beim Kaninchen. *Acta endocr., Copnh.* **29**, 27–32.

Kurosumi, K., Matsuzawa, T. and Fujie, E. (1962). Histological and histochemical studies on the rat pituitary pars intermedia. *Arch. histol. jap.* **22**, 209–227.

Kurosumi, K., Matsuzawa, T., Kobayashi, Y. and Sato, S. (1964). On the relationship between the release of neurosecretory substance and lipid granules of pituicytes in the rat neurohypophysis. *Gunma Symp. Endocr.* **1**, 87–118.

Kurosumi, K., Matsuzawa, T. and Shibasaki, K. (1961). Electron-microscope studies on the fine structures of the pars nervosa and pars intermedia, and their morphological inter-relation in the normal rat hypophysis. *Gen. comp. Endocr.* **1**, 433–452.

LaBella, F. S., Shin, S. H., Vivian, S. R. and Dular, R. (1971). Characterization of neurophysin polymorphs and trophin-releasing peptides associated with neurophysins. *Mem. Soc. Endocr.* **19**, 293–312.

Ladman, A. J. and Barrnett, R. J. (1956). Variations of the histochemically demonstrable protein-bound sulfhydryl and disulfide groups in cells of the anterior pituitary gland of the various endocrine conditions. *J. Morph.* **98**, 305–333.

Lagios, M. D. (1968). Tetrapod-like organization of the pituitary gland of the polypteriformid fishes, *Calamoichthys calabaricus* and *Polypterus palmas*. *Gen. comp. Endocr.* **11**, 300–315.

Lagios, M. D. (1970). The median eminence of the bowfin, *Amia calva* L. *Gen. comp. Endocr.* **15**, 453–463.

Lagios, M. D. (1972). Evidence for a hypothalamo-hypophysial portal vascular system in the coelacanth *Latimeria chalumnae* Smith. *Gen. comp. Endocr.* **18**, 73–82.

Landgrebe, F. W. and Mitchell, G. M. (1966). The function of the pars intermedia in lower vertebrates. In *The pituitary gland* (ed. G. W. Harris and B. T. Donovan), vol. III, pp. 41–58. London: Butterworths.

Landsmeer, J. M. F. (1963). A survey of the analysis of hypophyseal vascularity. In *Advances in neuroendocrinology* (ed. A. V. Nalbandov), pp. 29–57. Urbana: University of Illinois Press.

La Pointe, J. L. (1969). Effect of ovarian steroids and neurohypophysial hormones on the oviduct of the viviparous lizard, *Klauberina riversiana*. *J. Endocr.* **43**, 197–205.

Larsen, L. O. (1965). Effects of hypophysectomy in the cyclostome *Lampetra fluviatilis* (L.) Gray. *Gen. comp. Endocr.* **5**, 16–30.

Larsen, L. O. (1969). Hypophyseal functions in river lampreys. *Gen. comp. Endocr. Suppl.* **2**, 522–527.

Larsen, L. O., van Kemenade, J. A. M. and van Dongen, W. J. (1971). Localisation and identification of corticotropin-producing cells in the distal lobe of the *Rana temporaria* pituitary gland. *Gen. comp. Endocr.* **16**, 165–168.

Larsen, L. O. and Rosenkilde, P. (1971). Iodine metabolism in normal, hypophysectomized, and thyrotropin-treated river lampreys, *Lampetra fluviatilis* (Gray) L. (Cyclostomata). *Gen. comp. Endocr.* **17**, 94–104.

Larsen, L. O. and Rothwell, B. (1972). Adenohypophysis. In *The biology of lampreys* (ed. M. W. Hardisty and I. C. Potter), vol. 2, pp. 1–67. New York and London: Academic Press.

Laruelle, M. (1934). Le système végétatif méso-diencéphalique. *Rev. neurol.* **1**, 809–842.

Leatherland, J. F. (1969). Studies on the structure and ultrastructure of the intact and 'methallibure'-treated mesoadenohypophysis of the viviparous teleost *Cymatogaster aggregata* Gibbons. *Z. Zellforsch. mikrosk. Anat.* **98**, 122–134.

Leatherland, J. F. (1970*a*). Seasonal variation in the structure and ultrastructure of the pituitary of the marine form (*trachurus*) of the threespine stickleback, *Gasterosteus aculeatus* L. I. Rostral pars distalis. *Z. Zellforsch. mikrosk. Anat.* **104**, 301–317.

Leatherland, J. F. (1970*b*). Seasonal variation in the structure and ultrastructure of the pituitary gland in the marine form (*trachurus*) of the threespine stickleback, *Gasterosteus aculeatus* L. II. Proximal pars distalis and neuro-intermediate lobe. *Z. Zellforsch. mikrosk. Anat.* **104**, 318–336.

Leatherland, J. F. (1970*c*). Structure and ultrastructure of the neurohypophysis of the viviparous teleost, *Cymatogaster aggregata* Gibbons. *Canad. J. Zool.* **48**, 1087–1091.

Leatherland, J. F. and Dodd, J. M. (1969). Histology and fine structure of the preoptic nucleus and hypothalamic tracts of the European eel *Anguilla anguilla* L. *Phil. Trans. R. Soc. Ser. B* **256**, 135–145.

Lederis, K. (1962). Vasopressin and oxytocin in the mammalian hypothalamus. *Gen. comp. Endocr.* **1**, 80–89.

Lederis, K. (1967). Ultrastructural and biological evidence for the presence and likely functions of acetylcholine in the hypothalamo-hypophysial system. In *Neurosecretion* (ed. F. Stutinsky), pp. 155–164. Berlin, Heidelberg, New York: Springer-Verlag.

Lederis, K. (1969). Storage and release of neurohypophysial hormones with special reference to the fine structure of the vertebrate posterior pituitary. In *Physiology of adaptation mechanisms* (ed. E. Bajusz), pp. 237–264. Oxford and New York: Pergamon Press.

Lederis, K. and Heller, H. (1960). Intracellular storage of vasopressin and oxytocin in the posterior pituitary lobe. *Abst. 1st Int. Cong. Endocr.* 115–116.

Lederis, K. and Jayasena, K. (1970). Storage of neurohypophyseal hormones and the mechanism for their release. In *International encyclopaedia of pharmacology and therapeutics*, section 41, vol. I (ed. B. T. Pickering and H. Heller), pp. 111–154. Oxford and New York: Pergamon Press.

Lederis, K. and Livingston, A. (1966). Acetylcholine content of the rabbit neurohypophysis. *J. Physiol., Lond.* **185**, 37–38.

Legait, E. and Legait, H. (1964). Histophysiologie comparée de la pars intermedia de l'hypophyse. *Archs Biol.* **75**, 497–527.

Legait, E. and Legait, H. (1955). Modifications de structure du lobe distal de l'hypophyse au cours de la couvaison chez la poule Rhode-Island. *C. r. Ass. Anat.* **84**, 188–199.

Legait, H. (1964). *Recherches histophysiologiques sur le lobe intermédiaire de l'hypophyse*. Nancy: Société d'Impressions Typographiques.

Legait, H. (1969). Recherches expérimentales sur le lobe tubéral de l'hypophyse chez le rat impubère. *C. r. Séanc. Soc. Biol.* **163**, 714–715.

Legait, H. and Burlet, A. (1966). Recherches morphologiques et expérimentales sur les lobes tubéraux des amphibiens. *C. r. Séanc. Soc. Biol.* **160**, 2437–2439.

Leonhardt, H. (1966). Über ependymale Tanycyten des III. Ventrikels beim Kaninchen in elektronenmikroskopischer Betrachtung. *Z. Zellforsch. mikrosk. Anat.* **74**, 1–11.

Lerner, A. B. (1966). Possible physiological function of intermediate lobe hormones in mammals. In *The Pituitary gland* (ed. G. W. Harris and B. T. Donovan), vol. III, pp. 59–61. London: Butterworths.

Lerner, A. B. and McGuire, J. S. (1961). Effect of α- and β-melanocyte stimulating hormones on the skin colour of man. *Nature, Lond.* **189**, 176–179.

Leveque, T. F. and Small, M. (1959). The relationship of the pituicyte to the posterior lobe hormones. *Endocrinology* **65**, 909–915.

Leznof, A., Fishman, J., Goodfriend, L., McGarry, E., Beck, J. and Rose, B (1960). Localisation of fluorescent antibodies to human growth hormone in human anterior pituitary glands. *Proc. Soc. exp. Biol. Med.* **104**, 232–235.

Li, C. H. (1949). The chemistry of gonadotropic hormones. *Vitamins and Hormones* **7**, 223–252.

Li, C. H. (1969). β-Lipotropin, a new pituitary hormone. In *Colloque Internatl CNRS, Paris* **177**, 93–101.

Licht, P. (1970). Effects of mammalian gonadotropins (ovine FSH and LH) in female lizards. *Gen. comp. Endocr.* **14**, 98–106.

Licht, P. and Bradshaw, S. D. (1969). A demonstration of corticotropic activity and its distribution in the pars distalis of the reptile. *Gen. comp. Endocr.* **13**, 226–235.

Licht, P., Cohen, D. C. and Bern, H. A. (1972). Somatotropic effects of mammalian growth hormone and prolactin in larval newts, *Taricha torosa*. *Gen. comp. Endocr.* **18**, 391–415.

Licht, P. and Hartree, A. S. (1971). Actions of mammalian, avian and piscine gonadotrophins in the lizard. *J. Endocr.* **49**, 113–124.

Licht, P. and Nicoll, C. S. (1969). Localisation of prolactin in the reptilian pars distalis. *Gen. comp. Endocr.* **12**, 526–535.

Licht, P. and Papkoff, H. (1971). Gonadotropic activities of the subunits of ovine FSH and LH in the lizard *Anolis carolinensis*. *Gen. comp. Endocr.* **16**, 586–593.

Licht, P. and Pearson, A. K. (1969). Effects of mammalian gonadotropins (FSH and LH) on the testes of the lizard *Anolis carolinensis*. *Gen. comp. Endocr.* **13**, 367–381.

Licht, P. and Rosenberg, L. L. (1969). Presence and distribution of gonadotropin and thyrotropin in the pars distalis of the lizard *Anolis carolinensis*. *Gen. comp. Endocr.* **13**, 439–454.

Lisk, R. D. (1967). Neural control of gonad size by hormone feedback in the desert iguana *Dipsosaurus dorsalis dorsalis*. *Gen. comp. Endocr.* **8**, 258–266.

Livingston, A. and Lederis, K. (1971). The functional ultrastructure of the neurohypophysis. *Mem. Soc. Endocr.* **19**, 233–261.

Löfgren, F. (1961). The glial–vascular apparatus in the floor of the infundibular cavity. *Lunds Universitets Arsskrift.* **57**, No. 2.

Lothringer, S. (1886). Untersuchungen an der Hypophysis einiger Säugetiere und des Menschen. *Arch. mikrosk. Anat.* **28**, 257–292.

Lundin, P. M. and Schelin, U. (1964). Light and electron microscopic studies on thyrotrophic pituitary adenomas in the mouse. *Lab. Invest.* **13**, 62–68.

Luschka, H. (1860). *Der Hirnanhang und die Steissdrüse des Menschen.* Berlin.

McCann, S. M. (1962). A hypothalamic luteinizing hormone-releasing factor (LH–RF). *Am. J. Physiol.* **202**, 395–400.

McCann, S. M., Kalra, P. S., Donoso, A. O., Bishop, W., Schneider, H. P. G., Fawcett, C. P. and Krulich, L. (1972). The role of monoamines in the control of gonadotropin and prolactin secretion. In *Brain–endocrine interaction. Median eminence: structure and function* (ed. K. M. Knigge, D. E. Scott and A. Weindl), pp. 224–235. Basel: Karger.

McCann, S. M. and Porter, J. C. (1969). Hypothalamic pituitary stimulating and inhibiting hormones. *Physiol. Rev.* **49**, 140–284.

McConnell, E. M. (1953). The arterial blood supply of the human hypophysis cerebri. *Anat. Rec.* **115**, 175–203.

McDonald, R. K. and Weise, V. K. (1956). Effect of arginine-vasopressin and lysine-vasopressin on plasma 17-hydroxycorticosteroid levels in man. *Proc. Soc. exp. Biol. Med.* **92**, 481–483.

McGrath, P. (1968). Prolactin activity and human growth hormone in pharyngeal hypophysis from embalmed cadavers. *J. Endocr.* **42**, 205–212.

McGrath, P. (1971). The volume of the human pharyngeal hypophysis in relation to age and sex. *J. Anat.* **110**, 275–282.

McKeown, B. A. (1972). Prolactin and growth hormone concentrations in the plasma of the toad *Bufo bufo* (L.) following ectopic transplantation of the pars distalis. *Gen. comp. Endocr.* **19**, 167–174.

McKeown, B. A. and van Overbeeke, A. P. (1971). Immunohistochemical identification of pituitary hormone producing cells in the sockeye salmon (*Oncorhynchus nerka*, Walbaum). *Z. Zellforsch. mikrosk. Anat.* **112**, 350–362.

McManus, J. F. A. (1946). Histological demonstration of mucin after periodic acid. *Nature, Lond.* **158**, 202.

McShan, W. H. (1971). Secretory granules from anterior pituitary glands. *Mem. Soc. Endocr.* **19**, 161–184.

McShan, W. H. and Meyer, R. K. (1949). Gonadotrophic activity of granules isolated from rat pituitary glands. *Proc. Soc. exp. Biol. Med.* **71**, 407–410.

Markee, J. E., Sawyer, C. H. and Hollinshead, W. H. (1946). Activation of the anterior hypophysis by electrical stimulation in the rabbit. *Endocrinology* **38**, 345–357.

Marquet, E., Sobel, H. J., Schwarz, R. and Weiss, M. (1972). Secretion by ependymal cells of the neurohypophysis and saccus vasculosus of *Polypterus ornatipinnis* (Osteichthys). *J. Morph.* **137**, 111–130.

Marshall, A. J. (1964). *Bower birds. Their displays and breeding cycles.* Oxford University Press.

Marshall, J. M. (1951). Localisation of adrenocorticotrophic hormone by histochemical and immunochemical methods. *J. exp. Med.* **94**, 21–30.

Martinez, P. M. (1960). The structure of the pituitary stalk and the innervation of the neurohypophysis in the cat. Thesis, University of Leiden.

Martini, L. and De Poli, A. (1956). Neurohumoral control of the release of adrenocorticotrophic hormone. *J. Endocr.* **13**, 229–234.

Martinovitch, P. N. and Pavić, B. (1960). Functional pituitary transplants in rats. *Nature, Lond.* **185**, 155–156.

Masur, S. K. (1969). Fine structure of the autotransplanted pituitary in the red eft, *Notophthalmus viridescens. Gen. comp. Endocr.* **12**, 12–32.

Masur, S. K. and Holtzman, E. (1969). Lysosomes and secretory granules in the normal and autotransplanted salamander's pars distalis. *Gen. comp. Endocr.* **12**, 33–39.

Matsuo, H., Arimura, A., Nair, R. M. G. and Schally, A. V. (1971). Synthesis of the porcine LH- and FSH-releasing hormone by the solid-phase method. *Biochem. biophys. Res. Commun.* **45**, 822–827.

Matsuo, S., Vitum, A., King, J. R. and Farner, D. S. (1969). Light-microscope studies of the cytology of the adenohypophysis of the white-crowned sparrow, *Zonotrichia leucophrys gambelii*. *Z. Zellforsch. mikrosk. Anat.* **95**, 143–176.

Mattheij, J. A. M. (1968*a*). The cell types in the adenohypophysis of the blind Mexican cave fish, *Anoptichthys jordani* (Hubbs and Innes). *Z. Zellforsch. mikrosk. Anat.* **90**, 542–553.

Mattheij, J. A. M. (1968*b*). The ACTH cells in the adenohypophsis of the Mexican cave fish *Anoptichthys jordani*, as identified by metopirone (SU 4885) treatment. *Z. Zellforsch mikrosk. Anat.* **92**, 588–595.

Mattheij, J. A. M. (1969). The thyrotropin secreting basophils in the adenohypophysis of *Anoptichthys jordani*. *Z. Zellforsch. mikrosk. Anat.* **101**, 588–597.

Mattheij, J. A. M. (1970). The gonadotropic cells in the adenohypophysis of the blind Mexican cave fish, *Anoptichthys jordani*. *Z. Zellforsch. mikrosk. Anat.* **105**, 91–106.

Mattheij, J. A. M., Kingma, F. J. and Stroband, H. W. J. (1971). The identification of the thyrotropic cells in the adenohypophysis of the cichlid fish *Cichlasoma biocellatum* and the role of these cells and of the thyroid in osmoregulation. *Z. Zellforsch. mikrosk. Anat.* **121**, 82–92.

Mattheij, J. A. M. and Sprangers, J. A. P. (1969). The site of prolactin secretion in the adenohypophysis of the stenohaline teleost *Anoptichthys jordani*, and the effects of this hormone on mucous cell. *Z. Zellforsch. mikrosk. Anat.* **99**, 411–419.

Mattheij, J. A. M., Stroband, H. W. J. and Kingma, F. J. (1971). The cell types in the adenohypophysis of the cichlid fish *Cichlasoma biocellatum* Regan, with special attention to its osmoregulatory role. *Z. Zellforsch. mikrosk. Anat.* **118**, 113–126.

Maurer, S. and Lewis, B. (1922). The structure and differentiation of the specific cellular elements of the pars intermedia of the hypophysis of the domestic pig. *J. exp. Med.* **36**, 141–156.

Mazzi, V. (1969). Biologica della prolattina. *Boll. Zool.* **36**, 1–60.

Mazzi, V. (1970). The hypothalamus as a thermodependent neuroendocrine center in urodeles. In *The hypothalamus* (ed. L. Martini, M. Motta and F. Frashchini), pp. 663–676. New York and London: Academic Press.

Mazzi, V. (1971). Preliminary observations on the effect of subtotal adenohypophysectomy on some endocrine glands in the crested newt. Contribution to the pituitary histophysiology. *Atti. Accad. Sci., Torino* **105**, 639–645.

Mazzi, V., Peyrot, A., Anzalone, M. R. and Toscano, C. (1966). L'histophysiologie de l'adénohypophyse des tritons crêtés (*Triturus cristatus carnifex* Laur.). *Z. Zellforsch. mikrosk. Anat.* **72**, 597–617.

Mazzi, V., Vellano, C. and Colucci, D. (1971). Effects on the height of the newt (*Triturus cristatus*) caudal fin by prolactin contaminating the commercial growth hormone and by homologous prolactin purified by polyacrylamide gel disc electrophoresis. *Atti. Accad. Sci., Torino* **106**, 129–135.

Meites, J. (1972). Hypothalamic control of prolactin secretion. In *Lactogenic hormones* (ed. G. E. W. Wolstenholme and J. Knight), pp. 325–347. Edinburgh and London: Churchill Livingstone.

Mellinger, J. (1960*a*). Contribution à l'étude de la vascularisation et du développement de la région hypophysaire d'un sélacien, *Scyliorhinus caniculus* (L.). *Bull. Soc. Zool. France* **85**, 123–139.

Mellinger, J. (1960*b*). Esquisse structurale de l'appareil hypophysaire d'un sélacien, *Scyliorhinus caniculus* (L.), pour servir de base à une étude expérimentale des corrélations neuro-endocriniennes. *C. r. hebd. Séanc. Acad. Sci., Paris* **251**, 2422–2424.

Mellinger, J. (1960*c*). La circulation sanguine dans le complexe hypophysaire de la roussette. *Bull. Soc. Zool. France* **85**, 395–399.

Mellinger, J. (1962). Existence de plusieurs systèmes neurosécrétoires hypothalamo-hypophysaires chez les poissons élasmobranches *Scyliorhinus caniculus* et *Sc. stellaris*. Microscopie ordinaire et microscopie électronique. *C. r. hebd. Séanc. Acad. Sci., Paris* **255**, 1789–1791.

Mellinger, J. (1963). Étude histophysiologique du système hypothalamo-hypophysaire de *Scyliorhinus caniculus* (L.) en état de mélanodispersion permanente. *Gen. comp. Endocr.* **3**, 26–45.

Mellinger, J. (1964). Les relations neuro-vasculo-glandulaires dans l'appareil hypophysaire de la roussette, *Scyliorhinus caniculus* (L.). *Archs Anat. Histol. Embryol.* **47**, 1–201.

Mellinger, J. (1966). Variations de la structure hypophysaire chez les Chondrichthyens: étude de l'ange de mer (*Squatina*) et de la pastenaque (*Trygon*). *Annls Endocr., Paris* **27**, 439–450.

Mellinger, J. (1969). Développement post-embryonnaire de l'adénohypophyse de la torpille (*Torpedo marmorata*, Chondrichthyens); évolution du système des cavités et manifestations du dimorphisme sexuel. *Annls Université et A.R.E.R.S.* **7**, 33–48.

Mellinger, J. (1972). Types cellulaires et fonctions de l'adénohypophyse de la torpille (*Torpedo marmorata*). *Gen. comp. Endocr.* **18**, 608.

Mellinger, J., Follénius, E. and Porte, A. (1962). Présence de terminaisons neurosécrétoires sur les capillaires primaires du système porte hypophysaire de la roussette (*Scyliorhinus caniculus*). Étude au microscope électronique. *C. r. hebd. Séanc. Acad. Sci., Paris* **254**, 1158–1159.

Metuzals, J. (1956). The innervation of the adenohypophysis in the duck. *J. Endocr.* **14**, 87–95.

Meurling, P. (1962). The relations between neural and intermediate lobes in the pituitary of *Squalus acanthias*. *Z. Zellforsch. mikrosk. Anat.* **58**, 51–89.

Meurling, P. (1963). Nerves of the intermediate lobe of *Etmopterus spinax* (Elasmobranchii). *Z. Zellforsch. mikrosk. Anat.* **61**, 183–201.

Meurling, P. (1967*a*). The vascularisation of the pituitary in elasmobranchs. *Sarsia* **28**, 1–104.

Meurling, P. (1967*b*). The vascularisation of the pituitary in *Chimaera monstrosa*. *Sarsia* **30**, 83–106.

Meurling, P. (1972). Control of pars intermedia in large embryos of the spiny dogfish, *Squalus acanthias*. *Gen. comp. Endocr.* **18**, 609.

Meurling, P. and Björklund, A. (1970). The arrangement of neurosecretory and catecholamine fibres in relation to the pituitary intermedia cells of the skate, *Raja radiata*. *Z. Zellforsch. mikrosk. Anat.* **108**, 81–92.

Meurling, P., Fremberg, M. and Björklund, A. (1969). Control of MSH release in the intermediate lobe of *Raja radiata* (Elasmobranchii). *Gen. comp. Endocr.* **13**, 520.

Meurling, P. and Willstedt. A. (1970). Vascular connections in the pituitary of *Anolis carolinensis* with special reference to the pars intermedia. *Acta Zool., Stockh.* **51**, 211–218.

Mialhe-Voloss, C. and Benoit, J. (1954). L'intermédine dans l'hypophyse et l'hypothalamus du canard. *C. r. Séanc. Soc. Biol.* **148**, 56–59.

Midgley, A. R. (1964). Immunofluorescent localisation of human pituitary luteinizing hormone. *Expl Cell Research* **32**, 606–609.

Midgley, A. R. (1966). Human pituitary luteinizing hormone: an immunohisto-chemical study. *J. Histochem. Cytochem.* **14**, 159–166.

Mikami, S. (1969). Morphological studies of the avian adenohypophysis related to its function. *Gunma Symposia on Endocrinology* **6**, 151–168.

Mikami, S., Oksche, A., Farner, D. S. and Vitums, A. (1970). Fine structure of the vessels of the hypophysial portal system of the white-crowned sparrow, *Zonotrichia leucophrys gambellii. Z. Zellforsch. mikrosk. Anat.* **106**, 155–174.

Mikami, S., Vitums, A. and Farner, D. S. (1969). Electron microscopic studies on the adenohypophysis of the white-crowned sparrow, *Zonotrichia leucophrys gambellii. Z. Zellforsch. mikrosk. Anat.* **97**, 1–29.

Miller, M. R. (1948). The gross and microscopic anatomy of the pituitary and the seasonal histological changes occurring in the pars anterior of the viviparous lizard *Xantusia vigilis. Univ. Calif. Publ. Zool.* **47**, 225–246.

Millhouse, O. E. (1971). A Golgi study of third ventricle tanycytes in the adult rodent brain. *Z. Zellforsch. mikrosk. Anat.* **121**, 1–13.

Millot, J. and Anthony, J. (1965). *Anatomie de Latimeria chalumnae. II. Système nerveux et organes des sens.* Paris: CNRS.

Mira-Moser, F. (1969a). Histophysiologie de la fonction thyréotrope chez le crapaud *Bufo bufo* L. *Archs Anat. Histol. Embryol.* **52**, 87–182.

Mira-Moser, F. (1969b). Action de goîtrigènes sur le têtard de crapaud *Bufo bufo* L. *Archs Anat. Histol. Embryol.* **52**, 314–332.

Mira-Moser, F. (1970). L'ultrastructure de l'adénohypophyse du crapaud *Bufo bufo* L. I. Identification des types cellulaires et comparaison des resultats obtenus avec deux fixateurs différents. *Z. Zellforsch. mikrosk. Anat.* **105**, 65–90.

Mira-Moser, F. (1971). L'ultrastructure de l'adénohypophyse du crapaud *Bufo bufo* L. II. Étude de l'évolution des cellules glycotrotidiques de type II après thyroïdectomie chirurgicale. *Z. Zellforsch. mikrosk. Anat.* **112**, 266–286.

Mira-Moser, F. (1972a). L'ultrastructure de l'adénohypophyse du crapaud *Bufo bufo* L. III. Différentiation des cellules de la *pars distalis* au cours du développement larvaire. *Z. Zellforsch. mikrosk. Anat.* **125**, 88–107.

Mira-Moser, F. (1972b). Action des goîtrigènes sur le têtard de crapaud: étude des modifications ultrastructurales de la *pars distalis* de l'hypophyse. *Gen. comp. Endocr.* **18**, 609–610.

Molnár, B. and Szabó, Zs. (1968). Histological study of the hypophysis of the Transylvanian lamprey (*Eudontomyzon danfordi* Regan). *Acta biol. Acad. Sci. hung.* **19**, 373–379.

Monroe, B. G., Newman, B. L. and Shapiro, S. (1972). Ultrastructure of the median eminence of neonatal and adult rats. In *Brain–endocrine interaction. Median eminence: structure and function* (ed. K. M. Knigge, D. E. Scott and A. Weindl), pp. 7–26. Basel: Karger.

Monroe, B. G. and Scott, D. E. (1966). Ultrastructural changes in the neural lobe of the hypophysis of the rat during lactation and suckling. *J. Ultrastructure Res.* **14**, 497–517.

Morato, M. J. X. (1939). The blood supply of the hypophysis. *Anat. Rec.* **74**, 297–320.

Motta, M., Piva, F. and Martini, L. (1970). The hypothalamus as the centre of endocrine feedback mechanisms. In *The hypothalamus* (ed. L. Martini, M. Motta and F. Fraschini), pp. 463–490. New York and London: Academic Press.

Murakami, M. (1962). Neurosekretorische Zellen im Hypothalamus der Maus. *Z. Zellforsch. mikrosk. Anat.* **56**, 277–299.

Nagahama, Y. and Yamamoto, K. (1969a). Fine structure of the glandular cells in the adenohypophysis of the kokanee *Oncorhynchus nerka. Bull. Fac. Fish. Hokkaido Univ.* **20**, 159–168.

Nagahama, Y. and Yamamoto, K. (1969*b*). Basophils in the adenohypophysis of the goldfish (*Carassius auratus*). *Gunma Symp. Endocr.* **6**, 39–55.

Nagahama, Y. and Yamamoto, K. (1970). Morphological studies on the pituitary of the chum salmon, *Oncorhynchus keta*. (I). Fine structure of the adenohypophysis. *Bull. Fac. Fish. Hokkaido Univ.* **20**, 293–302.

Nair, R. M. G., Kastin, A. J. and Schally, A. V. (1971). Isolation and structure of hypothalamic MSH release inhibiting hormone. *Biochem. biophys. Res. Commun.* **43**, 1376–1381.

Nakai, Y. (1970). Electron microscopic observations on synapse-like contacts between pituicytes and different types of nerve fibres in the anuran pars nervosa. *Z. Zellforsch. mikrosk. Anat.* **110**, 27–39.

Nakai, Y. and Gorbman, A. (1969). Evidence for a doubly-innervated secretory unit in the anuran pars intermedia. II. Electron microscopic studies. *Gen. comp. Endocr.* **13**, 108–116.

Nayar, S. and Pandalai, K. R. (1963). Pars intermedia of the pituitary gland and integumentary colour changes in the garden lizard, *Calotes versicolor*. *Z. Zellforsch. mikrosk. Anat.* **58**, 837–845.

Nicoll, C. S. (1971). Aspects of the neural control of prolactin secretion. In *Frontiers in neuroendocrinology 1971* (ed. L. Martini and W. F. Ganong), pp. 291–330. Oxford University Press.

Nicoll, C. S. and Fiorindo, R. P. (1969). Hypothalmic control of prolactin secretion. *Gen. comp. Endocr. Suppl.* **2**, 26–31.

Nicoll, C. S. and Licht, P. (1971). Evolutionary biology of prolactins and somato-tropins. II. Electrophoretic comparison of tetrapod somatotropins. *Gen. comp. Endocr.* **17**, 490–507.

Nicoll, C. S. and Nichols, C. W. (1971). Evolutionary biology of prolactins and somatotropins. I. Electrophoretic comparison of tetrapod prolactins. *Gen. comp. Endocr.* **17**, 300–310.

Nikitovitch-Winer, M. (1962). Induction of ovulation in rats by direct intrapituitary infusion of median eminence extracts. *Endocrinology* **70**, 350–358.

Nikitovitch-Winer, M. and Everett, J. W. (1957). Resumption of gonadotrophic function in pituitary grafts following retransplantation from kidney to median eminence. *Nature, Lond.* **180**, 1434–1435.

Nikitovitch-Winer, M. and Everett, J. W. (1958). Functional restitution of pituitary grafts re-transplanted from kidney to median eminence. *Endocrinology* **63**, 916–930.

Nishioka, R. S. and Bern, H. A. (1966). Fine structure of the neurohaemal area associated with the hypophysis in the hagfish *Polistotrema stoutii*. *Gen. comp. Endocr.* **7**, 457–462.

Nouhouayi-Besnard, Y. (1966). Anatomie microscopique générale du complexe hypophyso-pituitaire de deux reptiles: *Varanus ex. exanthematicus* (Bosc) et *Varanus n. niloticus* (Linné). *C. r. Séanc. Soc. Biol.* **160**, 179–183.

Oboussier, H. (1947). Über die Grössenbeziehungen der Hypophyse und ihrer Teile bei Saügetieren und Vögeln. *Arch. EntwMech. Org.* **143**, 182–274.

Oboussier, H. (1956). Die hypophyse des Nashorns. *Zool. Anz.* **157**, 1–11.

O'Connor, W. J. (1947). Atrophy of the supraoptic and paraventricular nuclei after interruption of the pituitary stalk in dogs. *J. exp. Physiol.* **34**, 29–42.

Oehmke, H.-J., Priedkalns, J., Harnack, M. and Oksche, A. (1969). Fluoreszenz- und elektronenmikroskopische Untersuchungen am Zwischenhirn-Hypophysen-system von *Passer domesticus*. *Z. Zellforsch. mikrosk. Anat.* **95**, 109–133.

Oksche, A. (1962). The fine nervous, neurosecretory and glial structure of the median eminence of the white-crowned sparrow. *Mem. Soc. Endocr.* **12**, 199–208.

Oksche, A., Zimmermann, P. and Oehmke, H.-J. (1972). Morphometric studies of tubero-eminential systems controlling reproductive functions. In *Brain–endocrine interaction. Median eminence: structure and function* (ed. K. M. Knigge, D. E. Scott and A. Weindl), pp. 142–153. Basel: Karger.

Oldham, F. K. (1938). The pharmacology and anatomy of the hypophysis of the armadillo. *Anat. Rec.* **72**, 265–291.

Olivecrona, H. (1957). Paraventricular nucleus and pituitary gland. *Acta. physiol. scand.* **40**, *Suppl.* 136, 1–178.

Oliver, G. and Schäfer, E. A. (1895). On the physiological action of extracts of pituitary body. *J. Physiol., Lond.* **18**, 277.

Olivereau, M. (1954). Hypophyse et glande thyroïde chez les poissons. Étude histophysiologique de quelques corrélations endocriniennes, en particulier chez *Salmo salar* L. *Annls Inst. Océanogr. Monaco (NS)* **29**, 95–296.

Olivereau, M. (1967a). Observations sur l'hypophyse de l'anguille femelle, en particulier lors de la maturation sexuelle. *Z. Zellforsch. mikrosk. Anat.* **80**, 286–306.

Olivereau, M. (1967b). Notions actuelles sur le contrôle hypothalamique des fonctions hypophysaires chez les poissons. *Rev. europ. Endocr.* **4**, 174–196.

Olivereau, M. (1968). Étude cytologique de l'hypophyse du muge, en particulier en relation avec la salinité extérieure. *Z. Zellforsch. mikrosk. Anat.* **87**, 545–561.

Olivereau, M. (1969a). Activité de la pars intermedia de l'hypophyse autotransplantée chez l'anguille. *Z. Zellforsch. mikrosk. Anat.* **98**, 74–87.

Olivereau, M. (1969b). Complexe neuro-intermédiaire et osmorégulation: comparaison chez l'anguille européenne et chez l'anguille japonaise d'élevage au cours du transfert en eau de mer. *Z. Zellforsch. mikrosk. Anat.* **99**, 389–410.

Olivereau, M. (1970a). Coloration de l'hypophyse avec l'hématoxyline au plomb (H.Pb): données nouvelles chez les téléostéens et comparaison avec les résultats obtenus chez l'autres vertébrés. *Acta Zool., Stockh.* **51**, 229–249.

Olivereau, M. (1970b). Stimulation des cellules somatotropes de l'hypophyse de la carpe après un jeûne prolongé. *C. r. hebd. Séanc. Acad. Sci., Paris* D **270**, 2343–2346.

Olivereau, M. (1971). Elaboration d'intermédine par les cellules colorées avec l'hématoxyline au plomb dans la *pars intermedia* de l'anguille: preuves nouvelles et contrôle hypothalamique. *C. r. hebd. Séanc. Acad. Sci., Paris* D **272**, 102–105.

Olivereau, M. (1972). Identification des cellules thyréotropes dans l'hypophyse du saumon du Pacifique (*Oncorhynchus tschawytscha* Walbaum) après radiothyroïdectomie. *Z. Zellforsch. mikrosk. Anat.* **128**, 175–187.

Olivereau, M. and Ball, J. N. (1963). Fonction corticotrope et cytophysiologie hypophysaire chez deux téléostéens: *Mollienesia latipinna* Le Sueur et *Anguilla anguilla* L. *C. r. hebd. Séanc. Acad. Sci., Paris* **256**, 3766–3769.

Olivereau, M. and Ball, J. N. (1966). Histological study of functional ectopic pituitary transplants in a teleost fish (*Poecilia formosa*). *Proc. R. Soc. Lond. Ser. B* **164**, 106–129.

Olivereau, M. and Ball, J. N. (1970). Pituitary influences on osmoregulation in teleosts. *Mem. Soc. Endocr.* **18**, 57–85.

Olivereau, M. and Herlant, M. (1960). Étude de l'hypophyse de l'anguille mâle au cours de la réproduction. *C. r. Séanc. Soc. Biol.* **154**, 706–709.

Olsson, R. (1959). The neurosecretory hypothalamus system and the adenohypophysis of *Myxine. Z. Zellforsch. mikrosk. Anat.* **51**, 97–107.

Olsson, R. (1967). The exocrine pituitary region in primitive fishes. *Gen. comp. Endocr.* **9**, 478–479.

Olsson, R. (1969). General review of the endocrinology of the Protochordata and Myxinoidea. *Gen. comp. Endocr. Suppl.* **2**, 485–499.

van Oordt, P. G. W. J. (1963). Cell types in the pars distalis of the amphibian pituitary. *Colloq. Internat. CNRS, Paris* **128**, 301–313.

van Oordt, P. G. W. J. (1965). Nomenclature of the hormone-producing cells in the adenohypophysis. A report of the International Committee for Nomenclature of the Adenohypophysis. *Gen. comp. Endocr.* **5**, 131–134.

van Oordt, P. G. W. J. (1966). Changes in the pituitary of the common toad, *Bufo bufo*, during metamorphosis, and the identification of the thyrotropic cells. *Z. Zellforsch. mikrosk. Anat.* **75**, 47–56.

van Oordt, P. G. W. J. (1968). The analysis and identification of the hormone-producing cells of the adenohypophysis. In *Perspectives in endocrinology* (ed. E. J. W. Barrington and C. B. Jørgensen), pp. 405–467. New York and London: Academic Press.

van Oordt, P. G. W. J., van Dongen, W. J. and Lofts, B. (1968). Seasonal changes in endocrine organs of the male common frog, *Rana temporaria*. I. The pars distalis of the adenohypophysis. *Z. Zellforsch. mikrosk. Anat.* **88**, 549–559.

van Oordt, P. G. W. J. and De Kort, E. J. M. (1969). Functions of gonadotropins in adult male amphibians. *Colloq. Internat. CNRS, Paris* **177**, 345–350.

Ortman, R. (1961). Anterior lobe of pituitary of *Rana pipiens*. I. A cytological and cytochemical study. *Gen. comp. Endocr.* **1**, 306–316.

Ortman, R. (1964). Cytochemical study of the physiological activities in the pars intermedia of *Rana pipiens*. *Anat. Rec.* **119**, 1–9.

Ortman, R. and Etkin, W. (1963). The cytology of the pars distalis of metamorphosing and immature *Rana pipiens*. *Am. Zool.* **3**, 552–553.

Ortman, R. and Parker, M. I. (1968). Thyrotropic activity in separated rostral and caudal halves of the pars distalis of *Rana pipiens*. *Gen. comp. Endocr.* **11**, 139–150.

Ortmann, R. (1951). Über Experimentelle veranderungen der Morphologie des Hypophyse-Zwischenhirnsystems und die Beziehung der sog. 'Gomorisubstanz' zum Adiuretin. *Z. Zellforsch. mikrosk. Anat.* **36**, 92–140.

Oshima, K. and Gorbman, A. (1969). Evidence for a doubly innervated secretory unit in the anuran pars intermedia. I. Electrophysiological studies. *Gen. comp. Endocr.* **13**, 98–107.

van Overbeeke, A. P. and McBride, J. R. (1967). The pituitary gland of the sockeye (*Oncorhynchus nerka*) during sexual maturation and spawning. *J. Fish. Res. Bd Can.* **24**, 1791–1810.

Palay, S. L. (1945). Neurosecretion. 7. The preoptico-hypophysial pathway in fishes. *J. comp. Neurol.* **82**, 129–143.

Palay, S. L. (1955). An electron microscope study of the neurohypophysis in normal, hydrated and dehydrated rats. *Anat. Rec.* **121**, 348.

Palay, S. L. (1957). The fine structure of the neurohypophysis. In *Ultrastructure and cellular chemistry of neural tissue* (ed. H. Waelsch), pp. 31–49. New York: Hoeber.

Papkoff, H. and Hayashida, T. (1972). Pituitary growth hormone from the turtle and duck: purification and immunochemical studies. *Proc. Soc. exp. Biol. Med.* **140**, 251–255.

Papkoff, H. and Licht, P. (1972). On the purification of reptilian (turtle) pituitary gonadotropin. *Proc. Soc. exp. Biol. Med.* **139**, 372–376.

Parker, G. H. (1950). Chemical control of nervous activity. Neurohormones in lower vertebrates. In *The hormones* (ed. G. Pincus and K. V. Thimann), vol. ii, pp. 633–656. New York and London: Academic Press.

Pasteels, J. L. (1957). Recherches expérimentales sur le rôle de l'hypothalamus dans la différenciation cytologique de l'hypophyse chez *Pleurodeles Waltlii*. *Archs Biol., Liège* **68**, 65–114.

Pasteels, J. L. (1960). Étude expérimentale des différentes catégories d'éléments chromophiles de l'hypophyse adulte de *Pleurodeles Waltlii*, de leur fonction et de leur contrôle par l'hypothalamus. *Archs Biol., Liège* **71**, 409–471.

Pasteels, J. L. (1961). Premiers résultats de culture combinée *in vitro* d'hypophyse et d'hypothalamus, dans le but d'en apprécier la sécrétion de prolactine. *C. r. Séanc. Acad. Sci., Paris* **253**, 3074–3075.

Pasteels, J. L. (1972). Morphology of prolactin secretion. In *Lactogenic hormones* (ed. G. E. W. Wolstenholme and J. Knight), pp. 241–255. Edinburgh and London: Churchill Livingstone.

Paulesco, N. C. (1907). Recherches sur la physiologie de l'hypophyse de cerveau. L'hypophysectomie et ses effets. *J. Physiol. Path. gén.* **9**, 441 (Cited by Romeis, 1940.)

Payne, F. (1946). The cellular picture in the anterior pituitary of normal fowls from embryo to old age. *Anat. Rec.* **96**, 77–91.

Pearse, A. G. E. (1948). Cytochemistry of the gonadotropic hormones. *Nature, Lond.* **162**, 651.

Pearse, A. G. E. (1949). The cytochemical demonstration of gonadotropic hormone in the human anterior hypophysis. *J. Path. Bact.* **61**, 195–202.

Pearse, A. G. E. (1951). The application of cytochemistry to the localization of gonadotrophin in the pituitary. *J. Endocr.* **7**, xlviii–l.

Pearse, A. G. E. (1952). Observations on the localisation, nature and chemical constitution of some components of the anterior hypophysis. *J. Path. Bact.* **64**, 791–809.

Pearse, A. G. E. (1968). *Histochemistry: theoretical and applied.* 3rd edition, vol. I. Edinburgh and London: Churchill Livingstone.

Peczely, P. and Calas, A. (1970). Ultrastructure de l'éminence médiane du pigeon (*Columba livia domestica*) dans diverses conditions expérimentales. *Z. Zellforsch. mikrosk. Anat.* **111**, 316–345.

Pehlemann, F. W. and Hemme, L. (1972). Morphological transformation of TSH–cell granules in normal and thiouracil-treated *Xenopus laevis* larvae. *Gen. comp. Endocr.* **18**, 615.

Pelletier, G., Peillon, F. and Vila-Porcile, E. (1971). An ultrastructural study of sites of granule extrusion in the anterior pituitary of the rat. *Z. Zellforsch. mikrosk. Anat.* **115**, 501–507.

Pelletier, G. and Racadot, J. (1971). Identification des cellules hypophysaires sécrétant l'ACTH chez le rat. *Z. Zellforsch. mikrosk. Anat.* **116**, 228–239.

Peng, M.-T., Pi, W.-P. and Wu, C.-I. (1969). Growth hormone secretion by pituitary grafts under median eminence or renal capsule. *Endocrinology* **85**, 360–365.

Perdue, J. F. and McShan, W. H. (1962). Isolation and biochemical studies of secretory granules from rat pituitary glands. *J. Cell. Biol.* **15**, 159–172.

Peremeschko, P. (1867). Über den Bau des Hirnanhangs. *Virchows Arch. path. Anat. Physiol.* **38**, 329–342.

Perks, A. M. (1969). The neurohypophysis. In *Fish physiology* (ed. W. S. Hoar and D. J. Randall), vol. II, pp. 111–205. New York and London: Academic Press.

Peter, R. E. (1970). Hypothalamic control of thyroid activity and gonadal activity in the goldfish, *Carassius auratus*. *Gen. comp. Endocr.* **14**, 334–356.

Peter, R. E. (1971). Feedback effects of thyroxine on the hypothalamus and pituitary of goldfish, *Carassius auratus*. *J. Endocr.* **51**, 31–39.

Peterson, R. R. and Weiss, J. (1955). Staining of the adenohypophysis with acid and basic dyes. *Endocrinology* **57**, 96–108.

Peute, J. and Goos, H. J. T. (1970). Biogenic amines in the tuber cinereum of *Xenopus laevis* tadpoles. Electron and fluorescence microscopical observations.

In *Aspects of neuroendocrinology* (ed. W. Bargmann and B. Scharrer), pp. 112–117. Berlin, Heidelberg, New York: Springer-Verlag.

Peyrot, A. (1969). La fonction thyréotrope de l'adénohypophyse chez le triton crêté après lésion permanente de l'éminence médiale. *Gen. comp. Endocr.* **13**, 525–526.

Peyrot, A., Mazzi, V., Vellano, C. and Lodi, G. (1969). Prolactin activity of short-term and long-term autografted pituitaries of the hypophysectomized crested newt. *J. Endocr.* **45**, 515–530.

Peyrot, A., Pons, G., Biciotti, M. and Vottero, C. (1972). L'activité thyréotrope de l'autogreffe ectopique adénohypophysaire chez le triton crêté étudiée en fonction du temps. *Gen. comp. Endocr.* **18**, 616.

Peyrot, A., Vellano, C., Andreoletti, G. E., Pons, G. and Biciotti, M. (1971). On the activating effect of prolactin on thyroid metabolism in the crested newt. Comparison between the effect of prolactin and methylthiouracil. *Gen. comp. Endocr.* **16**, 524–534.

Philibert, R. I. and Kamemoto, F. I. (1965). The hypothalamo-hypophyseal neuro-secretory system of the ring-necked snake, *Diadophis punctatus. Gen. comp. Endocr.* **5**, 326–335.

Pickering, A. D. (1972). Effects of hypophysectomy on the activity of the endostyle and thyroid gland in the larval and adult river lamprey, *Lampetra fluviatilus* L. *Gen. comp. Endocr.* **18**, 335–343.

Pickford, G. E. and Atz, J. W. (1957). *The physiology of the pituitary gland of fishes.* New York: New York Zoological Society.

Pickford, M. (1939). The inhibitory effect of acetylcholine on water diuresis in the dog, and its pituitary transmission. *J. Physiol., Lond.* **95**, 226–238.

Pickford, M. (1947). The action of acetylcholine in the supraoptic nucleus of the chloralosed dog. *J. Physiol., Lond.* **106**, 264–270.

Pickford, M. and Richie, A. E. (1945). Experiments on the hypothalamic-pituitary control of water excretion in dogs. *J. Physiol., Lond.* **104**, 105–128.

Pietsch, K. (1930). Aufbau und Entwicklung der Pars tuberalis des menschlichen Hirnanhangs in ihren Beziehungen zu den übrigen Hypophysenteilen. *Z. mikrosk.-anat. Forsch.* **22**, 227–258.

Pines, L.-L. (1926). Über die Innervation der Hypophysis cerebri. II. Mitteilung. *Z. Neurol. Psychiat.* **100**, 123–138.

Polenov, A. L., Garlov, P. E., Konstantinova, M. S. and Belenky, M. A. (1972). The hypothalamo-hypophysial system in Acipenseridae. II. Adrenergic structures of the hypophysial neuro-intermediate complex. *Z. Zellforsch. mikrosk. Anat.* **128**, 470–481.

Polenov, A. L., Pavlovic, M. and Garlov, P. E. (1972). Preoptic nucleus and neuro-hypophysis in sturgeons (*Acipenser guldenstadti* Brand) in different stages of their life cycle and in experiments. *Gen. comp. Endocr.* **18**, 617.

Popa, G. T. (1937). Les vaisseaux portes hypophysaires. *Rev. frc. Endocrinol.* **15**, 122–135.

Popa, G. T. and Fielding, U. (1930). A portal circulation from the pituitary to the hypothalamic region. *J. Anat.* **65**, 88–91.

Popjak, G. (1940). The pathways of pituitary colloid through the hypothalamus. *J. Path. Bact.* **51**, 83–89.

Poris, E. G. (1941). Studies on the endocrines of reptiles. II. Variations in the histology of the hypophysis of *Anolis carolinensis,* with a note on the Golgi configuration in cells of the pars anterior and pars intermedia. *Anat. Rec.* **80**, 99–121.

Poris, E. G. and Charipper, H. A. (1938). Studies on the endocrine glands of reptiles. I. The morphology of the pituitary gland of the lizard (*Anolis carolinensis*) with special reference to certain cell types. *Anat. Rec.* **72**, 473–489.

Porte, A., Klein, M. J., Stoeckel, M. E. and Stutinsky, F. (1971). Sur l'existence de cellules de type 'corticotrope' dans la pars intermedia de l'hypophyse du rat. *Z. Zellforsch. mikrosk. Anat.* **115**, 60–68.

Porter, J. C., Dhariwal, A. P. S. and McCann, S. M. (1967). Response of the anterior pituitary-adrenocortical axis to purified CRF. *Endocrinology* **80**, 679–688.

Porter, J. C., Kamberi, I. A. and Ondo, J. G. (1972). Role of biogenic amines and cerebrospinal fluid in the neurovascular transmittal of hypophysiotrophic substances. In *Brain–endocrine interaction. Median eminence: structure and function.* (ed. K. M. Knigge, D. E. Scott and A. Weindl), pp. 245–253. Basel: Karger.

Purves, H. D. (1961). Morphology of the hypophysis related to its function. In *Sex and internal secretions*, 3rd edition (ed. W. C. Young), pp. 161–239. London: Baillière, Tindall and Cox.

Purves, H. D. (1966). Cytology of the adenohypophysis. In *The pituitary gland* (ed. G. W. Harris and B. T. Donovan), vol. I, pp. 147–232. London: Butterworths.

Purves, H. D. and Griesbach, W. E. (1951). The site of thyrotrophin and gonadotrophin production in the rat pituitary studied by the McManus–Hotchkiss staining for glycoprotein. *Endocrinology* **49**, 244–264.

Purves, H. D. and Griesbach, W. E. (1954). The site of follicle stimulating and luteinizing hormone production in the rat pituitary. *Endocrinology* **55**, 785–793.

Purves, H. D. and Griesbach, W. E. (1955). Changes in the gonadotrophs of the rat pituitary after gonadectomy. *Endocrinology* **56**, 374–386.

Purves, H. D. and Griesbach, W. E. (1956). Changes in the basophil cells of the rat pituitary after thyroidectomy. *J. Endocr.* **13**, 365–375.

Raftery, A. T. (1969). Enzyme histochemistry of the pars intermedia of the ox pituitary gland. *J. Anat.* **105**, 307–315.

Rahn, H. and Painter, B. T. (1941). A comparative histology of the bird pituitary. *Anat. Rec.* **79**, 297–311.

Ramirez, V. D. and Sawyer, C. H. (1965). Fluctuation in hypothalamic LH–RF (luteinizing hormone-releasing factor) during the rat estrous cycle. *Endocrinology* **76**, 282–289.

Rasmussen, A. T. (1938). Innervation of the hypophysis. *Endocrinology* **23**, 263–278.

Rastogi, R. K. and Chieffi, G. (1970*a*). A cytological study of the pars distalis of pituitary gland of normal, gonadectomized, and gonadectomized steroid hormone-treated green frog, *Rana esculenta* L. *Gen. comp. Endocr.* **15**, 247–263.

Rastogi, R. K. and Chieffi, G. (1970*b*). Cytological changes in the pars distalis of pituitary of the green frog, *Rana esculenta* L., during the reproductive cycle. *Z. Zellforsch. mikrosk. Anat.* **111**, 505–518.

Rastogi, R. K. and Chieffi, G. (1970*c*). Changes in the cytology of the pars distalis of pituitary of green frog, *Rana esculenta*, under laboratory confinement. *Gen. comp. Endocr.* **15**, 488–491.

Rastogi, R. K., Chieffi, G. and Marmorino, C. (1972). Effects of methallibure (ICI 33,828) on the pars distalis of pituitary, testis and thumb pads of the green frog, *Rana esculenta* L. *Z. Zellforsch. mikrosk. Anat.* **123**, 430–440.

Reddy, P. R. K. and Prasad, M. R. N. (1970). Hormonal control of the maintenance of spermatogenesis and sexual segment in the Indian house lizard *Hemidactylus flaviridis* Ruppell. *Gen. comp. Endocr.* **14**, 15–24.

Reese, J. B., Koneff, A. A. and Akimoto, M. B. (1939). Anterior pituitary changes following adrenalectomy in the rat. *Anat. Rec.* **75**, 373–403.

Reese, J. D., Koneff, A. A. and Wainman, P. (1943). Cytological differences between castration and thyroidectomy basophils in the rat hypophysis. In *Essays in biology*, pp. 471–485. University of California Press.

Rémy, C. (1969). Étude cytologique du lobe distal de l'hypophyse du têtard d'*Alytes obstetricans* Laur., au cours du développement larvaire. *Annls Endocr., Paris* **30**, 759–767.

Rennels, E. G. and Drager, G. A. (1955). The relationship of pituicytes to neuro-secretion. *Anat. Rec.* **122**, 193–203.

Retzius, G. (1894). Die Neuroglia der Neuro-Hypophyse der Säugethiere. *Biol. Untersuchungen, Neue Folge* **6**, 21–24.

Ribas-Mujal, D. (1958). Contribución al estudio de la inervación hypofisaria en el buey. *Z. Zellforsch. mikrosk. Anat.* **48**, 356–380.

Richerson, B. A. and deRoos, R. (1971). Comparative morphology of the neuro-hypophysis of the three life stages of the central newt (*Notophthalmus viridescens louisianensis*). *Gen. comp. Endocr.* **17**, 256–267.

Riddle, O., Bates, R. W. and Dykshorn, S. W. (1933). The preparation, identifica-tion and assay of prolactin – a hormone of the anterior pituitary. *Am. J. Physiol.* **105**, 191–216.

Rinehart, J. F. and Farquhar, M. G. (1953). Electron microscopic studies of the anterior pituitary gland. *J. Histochem. Cytochem.* **1**, 93–113.

Rinehart, J. F. and Farquhar, M. G. (1955). The fine vascular organization of the anterior pituitary gland. An electron microscopic study with histochemical correlations. *Anat. Rec.* **121**, 207–240.

Rinne, U. K. (1966). Ultrastructure of the median eminence of the rat. *Z. Zellforsch. mikrosk. Anat.* **74**, 98–122.

Rinne, U. K. and Kivalo, E. (1958). Effect of dehydration on the acid phosphatase activity of the hypothalamic magnocellular nuclei. *Annls Med. exp. Biol. Fenn.* **36**, 350–355.

Rioch, D. McK., Wislocki, G. B. and O'Leary, J. L. (1940). A précis of preoptic hypothalamic and hypophysial terminology with atlas. In *The hypothalamus* (ed. G. W. Harris and B. T. Donovan), pp. 3–30. London: Butterworths.

Rodríguez, E. M. (1966). Differences between median eminence and neural lobe in amphibians. *Z. Zellforsch. mikrosk. Anat.* **74**, 308–316.

Rodríguez, E. M. (1969). Ultrastructure of the neurohaemal area of the toad median eminence. *Z. Zellforsch. mikrosk. Anat.* **93**, 182–212.

Rodríguez, E. M. (1971). The comparative morphology of neural lobes of species with different neurohypophysial hormones. *Mem. Soc. Endocr.* **19**, 263–292.

Rodríguez, E. M. (1972). Comparative and functional morphology of the median eminence. In *Brain–endocrine interaction. Median eminence: structure and function* (ed. K. M. Knigge, D. E. Scott, and A. Weindl), pp. 319–334. Basel: Karger.

Rodríguez, E. M. and Dellman, H. D. (1970). Hormonal content and ultrastructure of the disconnected neural lobe of the grass frog (*Rana pipiens*). *Gen. comp. Endocr.* **15**, 272–288.

Rodríguez, E. M. and La Pointe, J. (1969). Histology and ultrastructure of the neural lobe of the lizard, *Klauberina riversiana. Z. Zellforsch. mikrosk. Anat.* **95**, 37–57.

Rodríguez, E. M. and La Pointe, J. (1970). Light and electron microscopic study of the pars intermedia of the lizard, *Klauberina riversiana. Z. Zellforsch. mikrosk. Anat.* **104**, 1–13.

Rodríguez, E. M., La Pointe, J. and Dellman, H. D. (1971). The nervous control of the pars intermedia of an amphibian and a reptile species. *Mem. Soc. Endocr.* **19**, 827–837.

Rodríguez, E. M. and Piezzi, R. S. (1967). Vascularization of the hypophysial region of the normal and adenohypophysectomized toad. *Z. Zellforsch. mikrosk. Anat.* **83**, 207–218.

Rodríguez, E. M., Vega, J. A. and La Malfa, J. A. (1970). The different origins of the neurosecretory hypothalamo-hypophysial tracts of the toad *Bufo arenarum* Hensel. *Gen. comp. Endocr.* **14**, 248–255.

Romeis, B. (1940). Innerskretorische Drüsen II. Hypophyse. *Handbuch der mikroskopischen Anatomie des Meschen* (ed. v. Möllendorff), vol. VI, Part 3. Berlin: Springer-Verlag.

Rosenkilde, P. (1972). Hypothalamic control of thyroid function in Amphibia. *Gen. comp. Endocr. Suppl.* **3**, 32–40.

Rühle, H. J. and Sterba, G. (1966). Zur histologie der Hypophyse des Flussneunauges (*Lampetra fluviatilis*). *Z. Zellforsch. mikrosk. Anat.* **70**, 136–168.

Russell, D. S. (1956). Effects of dividing the pituitary stalk in man. *Lancet* i, 466–468.

Sage, M. and Bern, H. A. (1971). Cytophysiology of the teleost pituitary. *Internat. Rev. Cytol.* **31**, 339–376.

Sage, M. and Bern, H. A. (1972). Assay of prolactin in vertebrate pituitaries by its dispersion of xanthophore pigment in the teleost *Gillichthys mirabilis*. *J. exp. Zool.* **180**, 169–174.

Sage, M. and Bromage, N. R. (1970). Interaction of the TSH cells and thyroid cells with the gonadotropic cells and gonads in poecilid fishes. *Gen. comp. Endocr.* **14**, 137–140.

Sage, M. and Purrott, R. J. (1969). The control of teleost ACTH cells. *Z. vergl. Physiol.* **63**, 85–90.

Saint-Girons, H. (1963). Histologie comparée de l'adénohypophyse chez les reptiles. *Colloq. Internat. CNRS, Paris* **128**, 275–285.

Saint-Girons, H. (1965). Données histologiques sur le lobe antérieur de l'hypophyse chez *Sphenodon punctatus*. *Archs Anat. microsc. Morph. exp.* **54**, 633–634.

Saint-Girons, H. (1967). Morphologie comparée de l'hypophyse chez les Squamata. *Annls Sci. Nat. (Zool.), Paris* 12 Sér. **9**, 229–308.

Saint-Girons, H. (1970). The pituitary gland. In *Biology of the Reptilia* (ed. C. Gans and T. S. Parsons), vol. III, pp. 135–199. New York and London: Academic Press.

Saland, L. C. (1968). Ultrastructure of the frog *pars intermedia* in relation to hypothalamic control of hormone release. *Neuroendocrinology* **3**, 72–88.

Sandman, C. A., Kastin, A. J. and Schally, A. V. (1971). Behavioural inhibition as modified by melanocyte-stimulating hormone (MSH) and light–dark conditions. *Physiol. Behav.* **6**, 45–48.

Sarkar, H. B. D. and Rao, M. A. (1971). Effect of thyroidectomy and administration of thyroxine on ovulation and spawning *in vivo, in vitro* and in transplantation in the skipper frog, *Rana cyanophlyctis* (Schn). *Gen. comp. Endocr.* **16**, 594–598.

Sathyanesan, A. G. (1963). On the structural peculiarities of the pituitary in some clupeoid fishes with a note on their probable evolutionary significance. *Anat. Rec.* **146**, 109–115.

Sathyanesan, A. G. (1965). The hypophysis and hypothalamo-hypophysial system in the chimaeroid fish *Hydrolagus colliei* (Lay and Bennett) with a note on their vascularization. *J. Morph.* **166**, 413–449.

Sathyanesan, A. G. (1972). Hypothalamo-hypophysial vascularization in a teleost fish with special reference to its tetrapodan features. *Acta Anat.* **81**, 349–366.

Sathyanesan, A. G. and Chavin, W. (1967). Hypothalamo-hypophyseal neurosecretory system in the primitive actinopterygian fishes (Holostei and Chondrostei). *Acta Anat.* **68**, 284–299.

Sathyanesan, A. G. and Haider, S. (1971). Tetrapod-like features of the hypothalamohypophysial vascularization in the air-breathing teleost, *Heteropneustes fossilis* (Bl.). *Gen. comp. Endocr.* **17**, 360–370.

Saunders, A. E. and Rennels, E. G. (1959). Evidence of the cellular source of luteotrophin derived from a study of rat pituitary autografts. *Z. Zellforsch. mikrosk. Anat.* **49**, 263–274.

Sawyer, C. H. (1959). Nervous control of ovulation. In *Recent progress in the endocrinology of reproduction* (ed. C. W. Lloyd), pp. 1–20. New York and London: Academic Press.

Sawyer, W. H. (1961). Neurohypophysial hormones. *Pharmacol. Rev.* **13**, 225–277.

Sawyer, W. H. (1969). The active neurohypophysial principles of two primitive bony fishes, the bichir (*Polypterus senegalis*) and the African lungfish (*Protopterus aethiopicus*). *J. Endocr.* **44**, 421–435.

Saxton, J. A. Jr (1941). The relation of age to the occurrence of adenoma-like lesions in the rat hypophysis and to their growth after transplantation. *Cancer Res.* **1**, 277–282.

Saxton, J. A. Jr and Graham, J. G. (1944). Chromophobe adenoma-like lesions of the rat hypophysis. *Cancer Res.* **4**, 168–175.

Scanes, C. G., Dobson, S., Follett, B. K. and Dodd, J. M. (1972). Gonadotrophic activity in the pituitary gland of the dogfish (*Scyliorhinus canicula*). *J. Endocr.* **54**, 343–344.

Schally, A. V., Arimura, A., Bowers, C. Y., Wakabayashi, I., Kastin, A. J., Redding, T. W., Mittler, J. C., Nair, R. M. G., Pizzolato, P. and Segal, A. J. (1970). Purification of hypothalamic releasing hormones of human origin. *J. clin. Endocr. Metab.* **31**, 291–300.

Schally, A. V., Arimura, A., Baba, Y., Nair, R. M. G., Matsuo, H., Redding, T. W., Debejuk, L. and White, W. F. (1971). Isolation and properties of the FSH and LH-releasing hormone. *Biochem. Biophys. Res. Commun.* **43**, 393–399.

Schelin, U. (1962). Chromophobe and acidophil adenomas of the human pituitary gland. *Acta path. microbiol. Scand., Suppl.* **158**, 1–80.

Schiebler, T. H. (1952). Cytochemische und elektronenmikroskopische Untersuchungen an granulären Fraktionen der Neurohypophyse des Rindes. *Z. Zellforsch. mikrosk. Anat.* **36**, 563–576.

Schönemann, A. (1892). Hypophysis und Thyreodea. *Virchows Arch. path. Anat. Physiol.* **129**, 310–336.

Schooley, J. P. and Riddle, O. (1938). The morphological basis of pituitary function in pigeons. *Am. J. Anat.* **62**, 313–349.

Scott, D. E., Dudley, G. K., Gibbs, F. P. and Brown, G. M. (1972). The mammalian median eminence. In *Brain–endocrine interaction. Median eminence: structure and function* (ed. K. M. Knigge, D. E. Scott and A. Weindl), pp. 35–49. Basel: Karger.

Serber, B. J. (1958). A cytological study of the anterior pituitary gland of the normal, gonadectomized and thyroid deficient hamster (*Mesocricetus auratus*). *Anat. Rec.* **131**, 173–191.

Severinghaus, A. E. (1938). The cytology of the pituitary gland. In *The pituitary gland. Res. Publs Ass. Res. nerv. ment. Dis.* **17**, 69–117.

Severinghaus, A. E., Smelser, G. K. and Clark, H. M. (1934). Anterior pituitary changes in the adult male rat following thyroidectomy. *Proc. Soc. exp. Biol. Med.* **31**, 1127.

Sharp, P. J. and Follett, B. K. (1968). The distribution of monoamines in the hypothalamus of the Japanese quail, *Coturnix coturnix japonica*. *Z. Zellforsch. mikrosk. Anat.* **90**, 245–262.

Sharp, P. J. and Follett, B. K. (1969). The blood supply of the pituitary and the basal hypothalamus in the Japanese quail (*Coturnix coturnix japonica*) *J. Anat.* **104**, 227–232.

Sheehan, H. L. (1954). The incidence of postpartum hypopituitarism. *Am. J. Obstet. Gynec.* **68**, 202–223.

Sheehan, H. L. and Stanfield, J. P. (1961). The pathogenesis of post-partum necrosis of the anterior lobe of the pituitary gland. *Acta endocrin. Copnh.* **37**, 479–510.

Sheela, R. and Pandalai, K. R. (1966). Blood supply of the pituitary gland with particular reference to pars intermedia control in the garden lizard, *Calotes versicolor. Neuroendocrinology* **1**, 303–311.

Sheela, R. and Pandalai, K. R. (1968). Reaction of the paraventricular nucleus to dehydration in the garden lizard, *Calotes versicolor. Gen. comp. Endocr.* **11**, 257–261.

Singer, C. (1952). *Vesalius on the human brain.* Publications of the Wellcome Historical Medical Museum. New Series No. 4. Oxford University Press.

Singh, T. P. (1969). Observations on the effect of gonadal and adrenal cortical steroids upon thyroid gland in hypophysectomized catfish, *Mystus vittatus* (Bloch). *Gen. comp. Endocr.* **12**, 556–560.

Sloper, J. C. (1954). Histochemical observations on the neurohypophysis in dog and cat with reference to the relationship between neurosecretory material and posterior lobe hormone. *J. Anat.* **88**, 576.

Sloper, J. C. (1955). Hypothalamic neurosecretion in the dog and cat, with particular reference to the identification of neurosecretory material with posterior lobe hormone. *J. Anat.* **89**, 301–316.

Sloper, J. C., Arnott, D. J. and King, B. C. (1960). Sulphur metabolism in the pituitary and hypothalamus of the rat: a study of radioisotope-uptake after the injection of ^{35}S DL–cysteine methionine and sodium sulphate. *J. Endocr.* **20**, 9–23.

Smith, P. E. (1926). Ablation and transplantation of the hypophysis in the rat. *Anat. Rec.* **32**, 221.

Smith, P. E. (1927). The disabilities caused by hypophysectomy and their repair. The tuberal (hypothalamic) syndrome in the rat. *J. Am. med. Ass.* **88**, 158–161.

Smith, P. E. (1930). Hypophysectomy and a replacement therapy in the rat. *Am. J. Anat.* **45**, 205–274.

Smith, P. E. (1932). The secretory capacity of the anterior hypophysis as evidenced by the effect of partial hypophysectomies in rats. *Anat. Rec.* **52**, 191–207.

Smith, P. E. and MacDowell, E. C. (1930). An hereditary anterior-pituitary deficiency in the mouse. *Anat. Rec.* **46**, 249–257.

Smith, P. M. and Follett, B. K. (1972). Luteinizing hormone releasing factor in the quail hypothalamus. *J. Endocr.* **53**, 131–138.

Smith, R. N. (1956). The presence of non-myelinated nerve fibres in the pars distalis of the pituitary gland of the ferret. *J. Endocr.* **14**, 279–283.

Smoller, C. G. (1966). Ultrastructural studies on the developing neurohypophysis of the Pacific treefrog, *Hyla regilla. Gen. comp. Endocr.* **7**, 44–73.

Solnitzky, O. (1939). The hypothalamus and sub-thalamus of *Sus scrofa. J. comp. Neurol.* **70**, 191–229.

Spanner, R. (1952). Die Bedeutung der Hypophysenpfortaden für die Blutströmungsmöglichkeiten zwischen Hypophyse und Hypothalamus im Hypophysenkreislauf. *Klin. Wschr.* **30**, 721–725.

Spatz, H., Diepen, R. and Gaupp, W. (1948). Zur Anatomie des Infundibulum und des Tuber Cinereum beim Kaninchen. *Dt. Z. NervenHeilk.* **159**, 229–268.

Stanfield, J. P. (1960). The blood supply of the human pituitary gland. *J. Anat.* **94**, 257–273.

Sterba, G. (1969). Endocrinology of the lampreys. *Gen. comp. Endocr. Suppl.* **2**, 500–509.

Sterba, G. (1972). Neuro- and gliasecretion. In *The biology of lampreys* (ed. M. W. Hardisty and I. C. Potter), vol. II, pp. 69–89. New York and London: Academic Press.

Sterba, G. and Bruckner, G. (1969). Elektronenmikroskopische Untersuchungen über die Reaktion der Pituizyten nach Hypophysenstieldurchtrennung bei *Rana esculenta. Z. Zellforsch. mikrosk. Anat.* **93**, 74–83.

Stoekel, M. E., Dellman, H.-D., Porte, A. and Gertner, C. (1971). The rostral zone of the intermediate lobe of the mouse hypophysis, a zone of particular concentration of corticotrophic cells. A light and electron microscopic study. *Z. Zellforsch. mikrosk. Anat.* **122**, 310–322.

Stutinsky, F. (1958). Rapports du neurosécrétat hypothalamique avec l'adénohypophyse dans des conditions normales et expérimentales. In *Pathophysiologia diencephalica*, pp. 78–102. Vienna: Springer-Verlag.

Sundararaj, B. I., Anand, I. C. and Sinha, V. R. P. (1972). Effects of carp pituitary fractions on vitellogenesis, ovarian maintenance, and ovulation in hypophysectomized catfish, *Heteropneustes fossilis* (Bloch). *J. Endocr.* **54**, 87–98.

Sundararaj, B. I. and Viswanathan, N. (1971). Hypothalamo-hypophyseal neurosecretory and vascular systems in the catfish *Heteropneustes fossilis* (Bloch). *J. comp. Neurol.* **141**, 95–106.

Szentágothai, J., Flerkó, B., Mess, B. and Halász, B. (1968). *Hypothalamic control of the anterior pituitary. An experimental-morphological study*, 3rd edition. Budapest: Akadémiai Kiadó.

Talanti, S. (1971). The incorporation of ^{35}S-labelled cysteine in the hypothalamic-hypophyseal neurosecretory system in the dehydrated rat. *Z. Zellforsch. mikrosk. Anat.* **115**, 110–113.

Taleisnik, S. and Orias, R. (1956). A melanocyte-stimulating hormone-releasing factor in hypothalamic extracts. *Am. J. Physiol.* **208**, 293–296.

Taleisnik, S. and Tomatis, M. E. (1968). The effect of copulation or vaginal stimulation on melanocyte-stimulating hormone content of the hypophysis. *Experientia* **24**, 143–144.

Tello, F. (1912). Algunas observaciones sobre la histologia de la hipófisis humana. *Trab. Lab. Invest. biol., Univ. Madr.* **10**, 145–183.

Thaon, P. (1907). L'hypophyse. (Thesis, cited by Landsmeer, 1963.)

Théret, C. and Tamboise, E. (1963). Étude ultrastructurale des rapports expérimentaux entre des cellules alpha et des fibres neurovégétatives dans l'adénohypophyse du rat. *Ann. Endocr., Paris* **24**, 421–440.

Thomson, A. P. D. and Zuckerman, S. (1954). The effects of pituitary stalk section on light-induced oestrus in ferrets. *Proc. R. Soc. Ser. B* **142**, 437–451.

Tixier-Vidal, A. (1965). Caractères ultrastructuraux des types cellulaires de l'adénohyphophyse du canard mâle. *Archs Anat. microsc. Morph. exp.* **54**, 719–780.

Tixier-Vidal, A. and Assenmacher, I. (1966). Étude cytologique de la préhypophyse du pigeon pendant la couvaison et la lactation. *Z. Zellforsch. mikrosk. Anat.* **69**, 489–519.

Tixier-Vidal, A. and Benoit, J. (1962). Influence de la castration sur la cytologie préhypophysaire du canard mâle. *Archs Anat. microsc. Morph. exp.* **51**, 265–286.

Tixier-Vidal, A., Chandola, A. and Franquelin, F. (1972). 'Cellules de thyroïdectomie' et 'cellules de castration' chez la caille japonaise *Coturnix coturnix japonica. Z. Zellforsch. mikrosk. Anat.* **125**, 506–531.

Tixier-Vidal, A., Follett, B. K. and Farner, D. S. (1967). Identification cytologique et fonctionnelle des types cellulaires de l'adénohypophyse chez la caille mâle *Coturnix coturnix japonica* soumise à différentes conditions expérimentales. *C. r. hebd. Séanc. Acad. Sci., Paris* **264**, 1739–1742.

Tixier-Vidal, A., Follett, B. K. and Farner, D. S. (1968). The anterior pituitary of the Japanese quail, *Coturnix coturnix japonica*. The cytological effects of photoperiodic stimulation. *Z. Zellforsch. mikrosk. Anat.* **92**, 610–635.

Trautmann, A. (1911). Hypophysis cerebri. In *Handbuch der vergleichenden mikroskopischen Anatomie der Haustiere* (ed. W. Ellenbeger), vol. II, pp. 148–169. Berlin: Paul Parey.

Trautmann, A. (1915). Hypophyse und Thyreoidektomie. *Frank. Z. Path.* **18**, 173–304.

Truscott, B. L. (1944). The nerve supply to the pituitary of the rat. *J. comp. Neurol.* **80**, 235–255.

Unsicker, K. (1971). On the innervation of mammalian endocrine glands (anterior pituitary and parathyroid). *Z. Zellforsch. mikrosk. Anat.* **121**, 283–291.

Urano, A. (1971a). Monoamine oxidase in the hypothalamo-hypophysial region of the brown smooth dogfish, *Triakis scyllia*. *Endocr. jap.* **18**, 37–46.

Urano, A. (1971b). Monoamine oxidase in the hypothalamo-hypophysial region of the teleosts, *Anguilla japonica* and *Oryzias latipes*. *Z. Zellforsch. mikrosk. Anat.* **114**, 83–94.

Urano, A. (1972). Monoamine oxidase in the neurohypophysis of the newt (*Cynops pyrrhogaster pyrrhogaster*), the toad (*Bufo bufo japonicus*) and the tortoise (*Clemmys japonica*). *Z. Zellforsch. mikrosk. Anat.* **126**, 454–465.

Van Dyke, H. B., Adamsons, K. and Engel, S. L. (1955). Aspects of the biochemistry and physiology of the neurohypophysial hormones. *Recent Prog. Horm. Res.* **11**, 1–41.

Van Dyke, H. B., Chow, B. F., Greep, H. O. and Rothen, A. (1942). Isolation of protein from pars neuralis of ox pituitary with constant oxytocic, pressor and diuresis-inhibiting activities. *J. Pharmacol.* **74**, 190–209.

Vanha-Perttula, T. and Arstila, A. U. (1970). On the epithelium of the rat pituitary residual lumen. *Z. Zellforsch. mikrosk. Anat.* **108**, 487–500.

Vellano, C. and Peyrot, A. (1970). La regolazione neuroendocrine dell'attività tireotropa dell'adenoipofisi negli anamni. *Boll. Zool.* **37**, 409–440.

Verney, E. B. (1947). The antidiuretic hormone and the factors which determine its release. *Proc. R. Soc. Ser. B* **135**, 25–106.

Vigh-Teichmann, I. and Vigh, B. (1970). Structure and function of the liquor contacting neurosecretory system. In *Aspects of neuroendocrinology* (ed. W. Bargmann and B. Scharrer), pp. 329–337. Berlin, Heidelberg, New York: Springer-Verlag.

Vijayakumar, S., Jørgensen, C. B. and Kjaer, K. (1971). Regulation of ovarian cycles in the toad *Bufo bufo* (L.): effects of autografting pars distalis of the hypophysis, of extirpating gonadotropic hypothalamic region, and of partial ovariectomy. *Gen. comp. Endocr.* **17**, 432–443.

Vila-Porcile, E. (1972). Le réseau des cellules folliculo-stellaires et les follicles de l'adénohypophyse du rat (pars distalis). *Z. Zellforsch. mikrosk. Anat.* **129**, 328–369.

Vitums, A., Mikami, S.-I., Oksche, A. and Farner, D. S. (1964). Vascularization of the hypothalamo-hypophysial complex in the white-crowned sparrow, *Zonotrichia leucophrys gambellii*. *Z. Zellforsch. mikrosk. Anat.* **64**, 541–569.

Voigt, A. (1939). Untersuchungen über die Cytogenese der Drüsenzellen im Hypophysen vorderlappen des Haushuns. *Z. Zellforsch. mikrosk. Anat.* **29**, 502–552.

Vollrath, L. (1966). The ultrastructure of the eel pituitary at the elver stage with special reference to its neurosecretory innervation. *Z. Zellforsch. mikrosk. Anat.* **73**, 107–131.

Vollrath, L. (1970). The origin of 'synaptic' vesicles in neurosecretory axons. In *Aspects of neuroendocrinology* (ed. W. Bargmann and B. Scharrer), pp. 173–176. Berlin, Heidelberg, New York: Springer-Verlag.

Vollrath, L. (1972). Morphological correlates of releasing factors in the pituitary of the eel, *Anguilla anguilla*. In *Brain–endocrine interaction. Median eminence: structure and function* (ed. K. M. Knigge, D. E. Scott and A. Weindl), pp. 154–163. Basel: Karger.

Weatherhead, B. (1969). Intra-ventricular ependymal processes in the pars nervosa of a chelonian, *Emys orbicularis. Gen. comp. Endocr.* **13**, 539–540.

Weatherhead, B. (1971). Cytology of the neuro-intermediate lobe of the tuatara, *Sphenodon punctatus* Gray. *Z. Zellforsch. mikrosk. Anat.* **119**, 21–42.

Weatherhead, B. and Whur, P. (1972). Quantification of ultrastructural changes in the melanocyte-stimulating hormone cells of the pars intermedia of the pituitary of *Xenopus laevis*, produced by change of background colour. *J. Endocr.* **53**, 303–310.

Weiss, M. (1965). The release of pituitary secretion in the platyfish, *Xiphophorus maculatus* (Guenther). *Z. Zellforsch. mikrosk. Anat.* **68**, 783–794.

Werff ten Bosch, J. J. van der and Donovan, B. T. (1957). Early onset of oestrus and puberty following hypothalamic lesions. *Acta physiol. pharmacol. neerl.* **5**, 490–495.

Westman, A. and Jacobsohn, D. (1940). Experimentelle Untersuchung über Hypophysentransplantate bei der Ratte. *Acta path. microbiol. scand.* **17**, 328–347.

Westwood, W. J. A. (1962). Anatomy of the hypothalamus of the ferret. *J. comp. Neurol.* **118**, 323–341.

Wheeler, R. S. (1943). Normal development of the pituitary in the opossum and its responses to hormonal treatments. *J. Morph.* **73**, 43–87.

Whitaker, S., LaBella, F. and Sanwal, M. (1970). Electron microscopic histochemistry of lysosomes in neurosecretory nerve endings and pituicytes of rat posterior pituitary. *Z. Zellforsch. mikrosk. Anat.* **111**, 493–504.

Willmer, E. N. (1970). *Cytology and evolution*, 2nd edition. New York and London: Academic Press.

Wilson, N. and Smith, M. (1971). Changes in oxytocic activity of the hypophysis during sexual maturation of Pacific salmon, *Oncorhynchus tschawytscha. Gen. comp. Endocr.* **16**, 395–397.

Wingstrand, K. G. (1951). *The structure and development of the avian pituitary*. Lund: Gleerup.

Wingstrand, K. G. (1956). The structure of the pituitary in the African lungfish *Protopterus annectens* (Owens). *Vidensk. Meddr dansk naturh. Foren.* **118**, 193–210.

Wingstrand, K. G. (1963). Comparative histology of the adenohypophysis of birds. In *Cytologie de l'adénohypophyse, Colloque Internatl. CRNS, Paris* **128**, 243–254.

Wingstrand, K. G. (1966*a*). Comparative anatomy and evolution of the hypophysis. In *The pituitary gland* (ed. G .W. Harris and B. T. Donovan), vol. I, pp. 58–126. London: Butterworths.

Wingstrand, K. G. (1966*b*). Microscopic anatomy, nerve supply and blood supply of the pars intermedia. In *The pituitary gland* (ed. G. W. Harris and B. T. Donovan), vol. III, pp. 1–27. London: Butterworths.

Wislocki, G. B. (1938*a*). The topography of the hypophysis in the Xenarthra. *Anat. Rec.* **70**, 451–471.

Wislocki, G. B. (1938*b*). Further observations on the blood supply of the hypophysis cerebri of the Rhesus monkey. *Anat. Rec.* **72**, 137.

Wislocki, G. B. and King, L. S. (1936). The permeability of the hypophysis and hypothalamus to vital dyes, with a study of the hypophyseal vascular supply. *Am. J. Anat.* **58**, 421–472.

Wolfe, J. M., Cleveland, R. and Campbell, M. (1933). Cyclic histological variation in the anterior hypophysis of the dog. *Z. Zellforsch. mikrosk. Anat.* **17**, 420–452.

Worthington, W. C. (1960). Vascular responses in the pituitary stalk. *Endocrinology* **66**, 19–31.

Worthington, W. C. (1963). Functional vascular fields in the pituitary stalk of the mouse. *Nature, Lond.* **199**, 461–465.

Wulzen, R. (1914). The pituitary body of the ox. *Anat. Rec.* **8**, 403–414.

Xuereb, G. P., Prichard, M. M. L. and Daniel, P. M. (1954*a*). The arterial supply and venous drainage of the human hypophysis cerebri. *Q. Jl exp. Physiol.* **39**, 199–217.

Xuereb, G. P., Prichard, M. M. L. and Daniel, P. M. (1954*b*). The hypophysial portal system of vessels in man. *J. exp. Physiol.* **39**, 219–230.

Yamada, T. (1959). Studies on the mechanism of hypothalamic control of thyrotrophin secretion: effect of intrahypothalamic thyroxine injection on thyroid hypertrophy induced by propylthiouracil in the rat. *Endocrinology* **65**, 216–224.

Yamada, K., Sano, M., Okumura, K. and Sakakura, K. (1960). Cellular changes in the mouse anterior pituitary from maturity· to senility. *Folia anat. jap.* **35**, 107–117.

Zambrano, D. (1970*a*). The nucleus lateralis tuberis system of the gobiid fish *Gillichthys mirabilis*. I. Ultrastructural and histochemical characterization of the nucleus. *Z. Zellforsch. mikrosk. Anat.* **110**, 9–26.

Zambrano, D. (1970*b*). The nucleus lateralis tuberis system of the gobiid fish *Gillichthys mirabilis*. II. Innervation of the pituitary, *Z. Zellforsch. mikrosk. Anat.* **110**, 496–516.

Zambrano, D. (1971). The nucleus lateralis tuberis system of the gobiid fish *Gillichthys mirabilis*. III. Functional modifications of the neurons and gonadotropic cells. *Gen. comp. Endocr.* **17**, 164–182.

Zambrano, D. and Iturriza, F. C. (1972). Histology and ultrastructure of the neurohypophysis of the South American lungfish, *Lepidosiren paradoxa*. *Z. Zellforsch. mikrosk. Anat.* **131**, 47–62.

Zambrano, D. and Iturriza, F. C. (1973). Hypothalamo-hypophysial relationships in the South American lungfish, *Lepidosiren paradoxa*. *Gen. comp. Endocr.* **20**, 256–273.

Zambrano, D. and De Robertis, E. (1967). Ultrastructure of the hypothalamic neurosecretory system of the dog. *Z. Zellforsch. mikrosk. Anat.* **81**, 264–282.

Zambrano, D. and De Robertis, E. (1968). Ultrastructure of the peptidergic and monoaminergic neurons in the hypothalamic neurosecretory system of anuran batracians. *Z. Zellforsch. mikrosk. Anat.* **90**, 230–244.

Zambrano, D., Nishioka, R. S. and Bern, H. A. (1972). The innervation of the pituitary gland of teleost fishes; its origin, nature and significance. In *Brain-endocrine interaction. Median eminence: structure and function* (ed. K. M. Knigge, D. E. Scott and A. Weindl), pp. 50–66. Basel: Karger.

Ziegler, B. (1963). Licht- und elektronenmikroskopische Untersuchungen an Pars intermedia und Neurohypophyse der Ratte. *Z. Zellforsch. mikrosk. Anat.* **59**, 486–506.

Zipser, R. D., Licht, P. and Bern, H. A. (1969). Comparative effects of mammalian prolactin and growth hormone on growth in the toads *Bufo boreas* and *marinus*. *Gen. comp. Endocr.* **13**, 382–391.

Zondek, B. and Krohn, H. (1932). Hormon des Zwischenlappens der hypophyse (Intermedin). *Klin. Wschr.* **11**, 405–408 and 849–853.

Zuber-Vogeli, M. (1953). L'histophysiologie de l'hypophyse de *Bufo vulgaris* L. *Archs Anat. Histol. Embryol.* **35**, 77–180.

Zuber-Vogeli, M. (1966). Les variations cytologiques de l'hypophyse distale du mâle de *Nectophrynoides occidentalis* au cours du cycle annuel. *Gen. comp. Endocr.* **7**, 492–499.

Zuber-Vogeli, M. (1968). Les variations cytologiques de l'hypophyse distale des femelles de *Nectophrynoides occidentalis*. *Gen. comp. Endocr.* **11**, 495–514.

Zuber-Vogeli, M. and Bihouès-Louis, M. A. (1971). L'hypophyse de *Nectophrynoides occidentalis* au cours de développement embryonnaire. *Gen. comp. Endocr.* **16**, 200–216.

Zuber-Vogeli, M. and Xavier, F. (1972). Les modifications cytologiques de l'hypophyse distale des femelles de *Nectophrynoides occidentalis* (Angel) castrées en début de gestation. *C. r. hebd. Séanc. Acad. Sci., Paris* **D 274**, 1361–1364.

INDEX

References to Figures are in italics

---

acetylcholine
and hypothalamic neurons 85, 305
in neurosecretory fibres 84, 139, 208, 229, 273, 276, 313, 314, 319
acidophilia *v.* basophilia 29, 32–3
acidophils *x*, 136–7, 164–6, 175–84, 242–6, 296–9
in avian pars distalis 328–30
in dwarf mice 52
mammalian 30–1, 40
ACTH (corticotropin) 11, 132–3, 145, 193–4, 267–8, 306
cells *x*, 40, 50, 132, 137, 146, 171, 172, 180–2, 194, 215, 217, 223, 258–9, 302–4, 346–7
and pars intermedia 60, 272
adenohypophysis 21
divisions of 5–9, *6*, 135, *136*, 141–4, *142*, *143*, *144*, *154*, *160*, *164*, 170–4, *172*, *222*, 230–2, *232*, 237, 238–41, *239*, *289*, 290–5, *292*
alcian blue
and pars distalis 38–9
and NSM 73–4
aldehyde fuchsin
and pars distalis 37–8
and NSM 73–4
amines, *see* catecholamines, monoamines
amphiphils, amphophils 146, 147, 165, 197, 247–8, 302–4
antidiuretic hormone (ADH) 12, 64–5
and NSM 73–7, 282–3, 313
and releasing factors 126–7
arcuate nucleus 124, 225, 277, 305, 343
arginine vasotocin (AVT) 65, 139, 156, 162, 166, 204, 206–7, 228, 229, 282–3, 313, 319
autoradiography
and pars distalis 49
and neurohypophysis 74–6

basophilia
in adenohypophysial cells 32–4
and RNA 34–5
basophils (cyanophils) 27–34, 40–1, 136–7, 165–6, 184–91, 245–9, 299–304, 339, 340–1
blood vessels of pituitary 9–11, *10*, 103–16, *104*, 134–5, 139–40, *149*, 151–2, 157–8, 162–3, 167–9, 211–14, *212*, *213*, 226, 228, 232–4, *284*, 285–7, 319–22, *321*, *335*, *336*,
arteries, hypophysial 211, *212*, *284*, 285, (inferior) 9, 101, (superior) 9, 101–4; hypothalamic *149*, 151, 211–12, *213*, 226; loral *104*, 105; of stalk (long) *104*, (short) *104*
capillaries of adenohypophysis 45, *46*, 56
(*see also* hypothalamo-hypophysioportal system)
buccal pars distalis (coelacanth) 144, *231*, 231

canal
cranio-pharyngeal 18
hypophysial (duct) 145, 153–5, *154*, *157*, 173–4, 339–41, 347
castration, *see* gonads
catecholamines 84, 148–9, 161–2, 199, 202, 208–11, 215–17, 220, 225, 229, 274–6, 277, 281, 285, 319
caudal aminergic nuclei
amphibians 275, 276, 343
teleosts, 202
cell types
distribution of *243*, *249*, *297*
illustrated *x*, *209*, *210*, *332*
nomenclature of 34–6
cerebrospinal fluid, and pituitary function 219–20, 278, 342–3
chrome alum haematoxylin (CAH) 73
chromophobes, and basophilia 34